ESSENTIALS OF
IMMUNOLOGY

EDITION 2

ESSENTIALS OF IMMUNOLOGY

BENJAMIN LEE GORDON, II,
M.D., Ph.D., F.A.C.A.

Director, Medical Research Department
Kuakini Hospital & Home
Honolulu, Hawaii

Associate Clinical Professor of Genetics
Associate Clinical Professor of Medicine
University of Hawaii School of Medicine
Honolulu, Hawaii

Consultant Clinical Immunologist
Departments of Medicine & Paediatrics
Tripler U.S. Army Medical Center
Honolulu, Hawaii

Formerly:
Assistant Professor of Paediatrics
Faculty of Medicine
University of British Columbia
Vancouver, Canada

Illustrated by:
BRUCE STEWART, SUSAN ANDERSON, KURT HENZE,
and BARDOLF PAUL

F. A. DAVIS COMPANY, Philadelphia, Pa.

ISBN 0-8036-0241-3
Library of Congress Catalog Card Number 74-75323

Dedicated in loving appreciation
to my wife

TRISNOWATI

for her patience and understanding
during the preparation of this book

List of Collaborators:

JULIA G. LEVY, Ph.D.

Professor of Microbiology
University of British Columbia

ALBERT A. BENEDICT, Ph.D.

Professor of Microbiology
University of Hawaii

DENYS K. FORD, M.D., F.R.C.P.(C)

Associate Professor of Medicine
University of British Columbia

DONNA GORDON BAIR, B.A.

Research Assistant
Kuakini Hospital & Home

WILLIAM H. CHASE, M.D., C.M.

Associate Professor of Pathology
University of British Columbia

SHELDON C. NAIMAN, M.D., F.R.C.P.(C)

Haematologist
Vancouver General Hospital

J. WALLACE THOMAS, M.D.

Haematologist
Vancouver General Hospital

PREFACE TO THE SECOND EDITION

More than two years have elapsed since the first edition of this book appeared in print. In that time, a number of people have communicated with the author regarding this book, and many helpful suggestions have been offered. As a result of these, a number of changes have been made, which, it is hoped, will improve its usefulness as an introductory textbook for medical and science students.

Division of the text into three sections, dealing with *basic immunology*, *clinical immunology*, and *molecular immunology* has been retained. A chapter on immunogens (antigens) has been added, and the original two chapters concerning basic aspects of cellular and humoral immune responses have been integrated into a single chapter in this edition.

The terminology used in discussing the basic organisation of the lymphoid system has been altered to conform with recommended terminology of the World Health Organisation.

A number of new illustrations and photographs have been added, which, it is hoped, will clarify certain concepts for the student.

The book has been extensively re-written, updated, and reorganised. The summary of principles of molecular biology has been removed from the text proper and placed in an appendix with the summary of methods used for primary structure analysis of proteins. This should give better continuity to the text.

The format has been altered to bring the book into conformity with others in the F. A. Davis "Essentials" series.

The author would like to express his sincere gratitude to the many people who offered criticisms or suggestions related to this book. Wherever possible, these suggestions have been incorporated into the second edition, and others will doubtlessly be incorporated into future versions, should the text survive.

A special debt of gratitude is owed to the medical students attending the author's lectures in Immunology at the University of British Columbia for providing most valuable critiques of these presentations.

The author also wishes to thank all of the members of the medical research department of Kuakini Hospital for their help in finishing this edition, especially Mrs. Kyoko Nakata and Mrs. Priscilla La Forte for typing the manuscript and for help in proof-reading.

Finally, the author wishes to thank his wife, Trisnowati, for her constant encouragement, and for her invaluable assistance with proof-reading, as well as his father, Maurice B. Gordon, M.D., and his mother, Muriel H. Gordon, for their encouragement when the going was rough, and the light at the end of the tunnel but dimly perceived.

PREFACE TO THE FIRST EDITION

Immunology is a rapidly-developing field of biomedical endeavour, in which it is impossible for any general text-book to be entirely up-to-date. However, where a firm foundation of basic principles is laid (and this is the primary function of an introductory text-book), it should be possible to assimilate new information with only minimal difficulty.

This text was prepared for the special needs of the undergraduate medical student. These needs include clinical orientation, with examples drawn from clinical situations wherever possible. Moreover, the writers have endeavoured to present essential material in as concise a form as possible.

The text has been presented in three sections, to allow the book to be adjusted to the needs of different medical schools.

Section I consists of "basic immunology", and the material contained therein is believed to represent the essential core knowledge necessary to understand the clinical aspects of immunology and modern "molecular immunology".

Section II presents the fundamental tenets of immunology as applied to medicine; thus it is of greatest direct concern to the medical student and clinician.

Sections I and II together constitute a "core curriculum" in undergraduate medicine.

Section III presents the modern molecular concepts of immunology that are developing at an exceedingly rapid rate, and have already begun to allow an understanding of the immune response at the biochemical and genetic levels. <u>It is not part of a "core curriculum" in undergraduate medicine</u>, but should enable the more advanced reader to understand certain aspects of clinical immunology which would otherwise remain enigmatic. Thus, this section was written primarily for physicians preparing for fellowship examinations or specialty certification in laboratory medicine, or for basic medical scientists and clinical immunologists.

The book is written in a didactic manner, and there are few references to individual researchers or to original work. This is in keeping with the aim of the book. Many excellent comprehensive text-books of immunology are available, which can be used to augment or complement this book; a list of these is presented at the end of Section III. It should be borne in mind by the reader that an approach of this type requires oversimplification of a complex subject.

The authors would like to acknowledge the invaluable assistance of the Departments of Medicine and Pathology at the University of British Columbia and the B. C. Division of the Canadian Arthritis and Rheumatism Society, without which this book would not have seen the light of day.

CONTENTS

SECTION I. BASIC IMMUNOLOGY

SECTION II. CLINICAL IMMUNOLOGY AND IMMUNOPATHOLOGY

SECTION I

BASIC IMMUNOLOGY

Chapter 1

INTRODUCTION

Immunology began as a branch of medical microbiology concerned with resistance to infectious diseases. Today, however, it is recognised as a field of biomedical endeavour in its own right - by no means restricted to the area of infection. In fact, the term immunity, as used by immunologists, no longer necessarily implies a response that is protective to the individual.

What, then, is immunity? No entirely satisfactory definition can be given without presupposing a considerable understanding of immune responses. Therefore, some initial ambiguity is inevitable. However, as the student's knowledge of basic immunologic phenomena increases, ambiguity will diminish, and a clearer idea of the uniqueness of these processes will emerge.

Immunity may be thought of as a state of altered responsiveness to a specific substance, induced by prior contact with that substance. From the outset, we will distinguish two broad categories of immune response - *i.e.*, those mediated by circulating humoral factors (classical serum antibodies) and those mediated by cells (cellular immunity). Although these types of immune response are almost entirely separable from one another, they are closely interrelated and frequently occur simultaneously.

Phylogeny of Immunity

Immunologic competence, *i.e.*, the ability to develop immunity upon appropriate stimulation, is an unique feature of vertebrate animals; no other group of organisms possesses this remarkable ability to recognise biochemically a seemingly limitless variety of extrinsic substances. Such recognition of extrinsic materials is by no means an academic matter; the possession of an immune system is a most powerful mechanism for survival against the incessant onslaught of parasitic invaders. Indeed, the primary adaptive function of any immune response appears to be to maintain the integrity of the body inviolate at all times. This is usually advantageous to both the individual and to the species, but there are circumstances under which immune responses can serve as pathogenetic mechanisms rather than as defensive reactions. Thus, immune responses, in common with many other important homeostatic mechanisms of the body (*e.g.*, blood clotting and fibrinolysis) possess ability both to harm and to protect the individual. They may thus be regarded as "double-edged swords".

Maintenance of the body's integrity, then, is the principal function of the immune system. This system has evolved mechanisms to repel and destroy invaders of extrinsic origin ranging from viruses through bacteria, fungi, protozoa, and even metazoa, such as the helminths. However, there is increasing reason to believe that at least part of the immune system may have evolved to deal primarily with a far more insidious type of parasite originating from within the body - *i.e.*, the neoplastic cell. Because neoplastic cells are derived from the body itself, it is a difficult problem for the body's immune system to recognise them as altered cells, dangerous to the body, which must be destroyed. Nevertheless, there is good reason to believe that powerful immunological surveillance mechanisms exist which are able to effect recognition and destruction of neoplastic tissue. Indirect evidence suggests that malignant new growths arise *de novo* many times during the life of every vertebrate, perhaps as an inevitable consequence of a high degree of cellular specialisation. In most cases, these new growths are intercepted and destroyed by the immune surveillance mechanisms before they are recognised clinically. More will be said about this aspect of immunity in later chapters.

The most primitive group of living vertebrates - the Cyclostomata, or jawless fishes - possess a fair degree of immunologic competence. Both suborders of cyclostomes - hagfishes (Myxinoidea) and lampreys (Petromyzontia) - are now recognised as possessing immunologic competence of a comparable degree, generally considerably less than that of higher vertebrates. Although concepts of the phylogeny of adaptive immunity are presently in a state of rapid flux, it appears safe to note that as one ascends the phyletic scale amongst vertebrates, the complexity of the lymphoid system as a morphologic entity and the versatility of immune responses as physiologic entities tend to increase in parallel. Both are developed maximally in homeothermic amniotes (*i.e.*, birds and mammals).

Some Basic Definitions

Antigen (*immunogen*)	Any substance capable of provoking an immune response

of any type in an immunologically-competent vertebrate. Antigens occurring in nature are substances of high molecular weight and usually are proteins or carbohydrates (or contain protein or carbohydrate components). Many components of parasitic organisms are antigenic; immune responses directed against these antigens may provide protection against disease and/or resistance to reinfections by the same type of parasite. However, it must be emphasised that functional protection is nowhere implicit in the definitions of antigen, immune response or antibody.

Hapten — Any incomplete antigen - *i.e.*, any substance not of itself capable of provoking an immune response, but able to serve as a partial immunogen when bound to another substance (usually of high molecular weight) denoted as a carrier molecule. Haptens are usually of low molecular weight and may be of relatively simple structure. For example, nickel may serve as a hapten if combined with structural proteins from skin; the complex is able to provoke an immune response which then no longer requires that the metal be associated with its carrier for recognition to occur. Another example is provided by a simple organic compound, 2,4-Dinitrophenol (2,4-DNP). Although not itself capable of provoking an immune response, 2,4-DNP will stimulate an immune response when it is coupled to a carrier protein. Individuals thus stimulated by the 2,4 DNP-Protein complex will produce plasma proteins capable of reacting with the complex, the carrier protein alone, and the simple (uncoupled) hapten alone.

Antibodies

Plasma proteins synthesised in (humoral) immune responses which are capable of combining with the provoking antigens. There are several types of plasma proteins with associated antibody activity and these are denoted collectively as immunoglobulins. More will be said about these in a later chapter.

Serological Specificity

A term used to express the specificity of antibodies for their provoking antigens. Antibodies in general will react strongly with the immunogen that stimulated their formation. They may, however, react less strongly with closely related antigens. Thus, the intensity of reaction is a measure of closeness of the test antigen to the original immunogen against which the antibodies are directed. Such comparative reactions have been used to determine the relationships of similar proteins.

Cellular Specificity

This term is the correlate of serological specificity when cellular immunity is involved. Immune cells, like antibodies, have a maximal reactivity with the specific antigen and a lessening reactivity with decreasingly-related compounds.

N.B.: The term immunological specificity can be used to include both of the terms above.

The Immune System — This term is used synonymously with the term lymphoid system in this text. Either term encompasses that system of the body which is responsible for all types of immune responses. The lymphoid system is divisible into two separate functional categories - the T-cell division and the B-cell division.

The "T-Cell" Division* — (or the cellular division) of the lymphoid system is defined functionally as the system responsible for the expression of cellular immunity. This division requires the presence of a thymus gland during embryogenesis for its development and maturation, as shown in Figure 1.

Fig. 1. SCHEMATIC ONTOGENY OF THE LYMPHOID SYSTEM.
(after R.A. Good, et al.)

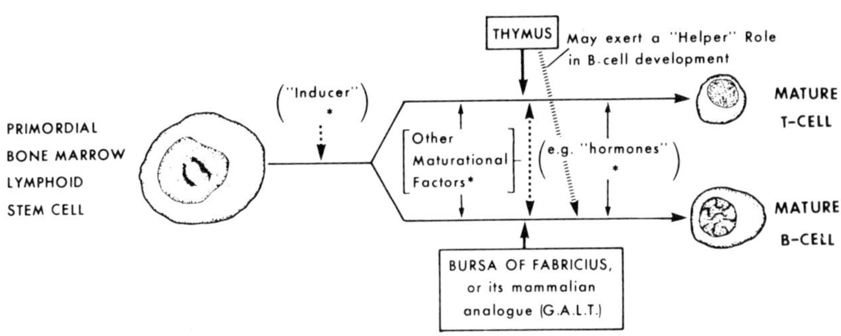

*(At present, these are purely hypothetical)

* *Designated as the "Lymphocytoid" Division of the lymphoid system in the first edition of this book, because of the morphology of the primary mediator cell.*

The "B-Cell" Division*

(or the humoral division) of the lymphoid system is defined functionally as the division responsible for the expression of humoral immunity (*i.e.*, antibodies) and for the synthesis of the immunoglobulins. In birds, this system depends on a hind-gut lymphoid organ termed the Bursa of Fabricius for its development and maturation. In mammals, a diffuse system of gut-associated lymphoid tissue (G.A.L.T.) (*e.g.*, Peyer's Patches, tonsils and the vermiform appendix) and/or bone marrow cells appear to serve as a Bursa-equivalent. It has not yet been possible to prove exactly which gut-associated (or bone marrow derived) lymphoid cells are essential for "B-cell" development in man, perhaps because of the diffuseness of these tissues and the difficulties inherent in human experimentation. It is permissible at present to refer to any type of mature immunocompetent lymphoid cell as an immunocyte.

* *Designated as the "Plasmacytoid" Division of the lymphoid system in the first edition of this book, because of the morphologic appearance of its primary effector cell.*

Chapter 2

BASIC ASPECTS OF IMMUNE RESPONSES

Physiology of Immune Responses

As noted in the introductory chapter, the immune system is functionally divisible into two parts. Contact with antigenic substances may activate either, or both divisions of the system. Antigenic stimulation of an immunologically-competent vertebrate may therefore result in the synthesis of humoral antibody against the antigen, the development of cellular immunity to the antigen, or (most likely) both types of response. This is illustrated in Figure 1.

Fig. 1 THE PHYSIOLOGY OF IMMUNITY

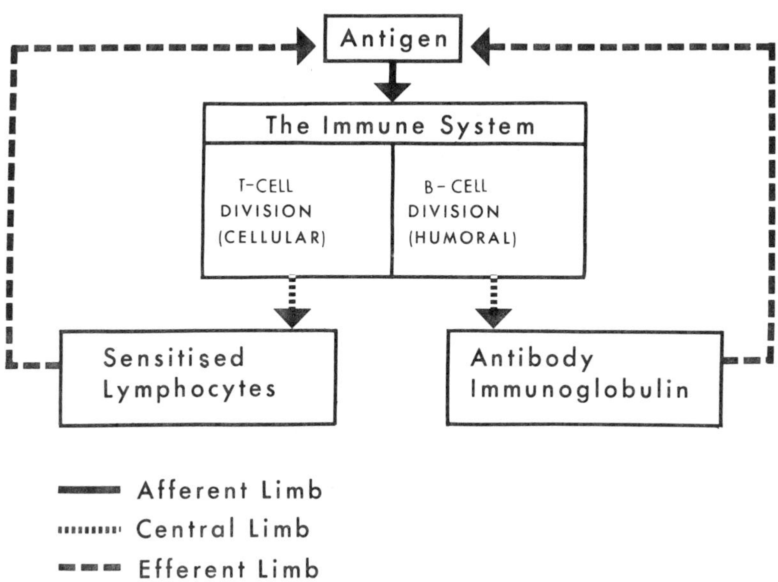

Both cellular and humoral immune responses have been arbitrarily divided into three physiological limbs. The afferent limb (I) comprises all processes involved in the transport of antigen to the immune system. The central limb (II) encompasses all processes (in both divisions of the immune system) culminating in production of the effectors of immunity (*i.e.*, sensitised cells or humoral antibodies). The effector limb (III)

comprises all processes occurring between the release of effectors and their ultimate actions upon the initiating antigen.

Each limb of the immune response is a highly complex series of events, still imperfectly understood. However, the physiological outline provided in Figure 1 is a useful concept in attempting to understand the complex events which follow the introduction of antigen into the vertebrate body.

The Divisions of the Immune System

Our present concepts of the immune system and its component divisions are derived from studies of certain human immune deficiency diseases viewed as Nature's Experiments in Immunity, and from a great number of experiments in laboratory animals. In depth studies of both types of data have led to the understanding of two divisions of the lymphoid system, functioning autonomously in many respects, yet interrelated in many ways.

The following examples will illustrate the interplay between the patient and the research laboratory which have led to our present concepts of the immune system.

A. B-Cell (Humoral) Division

(1) Removal of a central lymphoid organ called the Bursa of Fabricius from the hind-gut of neonatal chickens results in severe impairment of antibody synthesis. Neonatally-bursectomised chickens demonstrate a virtual absence of circulating immunoglobulins (agammaglobulinaemia), and failure of germinal centres to develop in central and peripheral lymphoid tissue. However, cellular immunity in bursectomised birds remains intact.

(2) The clinical disease seen in bursectomised chickens is virtually identical to that seen in male human infants suffering from a congenital sex-linked disease, Bruton's Agammaglobulinaemia. These children are unable to produce antibodies in response to antigenic stimulation, and, like bursectomised birds, also demonstrate other immunological abnormalities, such as (virtually total) plasmacytopenia and absence of germinal follicles in lymphoid tissue. In spite of these abnormalities, cellular immunity in infants with this disease remains intact.

Plasma-cells (or plasmacytes) represent the most important cell-type involved in the synthesis of humoral antibodies. However, cells of the plasmacytic series are not the only cells which synthesise antibodies and immunoglobulins; as will be seen, cells which can be described morphologically as lymphoblasts have been proven to synthesise antibodies in several studies with single cells in culture. These cells, because they synthesise antibodies, are classified physiologically as members of the B-Cell division of the lymphoid system, despite their morphologic dissimilarity from cells of the plasmacytic series. All cells capable of synthesising antibodies or immunoglobulins are thus designated as B-immunocytes.

B. T-Cell (Cellular) Division

(1) Removal of the thymus glands from neonatal mice results in a severe impairment of their ability to express cellular immunity. The lymphoid tissues of thymectomised mice are histologically abnormal; a selective small-to-medium lymphocyte deficit (*i.e.*, a selective T-immunocyte deficit) is seen at the corticomedullary junctions of lymph-nodes and at the penicilliary artery cuffs of the spleen. Germinal centres and plasma-cells, however, develop normally, but there are nevertheless variable deficiencies in humoral antibody production; thymectomised mice can respond almost normally to some antigens but poorly to others. It has thus been postulated that the thymus plays a definite role in certain humoral responses (*vide supra*, Figure 1, p.7). Immunoglobulin synthesis *per se* does not appear to be impaired by neonatal thymectomy, and the reason for the poor humoral responses observed with certain antigens is not understood. Severe lymphopenia occurs in the circulation of thymectomised animals.

(2) A congenital developmental anomaly occurring in man, Di George's IIIrd and IVth Pharyngeal Pouch Syndrome, results in the birth of infants totally lacking a thymus gland. Deficiency in the expression of cell-mediated immunities is a hallmark of these infants, and this defect is nearly identical to that seen in neonatally thymectomised mice - *i.e.*, severe (but not total) lymphopenia in the circulation and radical depression of small-to-medium lymphocytes in the lymph-nodes and spleen accompany the deficit in cellular immunities. Most humoral antibody responses are normal, as are the levels of circulating immunoglobulins. Normal numbers of plasma-cells and their precursors are present. Germinal centres develop normally in lymph-nodes, and spleen, and the tonsils also show numerous well-developed germinal follicles and a normal plasma-cell population.

By integrating the clinical and laboratory observations enumerated above, Dr. Robert A. Good and his colleagues at the University of Minnesota expanded the concept proposed originally by Szenberg and Warner of the lymphoid system being separable into two major divisions, corresponding to the two major types of immune responses. However, as will be seen, the autonomy of these two divisions is not complete; T-cell and B-cell function are frequently interdependent in naturally-occurring immune responses. Although B-cells alone are able to respond to many antigens with antibody synthesis, cooperation between T-cells and B-cells appears necessary to allow full expression of humoral immunity. The reasons why some antigens are T-cell independent and others T-cell dependent in initiating antibody production remains unclear at present.

The Lymphocyte and Cellular Immunity

Cell-mediated immunity (CMI) includes all immunological responses in which sensitised lymphoid cells (rather than serum antibodies) effect antigen recognition. Cellular immunity is an important defense mechanism against many types of extrinsic parasites, and against neoplastic growths from within (intrinsic parasites). Cellular immunity is important in the rejection of transplanted tissue by the host, and in the rejection of the host by transplanted tissues (*i.e.*, in allograft rejections and in graft-versus-host reactions). The phenomenon of delayed hypersensitivity is totally a cell-mediated reaction and certain autoimmune and neoplastic diseases are accompanied by abnormalities in cellular immunity.

The cells that mediate antigen-recognition in cellular immunity are small-to-medium lymphocytes belonging to the T-cell system that have become sensitised to the antigen by previous exposure. The molecular basis of antigen-recognition by sensitised lymphocytes is not at present understood. Immunoglobulins have not been demonstrated to have any role in this recognition, but, nonetheless, recognition of an antigen by the sensitised lymphocyte membrane is highly specific. Sensitised lymphocytes will not develop in individuals lacking functional thymus tissue during foetal development (as occurs in Di George's Syndrome) unless specific postnatal restitution is made, a procedure recently achieved by transplanting embryonic thymus tissue derived from abortuses into infants with Di George's Syndrome. Following thymus transplant, such infants rapidly develop normal populations of lymphocytes and normal CMI.

Fig. 2 THE CENTRAL LYMPHOID ORGANS

a) THYMUS

NORMAL THYMUS FROM A HUMAN INFANT

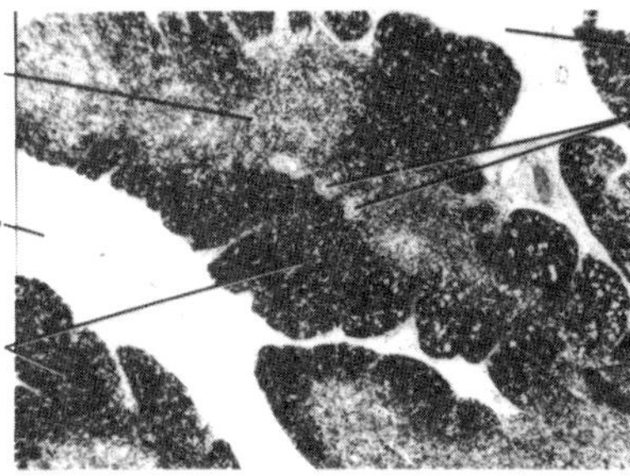

b) GUT ASSOCIATED

NORMAL HUMAN APPENDIX
(Juvenile)

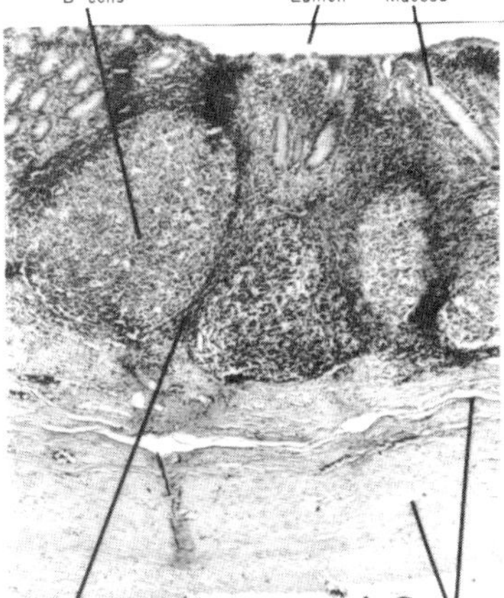

NORMAL HUMAN TONSIL
(Juvenile)

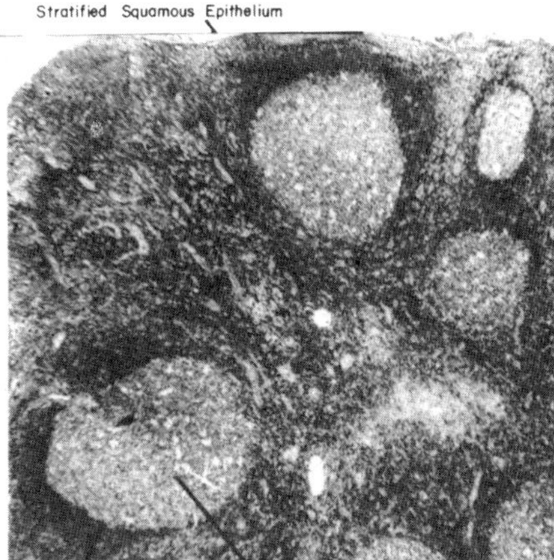

Fig. 3. THE PERIPHERAL LYMPHOID ORGANS

A Lymph Node

SCHEMATIC DIAGRAM OF A LYMPH NODE
(showing areas of T-cells and B-cells)

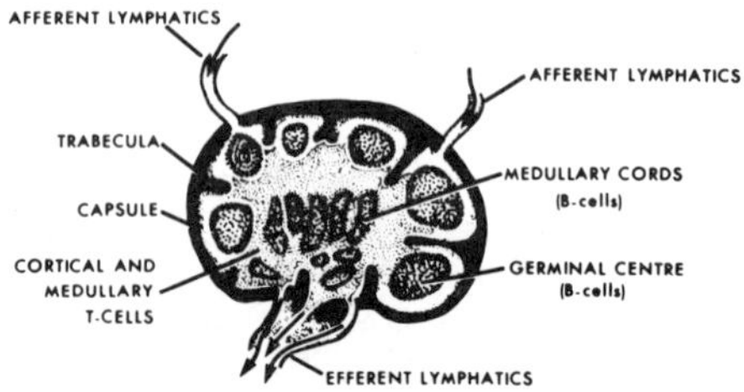

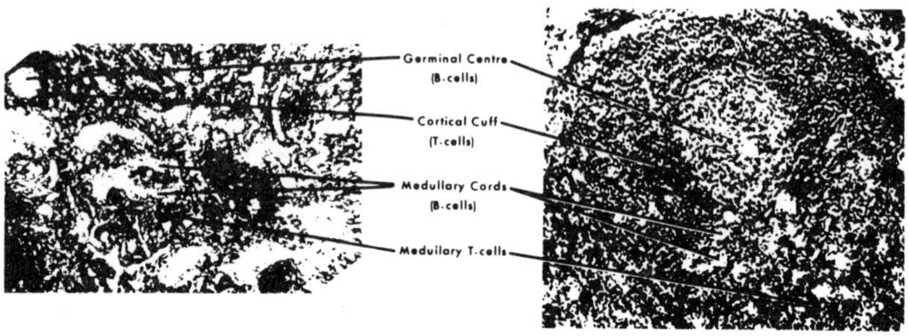

B Spleen

SCHEMATIC DIAGRAM OF A SECTION THROUGH AN IMMUNOLOGICALLY ACTIVE SPLEEN, SHOWING AREAS OF T-CELLS AND B-CELLS.

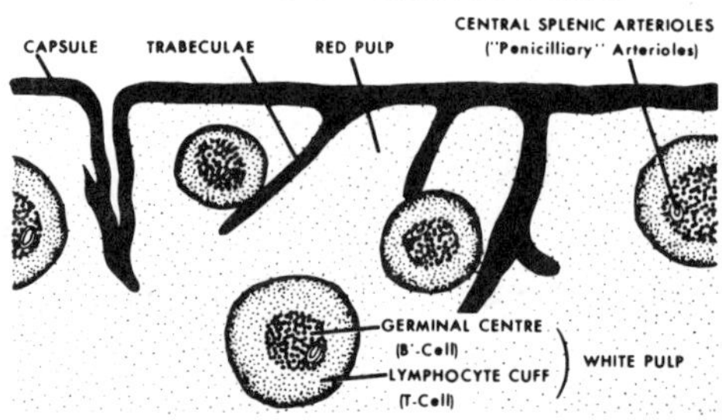

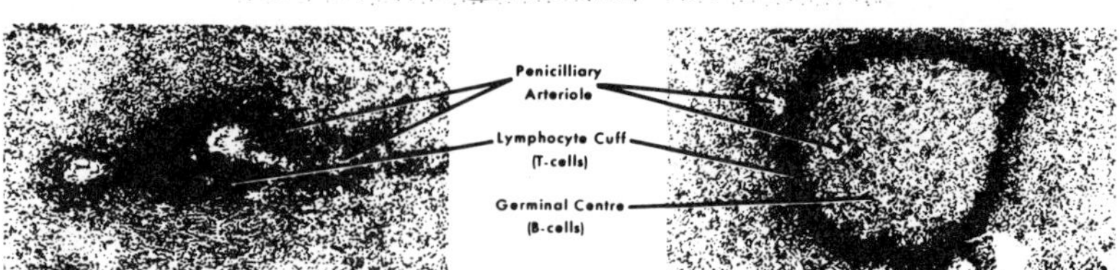

Cross- section through Lymphocyte Cuff

Cross-section through Germinal Centre

B-Cells and Antibody Synthesis

Plasma-cells and their precursors are not the only cells that synthesise immunoglobulins, as has been noted above. Review of the histology of lymphoid organs such as spleen and lymph-nodes will confirm that germinal follicle cells are not usually plasmacytic; they are best described as lymphoblastic. Lymphoblasts in the germinal centres have been shown to contain antibody; moreover, single-cell studies have established that such cells synthesise and release antibody. Some small-to-medium lymphocytes also have been shown to contain immunoglobulins, and to synthesise specific antibodies under experimental conditions. Several lines of evidence are now available that demonstrate unequivocally the existence of a population of B-lymphocytes whose morphology under light microscopy is very similar to that of T-lymphocytes. B-lymphocytes are also demonstrable clinically. For example, Di George patients always demonstrate some small and medium lymphocytes in the circulation and in lymphoid organs. Thus, although the lymphopenia in Di George's Syndrome is profound, it is never absolute, indicating that populations of cells classified morphologically as small or medium lymphocytes are not under control of the thymus. Despite the fact that these patients show absolutely no cellular immunity, they are reasonably immunocompetent with regard to antibody and immunoglobulin synthesis. It is extremely likely that the lymphocytes observed in these patients are members of the B-cell series.

In functional neoplasms of the humoral immune system (*e.g.*, multiple myeloma), the commonest cell type encountered is the plasma-cell. Some of these tumours, however, show neoplastic lymphoblasts synthesising immunoglobulin. Functional (immunoglobulin-producing) neoplastic cells with the morphology of mature small lymphocytes have not been demonstrated unequivocally in immunoglobulin-secreting neoplasms of this type.

In summary, we conclude that some cells with the morphology of mature small lymphocytes are members of the B-cell series, and thus involved in the expression of humoral immunity. Their total and precise role in humoral responses is not completely understood, although much evidence exists in favour of them serving the role of immunologic memory cells. Lymphoblasts are now well-established as immunoglobulin-synthesising cells, but are quantitatively of lesser importance than cells of the plasmacytic series, which represent the major cells involved in the synthesis of immunoglobulins. Follicular lymphoid tissue associated with the gut or even more primitive stem cells in bone marrow have been suggested as the source of mature B-cells in the mammal. However, the precise analogue of the avian Bursa of Fabricius in animals is still a matter of controversy-some workers favouring gut-associated lymphoid tissue ("GALT") and other favouring bone marrow. It is entirely possible that both bone marrow and GALT are sources of B-cells in mammalian species.

Macrophages in Immune Responses

The acquisition of systems of adaptive immunity by vertebrates has not lessened the importance of phagocytosis to these organisms as a mechanism of resistance to infectious disease. In fact, macrophages or mononuclear phagocytic cells were recognised as important elements in resistance to infectious diseases very early in the history of medical bacteriology. These cells are able to ingest and digest many types of organisms that gain entrance to the body, without requiring specific immunologic assistance from the lymphoid system. However, macrophages also play important (even essential) roles in immune responses of both cellular and humoral types.

Mononuclear phagocytes are involved in all three physiological limbs of immune responses.

In the afferent limb, they carry many phagocytosed antigens to the immunologically-competent cells of the lymphoid system. In fact, most antigens reach the immune system in the phagocytosed state.

Macrophages continue to function in the central limb of the immune response. There is a great deal of experimental evidence to support the view that macrophages are required to process antigens in some way that involves coupling the antigen to RNA. Although this processing reaction is not yet understood, it appears to result in activation of the antigen so that the immunocompetent lymphoid cells are better able to respond to it immunologically.

Macrophages also serve as important components of the efferent limb of many immune responses. For example, antibodies and macrophages interact in several ways. Certain antibodies, functionally categorised as opsonins*, increase the rate at which bacteria and

* *The term opsonin is derived from the Greek οψων meaning dressing or relish. Such antibodies serve to coat surface constituents of bacteria and render them more susceptible to phagocytosis.*

other infectious agents are phagocytosed. Opsonins also frequently confer on the macrophage an increased ability to digest and destroy microbial parasites.

Macrophages are able to interact with another type of antibody, which has affinity for certain receptors on the membranes of these phagocytic cells. This antibody is denoted as cytophilic for macrophages, because of its affinity for their membranes. In fact, the binding of this antibody to the macrophage membrane is so tight that repeated washings of suspended macrophages coated with cytophilic antibody *in vitro* fail to remove it from these cells. Heating the cell suspension to 56°C for one hour, or treatment of the cells with a proteolytic enzyme, appears to be necessary to detach cytophilic antibody from its macrophages. (These processes presumably destroy the receptor sites on the cell membrane). Macrophages containing cytophilic antibody have definitely enhanced abilities to recognise, engulf, and destroy antigenic microörganisms, or to restrict their intracellular growth.

Macrophages are also important components in the reactions which follow the contact of a sensitised lymphocyte with its provoking antigen. Reaction of a sensitised lymphocyte with its target antigen results in the activation of the sensitised cell, stimulating it to release biologically-active substances, denoted as "lymphokines", some of which affect the behaviour of macrophages. One of these substances is chemotactic for circulating blood monocytes, inducing these cells to emigrate through the walls of vessels and accumulate in the region of the activated lymphocyte, assuming the form of tissue macrophages or histiocytes. Another substance released from activated lymphocytes inhibits migratory activity of macrophages in proximity to the lymphocyte, thus preventing these cells from leaving the site. Histological sections of such sites show massive infiltrations of mononuclear phagocytes because of the activity of lymphokines which serve to concentrate them in the vicinity of antigen-activated lymphocytes. These macrophages are responsible for many of the features of cellular reactions, as will be seen presently.

The interactions of T-cells, B-cells, and macrophages in immune responses will be considered in more detail in chapter 8 (*vide infra*). This area has assumed great importance in immunobiology, and thus will be considered in some detail after certain basic concepts have been amplified in the next several chapters.

Chapter 3

EXAMPLES OF B-CELL AND T-CELL IMMUNE RESPONSES

A Model B-Cell Response: Immunity to Diphtheria

Acquired resistance to the toxic effects of a toxigenic bacterium, *Corynebacterium diphtheriae*, will serve as a type-example of a (B-cell dependent) humoral response. *C. diphtheriae* may infect the pharynx of a person who has not been infected previously by that organism and has not been immunised previously with diphtheria toxoid. Toxigenic *Corynebacteria* grow superficially on the pharyngeal mucous membranes. As they grow, they liberate a specific protein toxin, which has a necrotising effect on many kinds of mammalian cells. Since it is present in highest concentration in the vicinity of the growing bacteria, the first clinical effects are seen in the pharynx, where a pseudomembrane, composed of exuded fibrin and dead mucosal tissue, forms. As the *Corynebacteria* continue to grow, however, the constantly-accumulating toxin is disseminated via the blood and lymphatics to many different tissues at distant sites from the (still-localised) infection. The outcome of an untreated diphtheria infection depends on the celerity with which the toxin reaches susceptible tissue of critical importance (*e.g.*, myocardium) in contrast to the rapidity with which it acts as an antigen and stimulates B-cells to produce circulating antibodies capable of inactivating it. Where antitoxic antibodies are produced rapidly in sufficient quantity, the patient may recover from the infection.

Certain essential features of all humoral responses that are well illustrated by the response to diphtheria toxin follow:

(1) Antitoxic antibodies (or antitoxin) which circulate in the plasma and body fluids, can be produced in consequence of B-cells of the lymphoid system having been stimulated by contact with toxin-antigen.

(2) The antibodies thus produced are specific for the toxin that provoked their synthesis. Antibodies provoked by diphtheria toxin (or its formalin-inactivated product, denoted as toxoid) have no general antitoxic properties, and thus cannot inactivate other toxic substances - *e.g.*: tetanus toxin (*tetanospasmin*) or botulinus toxin (*botulin*). The antitoxic properties of these antibodies are absolutely specific for diphtheria toxin (the antigen that provoked their formation).

(3) The resistance conferred by antigenic exposure to diphtheria toxin is very long-lived (it often persists for life). Thus, a patient who has recovered from one attack of diphtheria or has been immunised by prophylactic injections of diphtheria toxoid, may be resistant to diphtheria for the rest of his life.

(4) Antisera from patients immune to diphtheria toxin can be used to confer short-term (passive) protection on another individual. Such serum, containing specific antitoxic antibodies, will protect any non-immune person into whom it is injected against diphtheria. Furthermore, similar antibody-containing sera (antisera) can be obtained from specifically-immunised animals, as well as humans; human recipients of a non-human antisera are also protected from the disease. However, the duration of protection in this instance is much shorter than when human antiserum is used.

Active and Passive Immunity

When an individual is stimulated to produce his own antibodies (*e.g.*, by toxoid injections or in diphtheria infections) he is said to be immunised actively. Active immunity is generally long-lived, as has been noted.

Conversely, when an individual is injected with antisera (containing pre-formed antibodies), the patient is said to be immunised passively. Passive immunity is short-lived, but nonetheless useful clinically when individuals require protection from a single exposure to an infectious disease like diphtheria.

A Model T-Cell Response: Immunity to Tuberculosis

The tuberculin reaction will serve as a type-example of a cell-mediated immune response - *i.e.*, a response predominantly involving T-cells. This reaction is utilised clinically as a screening test for persons infected with tuberculosis. Tuberculin sensitivity is an example of a cell-mediated immune (CMI) response known as delayed hypersensitivity*.

Individuals who have never been infected with tuberculosis do not react when given an intradermal injection of a bacteria-free filtrate of a broth culture of tubercle bacilli. The filtrate, called old tuberculin and abbreviated as OT, contains certain pro-

* *The prefix delayed is a clinical term used to distinguish this type of cell-mediated (T-cell) hypersensitivity response from antibody-mediated (B-cell) allergic responses, such as acute anaphylaxis, which develop more rapidly after sensitised patients contact their sensitising antigen (i.e., immediate or atopic hypersensitivity). The mechanism of immediate and delayed hypersensitivity reactions are entirely different, as will be seen.*

teins of tubercle bacilli in solution, although no whole tubercle bacilli are present. The tuberculoprotein can be injected in 0.1 cc. doses at 1:1000 dilution of the standardised OT; however, it is now more commonly administered in the form of a purified protein derivative of old tuberculin, designated PPD. Non—reactive (and therefore uninfected) individuals are designated as tuberculin negative.

An individual who has experienced a tuberculous infection (even without overt clinical disease), can be expected to react in a characteristic way to intradermal injections of OT or PPD. Reactive (and therefore at some time infected) individuals are designated as tuberculin positive. These individuals respond to the intradermal injection with a local reaction, which when especially severe, may be accompanied by systemic effects (such as pyrexia, malaise, arthralgia, and headache).

The Local Reaction

At the injection site, an area of erythema develops about six hours after injection. This is followed by the development of an indurated nodule over the next 18 to 48 hours. If this nodule is biopsied and examined histologically, a dense collection of perivascular mononuclear cells is seen. This consists primarily of lymphocytes and macrophages.

The tuberculin reaction, therefore, may be described as a specifically-provoked, slowly-evolving, mixed-cellular reaction, occurring in individuals who have been sensitised by prior infection with tubercle bacilli. Employed as a diagnostic tool, the reaction may be provoked by injection of tuberculoprotein (as in tuberculosis screening programmes). However, a similar sequence of events may be provoked by reinfection by tubercle bacilli or by reactivation of long-quiescent Mycobacteria within a dormant primary tubercle.

The tuberculin reaction (unlike the diphtheria antitoxic response) is not mediated by circulating antibodies. Consequently, non-sensitised (tuberculin-negative) individuals cannot be sensitised passively by injections of antiserum from sensitised (tuberculin-positive) persons. Tuberculin non-reactors can be sensitised passively to tuberculoproteins, however, by injecting them with lymphoid cells from tuberculin reactors. Sensitisation to tuberculoprotein is therefore a cellular phenomenon; the cells that mediate this reaction are referred to as sensitised lymphocytes, and are entirely members of the T-cells series - *i.e.*, thymus dependent.

The sensitised lymphocyte is the mediator of all CMI reactions, these cells both recognising and reacting with the antigens that stimulated their appearance. The molecular nature of the effector and the mechanism of antigen recognition by sensitised T-lymphocytes, however, remain unknown. The demonstrable independence of cellular immunity from serum antibodies suggests that if antibodies are the ultimate effectors of antigen-recognition, they are of a type that do not circulate in detectable quantities in the serum, and of a type that has a high affinity for the cell-membranes of lymphocytes*.

In spite of the fact that antibodies have not been demonstrated to play a role in the reactions of cellular immunity, the specificity of sensitised lymphocytes for antigen is very similar to that of serum antibodies. Like specific antibodies, sensitised T-cells are capable of a fine degree of discrimination between the sensitising antigen and closely-related substances.

The Passive Transfer of Specific Cellular Immunity to Tuberculin: Transfer Factor

It has been noted that sensitivity to tuberculin can be transferred by injecting non-sensitised recipients with lymphoid cells from sensitised donors, but not by injections of antiserum derived from sensitised donors. However, tuberculin sensitivity can also be transferred from sensitised human donors to non-sensitised recipients by means of a substance called transfer factor, prepared from sensitised lymphoid cells.

The chemical nature of transfer factor is not known at present. It is a relatively small molecule (molecular weight $\sim$10,000) which is readily dialysable. It is stable to heating to 56°C for six hours, and resistant to treatment with the hydrolytic enzymes DNA-ase, RNA-ase and trypsin. Although transfer factor has been isolated repeatedly from sensitised human lymphoid cells, a satisfactory animal model has not yet been developed. Thus, all of the above data derive from studies in man.

Activation of Sensitised Lymphocytes Following Contact with Specific Antigens: Lymphokine Release

When a sensitised T-lymphocyte contacts its antigen, the cell becomes activated. A series of

* *Antibodies with affinity for cell-membranes have been referred to as cytophilic (i.e., cell-loving) antibodies, as noted in Chapter 2.*

stereotyped biological processes is initiated within the lymphocyte, which ultimately results in the establishment of a delayed hypersensitivity reaction.

Physiologically-active substances, designated as "lymphokines", are synthesised and released by sensitised lymphocytes which have become activated by contact with antigens. A variety of lymphokines have now been identified. These include:

- A substance which inhibits the migratory activities of macrophages (designated as migration-inhibitory factor, or M.I.F.) in the vicinity of the sensitised, activated T-cell.
- A substance that is chemotactic to leucocytes (chemotaxin), and thus summons these cells into the vicinity of the activated T-lymphocyte.
- A substance that has non-specific toxic activity on living cells (cytotoxin).
- A substance that will induce non-sensitised lymphocytes to undergo blastogenic transformation, and to undergo repeated cell division (blastogen-mitogen).
- A non-specific inhibitor of virus replication (interferon).

M.I.F.: Macrophages placed in a capillary tube within a tissue-culture chamber will migrate out of the tube, and spread out over the glass walls of the chamber. If, however, a small number of sensitised T-lymphocytes are present within the chamber, and a small amount of antigen is then added, the migration of macrophages out of the capillary tube will be prevented. This is a consequence of the synthesis and release of M.I.F. by sensitised lymphocytes following contact with antigen, and is illustrated in Figure 1. M.I.F. is a biological effector which inhibits migratory activities of macrophages and other leucocytes present in the area of the sensitised lymphocyte. It is a protein (molecular weight $\sim$ 80,000), stable at 56°C for 30 minutes, but rapidly inactivated by trypsin, and close to albumin in its electrophoretic mobility. M.I.F. has not yet been purified entirely. However, relatively-pure preparations have been prepared with very high biological activity, and injection of such preparations intradermally will induce the development of a typical delayed-hypersensitivity reaction *in situ*, except that the development of the lesion is somewhat accelerated. Thus, M.I.F. is thought to favour the accumulation of mononuclear phagocytes in the vicinity of an activated T-lymphocyte, and the localisation of these cells at sites of antigenic stimulation *in vivo*.

Cytotoxin: A non-specific cytotoxic effect on living cells is produced when such cells are incubated with cell-free medium from leucocyte cultures contain-

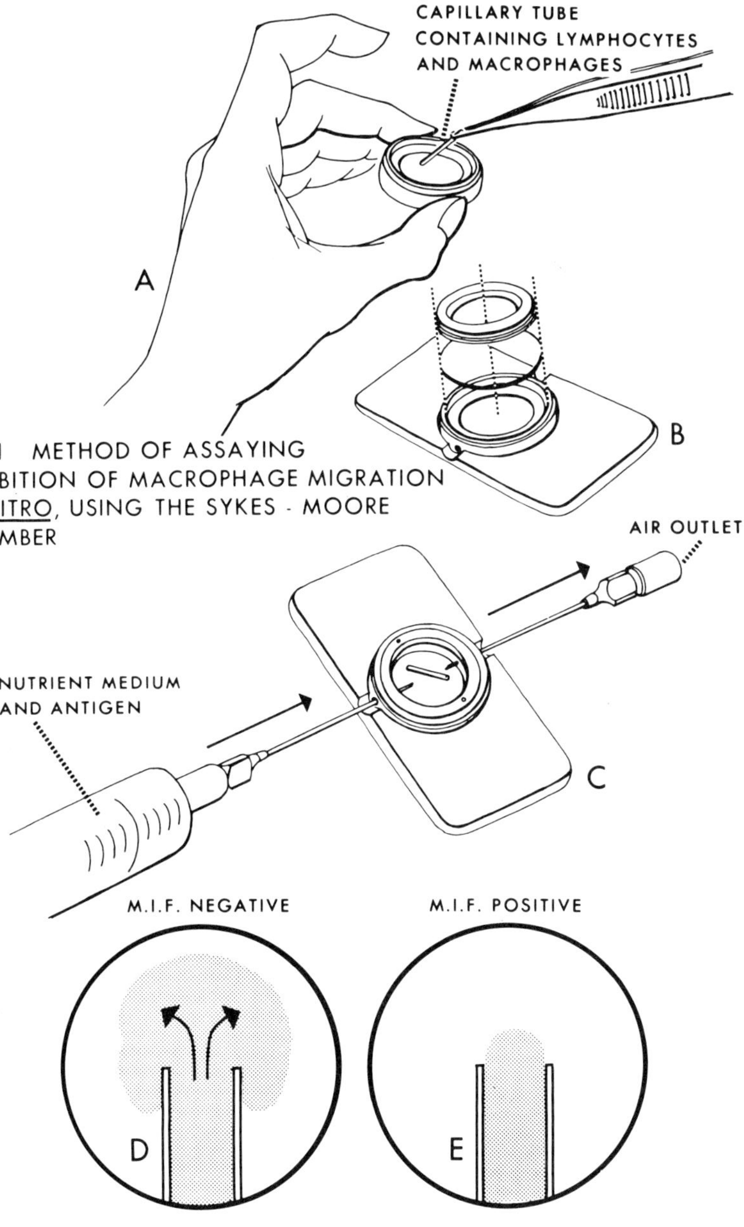

Fig. 1 METHOD OF ASSAYING INHIBITION OF MACROPHAGE MIGRATION IN VITRO, USING THE SYKES - MOORE CHAMBER

ing antigen-activated T-lymphocytes. The cytotoxin produced by activated T-lymphocytes has been separated clearly from M.I.F. activity. It is readily inactivated by heating to 80°C for 30 minutes, and migrates electrophoretically in the slow-β-to-fast-γ-region.

Chemotaxin: Cell-free media from activated lymphocyte cultures are chemotactic to mononuclear phagocytes. This chemotaxin has not yet been adequately characterised, but preliminary studies have indicated that it has a molecular weight of ∿ 80,000 and migrates electrophoretically with albumin. Chemotactic and migration-inhibiting activities have been separated by the use of polyacrilamide gel electrophoresis. The two activities would appear to act synergistically *in situ* to favour the accumulation of inflammatory cells characteristic of delayed hypersensitivity.

Blastogen-Mitogen: Cell-free media from activated lymphocyte cultures exert a blastogenic and mitosis-stimulating effect on non-sensitised small lymphocytes. Blastogenic (and mitogenic) activities have not yet been separated clearly from M.I.F.

Blast Transformation by Activated Lymphocytes

In addition to the synthesis and release of biologically-active compounds, activated lymphocytes themselves transform into large metabolically-active cells which have the morphology of lymphoblasts. This process is termed blast cell transformation. It is accompanied by demonstrable synthesis of DNA, RNA and protein, and also by mitotic activity.

In vitro transformation of lymphocytes can be used to assess the degree of sensitisation of a lymphocyte population. The parameters used to measure transformation in the laboratory include:

(a) counting the proportion of the cells that undergo morphological alterations, such as increase in size,

(b) counting the number of dividing cells (the mitotic-index count), expressed as a fraction over the total number of cells, and,

(c) measuring DNA synthesis by the uptake of tritium (H^3)-labelled thymidine.

Method (c) is the one now most commonly employed, and peripheral blood lymphocytes are usually the cells which are studied.

A blood sample is taken and the white cells of the buffy-coat are placed in replicate tubes for culture. The antigen is added to some of the tubes, whilst others serve as controls. After five-to-seven days of culture in the presence of the antigen, H^3-thymidine is added for a two-to-twelve hour period, and the incorporation of isotopically-labelled thymidine into DNA is determined.

If T-lymphocytes are present which have been sensitised previously to the antigen under test, the cultures to which the antigen was added will incorporate significantly larger amounts of the radioactive tracer then will the controls to which no antigen was added.

M.I.F. can be detected within six hours after contact of sensitised cells with antigen, whilst transformation does not occur for some time thereafter. However, cells which release M.I.F. usually undergo transformation as well, and both processes may be regarded as consequences of the general process of lymphocyte activation.

Activation of Lymphocytes Following Contact With Non-Specific Mitogens

It is interesting to note that many of the biological activities discussed above can be induced in two ways, as shown in Figure 2.

Firstly, lymphocytes can be activated specifically by contact with the antigen to which they are sensitised, as has been noted in the discussion above.

Secondly, non-sensitised lymphocytes can be activated non-specifically by treatment with any of several types of non-specific activators - including such plant-derived agents ("lectins") as phytohaemagglutinin (PHA), poke-weed mitogen, and concanavallin-A. Although the biological effects on lymphocytes induced by these non-specific mitogens are generally similar to specific antigen-induced blast transformation, minor differences do exist. For example, the degree of blast transformation is usually much greater when the non-specific mitogens are employed than during specific antigenic stimulation of previously-sensitised cells. However, the ability of lymphocytes in culture to respond to plant mitogens like PHA correlates well with *in vivo* T-cell immunocompetence. Hence, such cultures are frequently employed in the clinical laboratory as an aid in the diagnosis of T-cell dysfunction, such as may occur in a variety of clinical diseases.

Fig. 2 SCHEMA OF LYMPHOCYTE ACTIVATION BY SPECIFIC AND NON-SPECIFIC ACTIVATORS

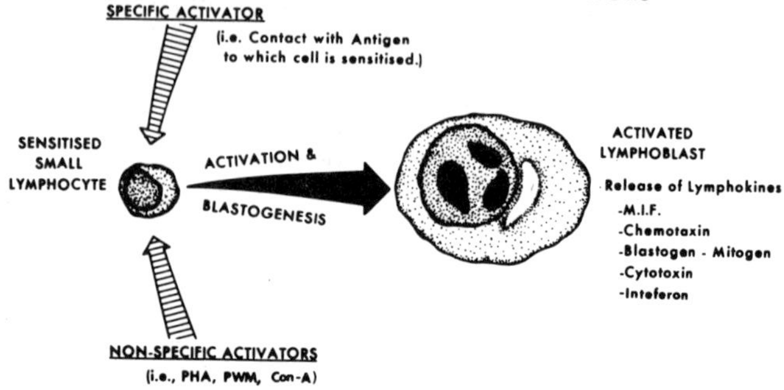

Tuberculin Sensitivity as a Defense Mechanism in Tuberculosis

Tuberculin sensitivity (like diphtheria antitoxin) may assist individuals who have recovered from an infection with *M. tuberculosis* in resisting subsequent attacks or reinfections by this agent. When a tuberculin-positive patient is reinfected with tubercle bacilli, the intense cellular infiltrate stimulated by contact with the bacilli often walls off the focus of infection before it can establish itself fully. This same reaction may also prevent the establishment of satellite lesions in adjacent or distant sites by bacilli shed from a primary focus of infection.

However, tuberculin sensitivity is by no means an unmixed blessing, since massive destruction of tissue consequent upon this reaction may itself cause severe clinical disease. For example, a reaction of this type occurring in the lungs may lead to the development of caseous pneumonia (phthisis). A common condition in past years, phthisis often had a fulminating, fatal course. (Its present rarity is due primarily to the widespread availability of potent chemotherapeutic agents for tuberculosis). Tuberculin hypersensitivity thus has potential value in containing infection, but such sensitivity also carries potential threat to the host. Perhaps it is best viewed as a double-edged sword, which may be helpful or harmful in differing circumstances.

Summary and Concluding Remarks

Although there are still large gaps in our understanding of the mechanisms of cellular immunity, a pattern is beginning to emerge which may ultimately tie many isolated facts and interpretations of fact into a logical mechanistic sequence. Let us see how this might occur:

Intradermal injection of PPD into a tuberculin-sensitised patient causes a small number of sensitised lymphocytes at the site of injection to become activated. These activated cells release into the surrounding extracellular fluids several physiologically-active effectors, including M.I.F., chemotaxin, blastogen-mitogen, cytotoxin, and interferon. These processes are diagrammed in Figure 2 (*vide infra*). The substances released following antigen-activation of a T-lymphocyte cause monocytes, macrophages, polymorphonuclear cells, and other (non-sensitised) lymphocytes to accumulate at the injection site. Non-sensitised lymphocytes accumulating in the reaction site become transformed into blast cells, and liberate more biological effectors, *i.e.*, lymphokines, into the area. These effectors amplify the initial effects and result in larger accumulations of mononuclear cells into the area of injection. Only the initial antigen-binding by the T-lymphocyte membrane is specific; this specific process serves primarily in the role of an initiator of the subsequent cycle of non-specific effects. The end-result is the development of a delayed hypersensitivity reaction at the site of antigen deposition.

Evidence exists that the list of lymphokines presented here is not complete. However, the addition of more soluble factors with non-specific biological amplifier properties produced by activated lymphocytes to the already formidable list of lymphokines presented herein, does not seem didactically advantageous to the author.

Chapter 4

THE NATURE OF ANTIGENS

An antigen (or immunogen) is defined as any molecule which elicits either a cellular or humoral immune response. Although either T-cell or B-cell stimulation may predominate in any given circumstance, usually both types of lymphoid cells are stimulated to some degree by most antigens. Whilst the most significant antigens are proteins, certain highly polymerised carbohydrates may elicit immune responses of either or both types. Other biological macro-molecules, such as nucleic acids and polymerised fatty acids, have not been shown conclusively to be immunogenic (antigenically-active) when administered by themselves in highly purified states. However, these molecules, though inactive when administered alone, may elicit specific antibody formation (or specific cellular immunity) when adminstered as protein conjugates. In other words, these molecules are capable of acting as haptens. Moreover, much smaller and simpler chemicals exhibit haptenic properties.

For example, simple chemical haptens such as aminobenzene sulphonate linked covalently to carrier proteins, elicit antibodies highly specific for the steric structure of the hapten employed (*e.g.*, antibodies directed against meta-aminobenzene sulphonate obtained by immunising with a diazo-protein derivative of this hapten cross-react poorly with different hapten isomers such as the ortho-or para-forms, as may be seen in Fig. 1). Furthermore, the experimental work that established isomer binding specificity of antibodies suggested that these antibodies were directed against relatively small areas on the antigen molecule. In other words, haptenic groups could be of small molecular size; were this not the case, it would be impossible to explain the steric specificity of antibodies in the situation illustrated in Fig. 1. Further substantiation of this point was achieved by demonstrating that antibodies directed against polysaccharide antigens were fully reactive with oligosaccharide (hapten) derivatives of the parent polysaccharide consisting of 5 sugar residues.

Studies with protein immunogens have established that antibodies to these will also react with small oligopeptide segments of these proteins, comprising only 5 to 6 amino-acid residues. In these cases the determinants are most likely sequential. However, for most proteins the determinants are conformational. Recognition of either certain oligopeptide sequences or conformations on protein antigens is not random; the same sequences or shapes can be recognised as antigens

Fig. I STERIC SPECIFICITY OF ANTIBODIES

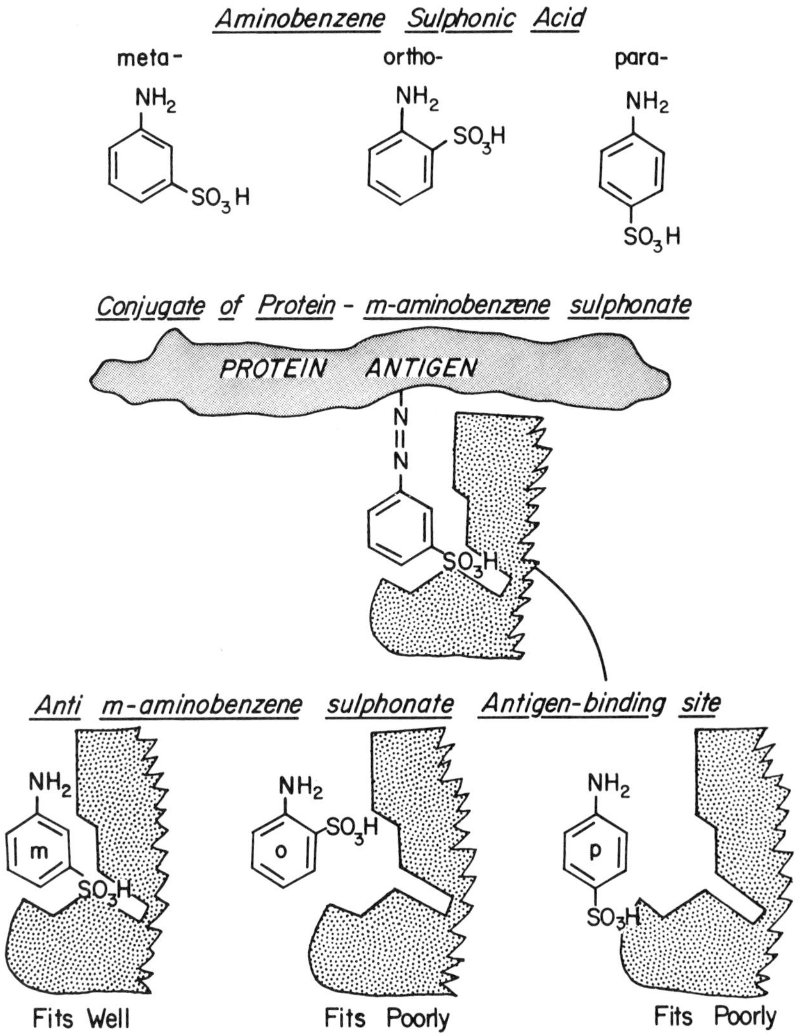

in a wide variety of animals, and furthermore, only a limited number of sequences can be so recognised. Such immunologically recognisable haptenic regions on antigen molecules are defined as antigenic determinants.

Thus, protein antigens may be regarded as possessing a relatively small number of *immunologically-reactive* regions (antigenic determinants) joined together by (much larger) sequences of *immunologically-inert* polypeptides.

Methods of Demonstrating Haptenic Regions on Protein Antigens

Since proteins represent the major naturally-occurring complete immunogens, special emphasis is placed on approaches to haptens derived from studies of protein molecules. Definition of the antigenic determinants of a protein or peptide involves localisation of these regions against which antibodies are directed. Three major methods of approach to this problem have been utilised in the laboratory.

(1) Certain amino-acids (*e.g., tyrosine* and *tryptophane*) can be modified by treating the protein with appropriate chemical reagents. Subsequent to modification, antigenic determinants containing such altered amino-acid residues will have different affinities for antibody binding sites than did the original antigenic determinant. In this way, the regions against which antibody activity is directed (antigenic determinants) can be identified and localised to some extent. However, the results obtained by this method may be misleading, because of the fact that modification of amino-acid residues on the surface of a protein or peptide may mask old or uncover new antigenic determinants by altering the tertiary structure of the entire molecule (Fig. 2). One cannot therefore conclude that peptides which contain modified amino-acids and altered antibody combining activity are functional antigenic determinants in the native protein.

(2) Antigenic determinants on polypeptides or proteins may be studied in a more precise manner, wherein controlled partial cleavage of the protein antigen (either with proteolytic enzymes or chemicals like cyanogen bromide*) is initially accomplished, followed by isolation of the resultant peptides, and subsequent testing of these for their reactivity with antibodies directed against the intact antigen.

* *Vide infra, appendix B.*

Fig. 2

ANALYSIS OF THE STRUCTURE OF PROTEIN ANTIGEN BY CHEMICAL MODIFICATION OF COMPONENT RESIDUES

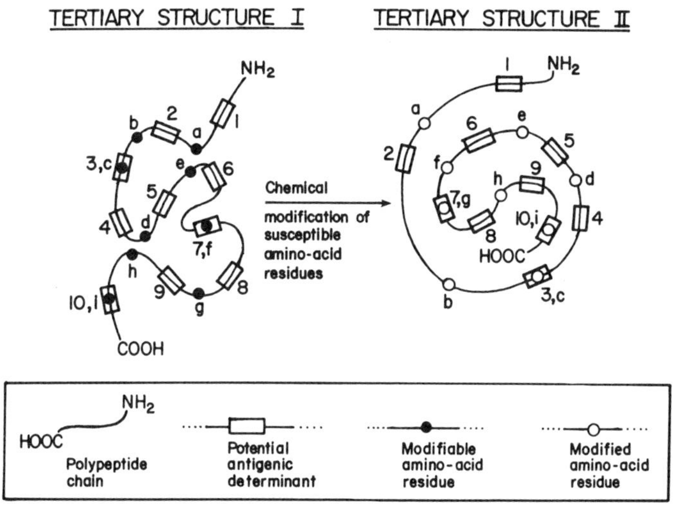

Where this situation (····—▭●▭—····) occurs, this technique may be employed

On this protein, potential antigenic determinants 3, 7 and 10 have modifiable key amino-acid residues.

Structure I (Prior to treatment):

Determinants 1, 2, 3, 4, 6, 8, 10 are accessible to antibody.

Structure II (Following treatment):

Determinants 1, 2, 3, 4, 5 are accessible to antibody.

∴ Only Determinants 1-4 are accessible in both forms.
Of these, only Determinant 3 has modified residue within it.

Thus, in this situation, only 1 residue (Nº 3, containing modified amino-acid residue c) can be studied by this technique.

Susie Anderson

(3) Considerable use has been made of synthetic polypeptides for determining the structure of antigenic determinants. The synthetic approach offers the advantage that once a biological property has been unequivocally demonstrated, a number of analogs may be prepared and tested. For example, the effects of the following variables may be studies: amino-acid substitution, conformational changes, differences in electrostatic charge, etc.

By these kinds of studies, definitive information on the nature of antigenic determinants of proteins is currently coming to light.

Methods for Measuring Primary Interactions Between Antigens and Antibodies: Peptide Antigens and Haptens

Inhibition of Agglutination and Precipitation

Since antibodies to protein immunogens are directed against small peptides, these peptides retain their affinity for antibodies produced in response to the intact protein, even following isolation from the parent molecule. Because such isolated antigenic determinants are non-precipitating, antigen-antibody reactions which require multivalent antigens (see chapters 6 and 7) for measurement of the interaction cannot be employed in such studies. Nonetheless, these "monovalent" antigenic determinants, when combined with specific antibody, block the antibody's ability to bind complete antigen. This mechanism, *i.e.*, inhibition of precipitation or agglutination reactions, is the basic principle utilised by all indirect methods for measuring binding activity. When conducting inhibition studies, virtually any standard system may be employed to measure antigen-antibody binding following inhibition. An example of a typical inhibition test follows:

A. Antiserum to bovine serum albumin (BSA) is titred using an agglutination reaction with latex particles or specially prepared sheep red cells in which the antigen (BSA) is bound to the surfaces of the particles or cells.

B. The titred antiserum is then mixed and incubated with antigenic peptide derived from BSA to allow hapten binding to occur.

C. The reactant mixture (containing antigen fragments bound to the antiserum) is then diluted into a series of test tubes, in parallel to a series of control tubes containing the same amount of antiserum, but no antigenic fragments. A fixed amount of BSA-coated particles is added to each control and experimental tube. The control series and the test series are then incubated with the antigen-coated particles or cells to allow both series to reach a state of reaction equilibrium.

D. The end-points in both series are observed and compared. If the experimental mixture did contain the inhibiting peptide bearing antigenic determinants for anti-BSA antibodies prior to the addition of BSA-coated particles, the apparent titre (end-point) of the experimental series will be lower than that of the control series (*i.e.*, the binding sites which are occupied by inhibitor in the experimental series will reflect the apparent fall in titre over the control series, in which no sites are bound prior to mixture with antigen-coated particles, *vide infra*, Chapter 6, discussion of agglutination reactions). The technique is similar to that employed in the pregnancy test illustrated in Fig. 13.

The Ammonium Sulphate Precipitation Method (Farr Technique)

A radioactively-labelled peptide prepared from BSA is mixed with antiserum to the intact protein, and incubated for an appropriate length of time. The immune (antibody-peptide) complexes are then precipitated with 50% saturated ammonium sulphate. The precipitate is washed and its radioactivity measured. The presence of radioactivity in the precipitate indicates binding of peptide by the antibody immunoglobulin, since this concentration of ammonium sulphate will precipitate immunoglobulins and antigen-antibody complexes but not peptide alone. A control test, wherein radioactive peptide is mixed with normal serum and the precipitated with 50% ammonium sulphate, will not show radioactivity in the washed precipitate.

Equilibrium Dialysis: This method, developed by Karush, enables us to quantitate the actual amount of a hapten bound by an antibody, and also to measure the affinity with which the antibody binds the hapten, by calculating the dissociation constant of the reaction. The technique is performed as follows:

a. Previously purified specific antibody to the complete antigen, the immunoglobulin fraction of nonspecific serum and suspending buffer, are placed in separate dialysis chambers and suspended in a solution of the radioactively-labelled haptenic peptide. This test is usually run using a range of hapten concentrations of about 100 fold and a number of separate preparations are thus set up.

b. The containers (with the dialysis chambers and the hapten solution) are shaken gently until counts from the peptide are equal in the outside solution to those in the dialysis chamber containing the suspending buffer. At this time it can be assumed that the peptide has reached equilibrium with the fluids inside the dialysis chambers.

c. Samples from the specific antibody and the non-specific immunoglobulin dialysis preparations are taken, as well as from the peptide solutions, and aliquots are counted for radioactivity. Specific antibody combines (depending on the concentration of the hapten and the dissociation constant of the reaction) with the hapten, and once combined, the hapten is no longer in equilibrium with the free hapten on either side of the dialysis membrane. Consequently, *more* hapten will be present in the dialysis chambers containing specific antibody, since this will contain an equivalent amount of free hapten (both inside and outside at equilibrium) *plus* the amount bound to specific antibody. Moreover, an antibody with a high binding-affinity for the hapten will show a great deal of binding even at a low hapten concentration. The use of non-specific immunoglobulin in such tests merely serves as a negative control to demonstrate that the hapten under test does not bind non-specifically to immunoglobulin molecules.

Equilibrium dialysis studies carried out on chemical haptens decades ago demonstrated clearly that antigen-antibody reactions occur only over a pH range of about 4 - 9, and are optimal in solutions in which the ionic strength approaches those of physiological fluids, within a temperature range of 4 to 40°C. Studies using equilibrium dialysis also indicated the bivalence to the antibody molecule and the heterogeneity of so-called "pure" populations of antibodies long before rigorous chemical means were available to confirm these concepts.

The Present State of Knowledge of Protein Antigens

To date, there is still relatively little information regarding the nature of the antigenic determinants on protein antigens. However, certain general observations may be summarised:

1. When undenatured proteins, which retain their tertiary structures, are used as antigens, active anti-

genic determinants appear to encompass either external sequences or regions located on the "corners" of the molecule. Potentially-immunogenic regions inaccessible to the lymphoid system do not stimulate immunologic reactions unless they are externalised by denaturation or by partial hydrolysis of the molecule.

2. When a protein is denatured, and its tertiary structure destroyed before it is used as an antigen, the antibody molecules produced against the denatured protein frequently fail to react with the "undenatured" form of the molecule and *vice versa*. However, the amino-acid sequences of the antigen which can stimulate and react with antibody in either the natural or denatured protein often appear to be the same. Immunogenic activity in a given situation appears to be largely a matter of accessibility of potential antigenic determinants.

3. The maximum size of an antigenic determinant on a protein antigen is probably four to five amino-acid residues in length.

4. Both charge and hydrophobicity of polypeptide regions within a protein antigen molecule may contribute to the specificity and reactivity of that molecule's antigenic determinants. These non-covalent intramolecular bonds affect the ability of the molecule to combine with antibody by conferring a fixed, specific tertiary structure on the antigen molecule, which governs the accessibility of antigenic determinants to the antigen-binding sites of antibodies, as well as the 3-dimensional structure of the antigenic determinants themselves.

(Review of the methods employed in studying the primary structure of proteins are presented in appendix B).

Chapter 5

THE IMMUNOGLOBULINS

Human antibody molecules can serve as antigens to other animals; therefore, antibody molecules can be characterised according to their antigenic structure.

In the introductory chapter, it was noted that plasma proteins with antibody activity are classified as immunoglobulins. A more precise definition of immunoglobulins is now required. Immunoglobulins include all plasma proteins with demonstrable antibody activity and any other plasma proteins that have antigenic determinants in common with any known antibody. Thus, a plasma protein possessing no demonstrable antibody activity is considered an immunoglobulin if it shares any antigenic determinant with any known antibody.

The immunoglobulins of man have been shown to include five antigenically-distinct classes of molecules. That is, although each class of proteins bears certain antigenic determinants which are common to all immunoglobulins, they are divisible into classes by virtue of other antigenic determinants which fall into five unique groups. The nomenclature of these classes is presented in Figure 1.

Fig. 1 NOMENCLATURE OF IMMUNOGLOBULINS

	Immunoglobulin (Ig) Class	*Established Antibody Activity*	*Ultracentrifugal Sedimentation*
Major Classes	IgG (γG)	+	7S
	IgA (γA)	+	7S - 11S
	IgM (γM) (macroglobulin)	+	19S
Minor Classes	IgD (γD)	+	7S
	IgE (γE) (reagin)	+	7.8S

The Structure of Immunoglobulins

All immunoglobulins, irrespective of class, are composed of similar basic structural units having four polypeptide chains per unit as indicated in Figure 2. The polypetide chains in any immunoglublin molecule are of two kinds, denoted as H-chains (heavy-chains, molecular weight ~ 50,000) and L-chains (light-chains, molecular weight ~ 20,000).

Fig. 2 THE BASIC STRUCTURAL UNIT OF IMMUNOGLOBULINS

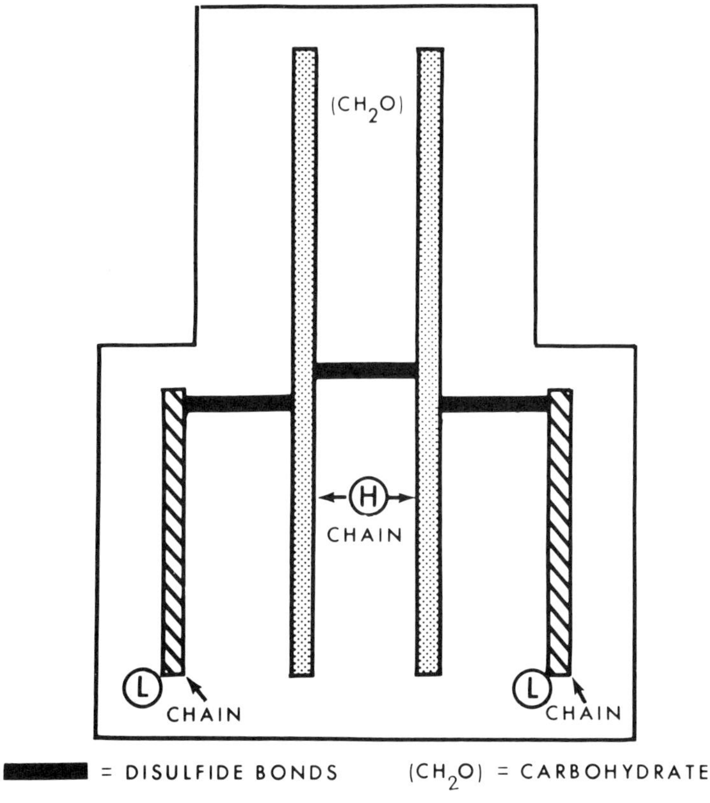

All classes of immunoglobulins are glycoproteins of similar basic structure. The basic structural units are composed of two kinds of polypeptide chains, denoted as *H-* and *L-chains*. The chains are interconnected with each other by a combination of covalent disulfide bonds and non-covalent bonds of various sorts, so that they form basic 4-chain units, as shown. The two *H-chains* and the two *L-chains* that occur in any given immunoglobulin molecule are always duplicates (*i.e.*, of identical structure). Thus, a 4-chain basic unit can be split into two identical (2-chain) half-molecules, comprised of one *H-chain* and one *L-chain* in each half.

H-chains contain the class-specific antigenic determinants. They are of five separate antigenic types, and they specify the antigenic class to which an immunoglobulin molecule belongs. The antigenic types of H-chains are denoted by Greek-letter equivalents for the letters used to express the corresponding immunoglobulin class. For example, the H-chains of IgM molecules are denoted as μ-chains, the H-chains of IgG molecules as γ-chains, the H-chains of IgA molecules as α-chains, the H-chains of IgD as δ-chains, and the H-chains of IgE as ε-chains.

L-chains, on the other hand, occur in two principal antigenic types, denoted as κ- and λ-, in all classes of immunoglobulins. However, a single immunoglobulin molecule may have either two κ-chains or two λ-chains - never one of each. Molecules with κ-chains and molecules with λ-chains occur in all of the immunoglobulin classes. The former type of molecule is denoted as a K-type immunoglobulin, and the latter type of molecule as an L-type immunoglobulin.

The above remarks are summarised in Figure 3.

Fig. 3 ANTIGENIC CLASSES OF IMMUNOGLOBULINS

Ig Class	*Class-Specific H-chain*	NOTE: Each class of immunoglobulin is subdivided into K-type molecules and L-type molecules depending on the type of L-chain occurring in each molecule.
IgG	γ-	
IgA	α-	
IgM	μ-	
IgD	δ-	
IgE	ε-	

Thus, we see that K-type IgG would be composed of two κ-chains, and two γ-chains, whilst L-type IgG would be composed of two λ-chains and two γ-chains.

Immunoglobulin Heterogeneity

The preceding remarks have indicated that immunoglobulins are heterogeneous entities. Five basic classes of molecules, each antigenically distinct by virtue of H-chain determinants, but sharing common antigenic determinants on the L-chains, have been defined. This means that antiserum prepared in a rabbit, for example, directed against human α-chains will distinguish immunoglobulins of the IgA class from all other classes of immunoglobulins. Rabbit antiserum prepared against human κ-chains, however, will react with all immunoglobulins of the K-type, irrespective of their H-chain class.

The foregoing, however, only illustrates the most basic degree of heterogeneity in immunoglobulins - the complexity of these proteins is far greater than has been indicated. In addition to the classes and types mentioned, antigenic subclasses have been demonstrated within the IgG, IgM, and IgA classes of human immunoglobulins. Antigenic subclasses are defined as variations in antigenic type which occur within a given class of H-chains. That is, in addition to the class-specific antigenic determinants which are present on H-chains, the heavy chains possess other antigenic determinants which specify subclasses. All subclasses of immunoglobulins are found in the sera of all normal patients. They are denoted by Arabic numeral subscripts following the Greek letter specifying the H-chain class (*e.g.*, γ_1, γ_2, etc.).

Refined antigenic analysis of human immunoglobulins has revealed four subtypes of γ-chains (IgG), two subtypes of α-chains (IgA), and two subtypes of μ-chains (IgM). It is likely that subclasses will be recognised for the minor classes of immunoglobulins (IgD and IgE) in the near future, and that more subclasses will be recognised similarly within the major classes of immunoglobulins (IgG, IgM and IgA).

A tabular summary of the heterogeneities of human immunoglobulins that have been discussed thus far is presented in Figure 4.

All of the antigenic determinants in Figure 4, being found in the sera of all normal persons, are designated as immunoglobulin isotypes. In contrast to these isotypic determinants, certain other antigenic determinants have been described which occur in the immunoglobulins of some - but not all - normal individuals. These antigenic determinants have been designated as allotypes. Thus, allotypes represent genetic variations in immunoglobulins occurring within the normal population (*i.e.*, the phenotypic markers for allelic genes).

Fig. 4 THE SUBCLASSES AND TYPES OF HUMAN IMMUNOGLOBULIN MOLECULES

H-chain Class	*H-chain Subclass*	*L-chain Type*	*Molecular Formula*	*Alternate Notation*
γ-	γ1	κ-	$(\gamma 1)_2\kappa_2$	G1K
		λ-	$(\gamma 1)_2\lambda_2$	G1L
	γ2	κ-	$(\gamma 2)_2\kappa_2$	G2K
		λ-	$(\gamma 2)_2\lambda_2$	G2L
	γ3	κ-	$(\gamma 3)_2\kappa_2$	G3K
		λ-	$(\gamma 3)_2\lambda_2$	G3L
	γ4	κ-	$(\gamma 4)_2\kappa_2$	G4K
		λ-	$(\gamma 4)_2\lambda_2$	G4L
α-	α1	κ-	$(\alpha 1)_2\kappa_2$	A1K
		λ-	$(\alpha 1)_2\lambda_2$	A1L
	α2	κ-	$(\alpha 2)_2\kappa_2$	A2K
		λ-	$(\alpha 2)_2\lambda_2$	A2L
μ-	μ1	κ-	$(\mu 1)_2\kappa_2$	M1K
		λ-	$(\mu 1)_2\lambda_2$	M1L
	μ2	κ-	$(\mu 2)_2\kappa_2$	M2K
		λ-	$(\mu 2)_2\lambda_2$	M2L
δ-	(δ-)	κ-	$\delta_2\kappa_2$	DK
		λ-	$\delta_2\lambda_2$	DL
ε-	(ε-)	κ-	$\varepsilon_2\kappa_2$	EK
		λ-	$\varepsilon_2\lambda_2$	EL

Three independently-assorting genetic loci regulate human allotype markers. These three sets of allelic genes are designated as *Gm*, *Am* and *InV*.*

The *InV* locus controls inheritable antigenic differences in the κ-type of L-chain.

The *Am* locus regulates an antigenic determinant which is present only on α_2-chains. *Am* genes segregate and assort independently of *Gm* and *InV* genes.

The *Gm* locus specifies inherited antigenic variants occurring amongst the γ-chains of man. Twenty-three *Gm* allotypes are presently known.

Definition of antigenic markers in terms of primary structural variations is proceeding rapidly at present. For example, *InV* alleles have been shown to regulate a single amino-acid substitution in κ-chains. Although *Gm* and *Am* allotypes are not yet this clearly defined in terms of primary structure, they are being

* *A fourth antigen, the Oz factor, and a fifth, the Kern factor, were originally thought to represent allotypic markers. They are now generally regarded as isotypic markers related to L-type immunoglobulins, since all sera studied from normal individuals appear to have all four forms of λ-chain. These genes regulate two pairs of alternative amino-acid residues on λ-chains, which determine the alternative antigenic determinants for each phenotypic factor.*

intensively investigated at present, and further definition can be expected in the near future.

The Chemistry of Immunoglobulin Molecules

(1) IgG: It has been noted already that all immunoglobulins are made up of basic units with similar structure, containing four polypeptide chains and some associated carbohydrate.

Since IgG is quantitatively the most important class of immunoglobulin in human serum (accounting for well over 80% of total serum immunoglobulin) it has been the most extensively studied of the immunoglobulins.

The four-chain molecular model for IgG, illustrated in Figure 5, was proposed originally by Dr. R. R. Porter, in 1962. Because the derivation of this model is easily understood, and basic to the understanding of many aspects of immunoglublin structure and function, a *precis* of it is presented here.

Porter derived the model represented in Figure 5 from the following data:

(a) IgG antibodies, treated with the proteolytic enzyme papain, yielded two moles of antigen-binding

Fig. 5 PORTER MODEL FOR THE IgG MOLECULE

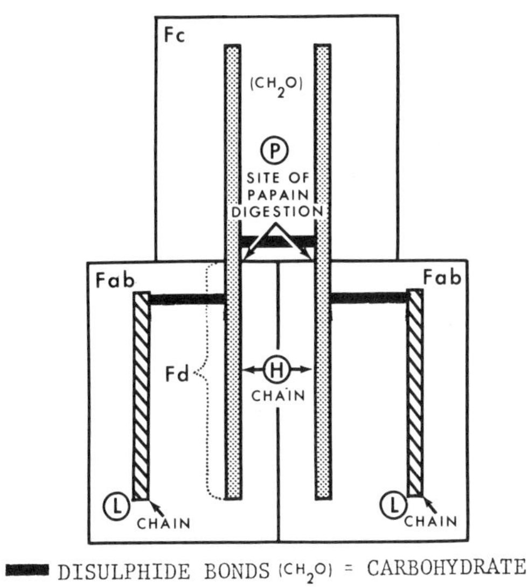

Note: The model has been modified slightly to conform to newer data, but is essentially similar to Porter's.

fragment (denoted *Fab*) and one mole of a crystalline fragment (denoted *Fc*) per mole of antibody. The *Fc*-fragment was necessary to allow the activation of complement. Alternatively, the splitting off of a bivalent antigen-binding fraction could be accomplished by the use of the proteolytic enzyme pepsin. Pepsin digestion resulted in a 5S molecule, having a molecular weight of about 100,000 and still retaining its bivalence in antigen-binding (*i.e.*, one mole of pepsin-digested antibody fragment could bind two moles of antigen). This (5S) bivalent fragment could be broken into two univalent halves (analogous to *Fab*-fragments in papain-digestion) by a reducing agent. The bivalent pepsin fragment is referred to as $(Fab')_2$.

(b) Treatment of monoclonal (homogeneous) preparations (derived from the sera of patients with multiple myeloma) with reagents that destroy disulphide bonds and dissociate polypeptide chains from each other resulted in a reaction mixture that contained four moles of polypeptide per mole of immunoglobulin. The reagents employed for these purposes were a reducing agent (mercaptoethanolamine), a dissociating agent (6-molar urea), and an alkylating agent (iodacetamide), to prevent spontaneous reassociation of the separated polypeptide chains.

The products of reduction and alkylation of IgG molecules were separated by gel-filtration on G-75 Sephadex® to ascertain the sizes of the dissociated polypeptide chains. Gel-filtration demonstrated that each mole of IgG starting material yielded two moles of light-chain and two moles of heavy-chain.

Sephadex® gels are hydrated matrices of cross-linked dextrans which can be employed as "molecular sieves" to separate molecules of different sizes. They are obtainable with different known distances between cross-linkages, which result in the hydrated gels having different-sized pores, through which mixtures of molecules can be passed. When a Sephadex® preparation is chosen with a pore size sufficient to allow the smaller of two types of molecules in a mixture to pass into the interstices of the Sephadex® "beads", but to preclude the passage of the larger molecules, the larger molecules will separate from the smaller ones *in transit* through the column. That is, molecules larger than the pores in the Sephadex® beads will not be retarded by the column, but will pass through it by circumventing the Sephadex® beads. Conversely, molecules smaller than the pore size will pass into the interstices of the Sephadex® beads, retarding their transit through the column. Thus, the larger molecules are eluted from the column with the first (exclusion) peak, whilst the smaller molecules are eluted with the second (inclusion) peak, as illustrated in Figure 6.

When monoclonal (homogeneous) IgG preparations were employed, the two L-chains could not be distinguished from each other by any of the physico-

Fig. 6 THEORY OF SEPHADEX® GEL FILTRATION: SEPARATION OF A MIXTURE OF TWO PROTEINS BY THEIR DISPARITY OF MOLECULAR SIZE

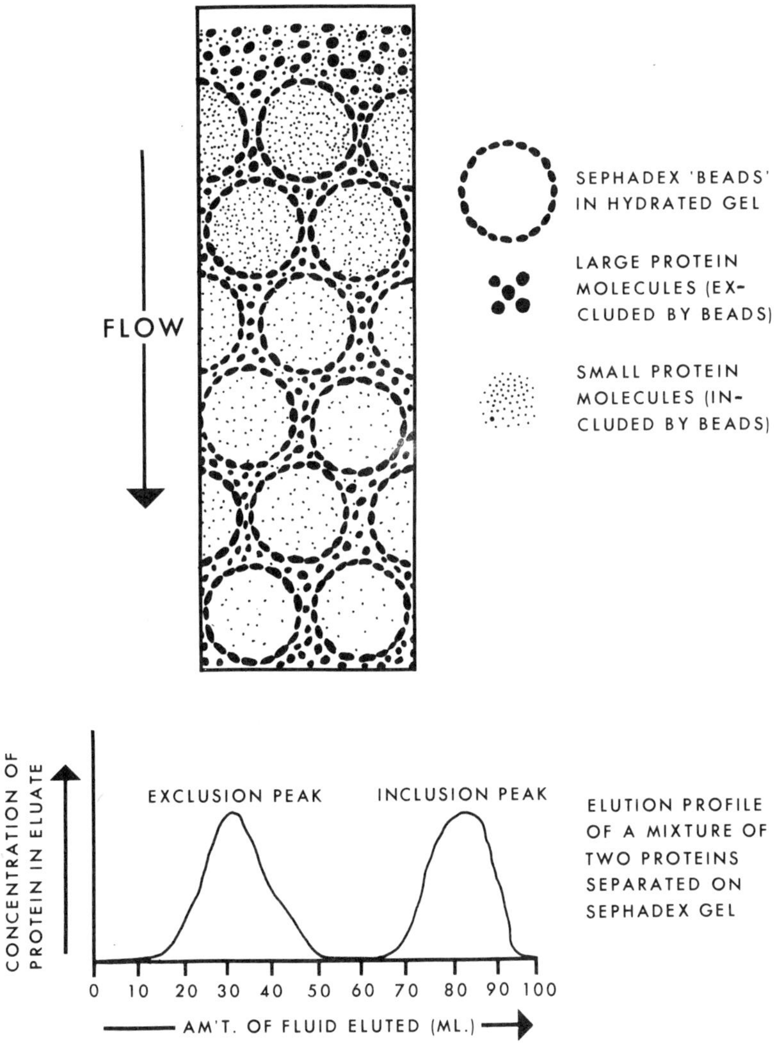

chemical methods employed. The two H-chains likewise could not be distinguished from each other. Thus, it was concluded that monoclonal IgG was composed of two identical L-chains and two identical H-chains.

(c) Antiserum directed against *Fab* reacted with both H-chains and L-chains; antiserum directed against *Fc* reacted only with H-chains. Therefore, it was concluded that *Fc* was composed only of H-chains, whilst *Fab* was composed of both L-chains and H-chains. The portion of H-chains located within the *Fab*-fragment was denoted as *Fd*.

(2) <u>IgA</u>: IgA is the principal immunoglobulin class found in seromucous secretions, where much of it is produced locally. It also occurs in serum, however - primarily in the form of a 7S molecule of molecular weight ~ 170,000. Serum IgA occurs as basic four-chain (monomeric) units, consisting of two α-chains (class-specific H-chains) and two L-chains (of either κ- or λ-type). Each IgA monomer is similarly divisible into two *Fab* and one *Fc* by the action of papain. Serum IgA may also occur as dimers and trimers of the basic 4-chain unit. Secretory IgA, however, occurs principally in the form of an 11S molecule of molecular weight ~ 400,000, which represents a complex of two basic units attached to a β-globulin of molecular weight ~ 50,000, called the T-piece, (Transport-piece), or alternatively, the S-piece (Secretory-piece). The T-piece is secreted by the epithelial cells of the

Fig. 7 MOLECULAR MODEL FOR SECRETORY IgA (11S) (adapted from Alexander and Good)

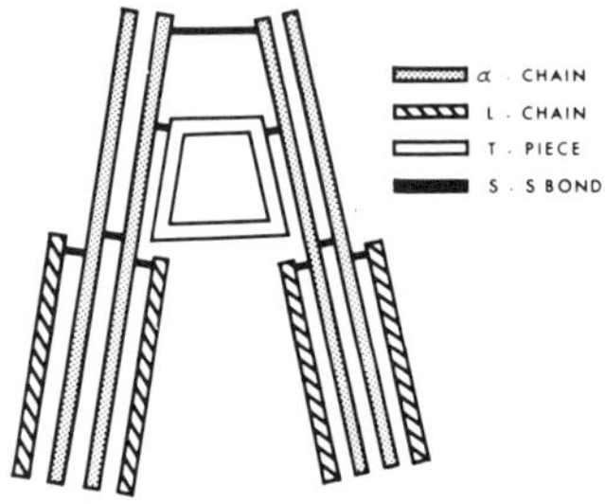

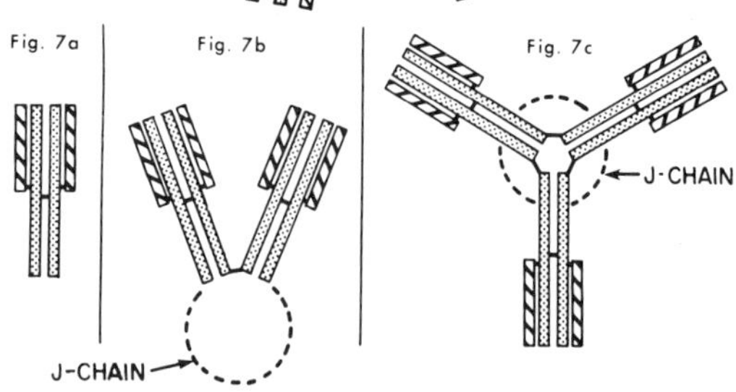

EXACT LOCATION OF J-CHAIN IS UNKNOWN AT PRESENT

gland producing the secretion containing the IgA. IgA is conjugated to the T-piece whilst passing through the cell into the acinar lumen; the secretion product occurs as a conjugate of two IgA units to one T-piece, as is shown in Figure 7. Affinity of IgA for the T-piece resides in the *Fc*-portion of the molecule.

Another polypeptide chain, approximately the same size as an L-chain, is associated with polymeric *serum* IgA and with pentameric IgM (*vide infra*). This has been designated as the J-chain, because it is thought to be involved with joining the monomeric units together.

(3) IgM: IgM, the largest of the immunoglobulins, is composed of 5 basic (4-chain) units attached to each other by their *Fc*-fragments via disulphide bridges to form a 19S pentamer. This is illustrated in Figure 8.

Fig. 8
MOLECULAR MODEL FOR
PENTAMERIC IgM (19 S)

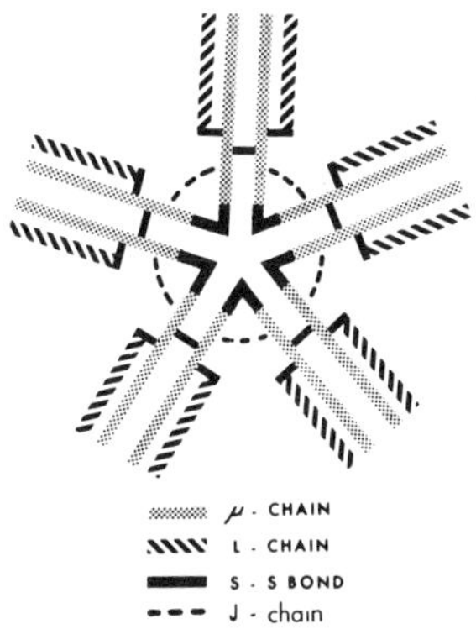

(19S) IgM molecules can be subjected to partial reduction/alkylation to yield five (7S) basic units. Each basic unit can be treated with proteolytic enzymes to yield 2 *Fab*-fragments and 1 *Fc*-fragment (as for IgA and IgG), or further reduced and alkylated to yield 2 μ-chains and 2 L-chains per unit. However, in spite of the theoretical antigen-binding valence of 10 antigen-binding sites/19S IgM pentamer (2 binding sites per 7S monomer), stoichiometric studies of antigen-binding by IgM antibodies have indicated ~ 5 antigen-binding sites per 19S molecule. This is now known to be due to the fact that each basic monomeric unit contains 1 *Fab*-unit (with 1 binding-site) of high affinity for antigen (*i.e.*, 1 avid site) and 1 *Fab*-unit (with 1 antigen-binding site) of low affinity for antigen (avidity ~ 1/100 of avid site). The reason for the disparity in antigen-binding avidity is not yet clear, but it is thought that the non-avid sites are blocked in some way that prevents the access of antigen to them. However, a monoclonal IgM protein, with antibody activity for the hapten *2,4-dinitrophenol (DNP)* has been shown by equilibrium dialysis studies (*vide supra*, chapter 4) to possess an antigen-binding valence of 10 sites per 19S molecule.

(4) IgD and IgE: The minor classes of immunoglobulin have not yet been sufficiently studied to warrant detailed comments on their structure. Immunoglobulins of the IgD and IgE classes occur as basic units, composed of 2 L-chains and 2 class-specific H-chains (*i.e.*, δ- or ε-) per unit, constituted in analogous manner to immunoglobulins of the other classes.

IgD has a sedimentation coefficient of 7S, and an estimated molecular weight of ~ 185,000. Antibody activity has been established indirectly for IgD immunoglobulins. IgD is present in all normal sera, but at very low levels (~ 3mgm%). Monoclonal IgD occurs rarely in multiple myeloma; about 40 such monoclonal proteins have been described. This immunoglobulin class is extremely susceptible to degradation by heat and by serum proteins such as plasmin.

IgE has a sedimentation coefficient of 8S, a molecular weight of ~ 200,000 and contains 10.7% carbohydrate. This immunoglobulin occurs in extremely low levels in normal sera (an average value for serum IgE is 33μmg%). Two cases of monoclonal IgE have been reported in patients with multiple myeloma. IgE antibodies possess reaginic activity (*vide infra*), and appear to have an antigen-binding valence of two (*i.e.*, IgE antibodies possess 2 antigen-binding sites per 8S unit).

Biological Properties of Immunoglobulins

IgG and IgM Antibodies: IgG and IgM antibodies together constitute 85 - 90% of the total serum antibody activity. IgG antibodies alone account for 80%, whilst IgM antibodies account for 5 - 10%. These antibodies are important in host defenses against infection. For example, IgG and IgM antibodies to certain surface antigens of many gram-negative bacteria can exert specific antibacterial activity in the presence of complement*. IgM and IgG antibodies to viral receptor

* *Complement is a complex series of serum proteins activated by the interaction of IgG or IgM antibodies with their provoking antigens. Complement serves as a biological amplifier of antibodies capable of activating it. It will be discussed in more detail in Chapter 7.*

proteins will neutralise the ability of that virus to infect susceptible cells. Antibodies of the IgG and IgM classes can serve as specific antitoxins against bacterial and other toxins (*e.g.*, diphtheria, tetanus, botulism, gas gangrene, anthrax, snake venoms, etc.). These antibodies can also serve as specific *opsonins*, which promote the phagocytosis of bacteria such as *Pneumococci*.

In fact, IgG or IgM antibodies are responsible for most of the specific activities classically associated with antibodies in general (*e.g.*, precipitation, agglutination, haemolysis, complement-fixation, immune cytotoxicity reactions, transfusion reactions, haemolytic disease of the newborn (*erythroblastosis foetalis*), and many others). These reactions are discussed individually in later chapters.

IgA Antibodies: Secretory IgA antibodies are believed to comprise an important defense mechanism against local infections of the mucous membranes of the body. The importance of secretory IgA antibodies has been stressed in resistance to respiratory tract infections, gastrointestinal infections, and genitourinary infections, because large amounts of secretory IgA (often with established antibody activity against local microbial flora) have been found in parotid saliva, tears, nasal mucus, bronchial secretions, prostatic fluid, vaginal secretions, and the mucous secretions of the small intestine. In the latter site, secretory IgA constitutes the bulk of the so-called copro-antibodies*.

The consistent presence of secretory IgA in human colostrum and amniotic fluid further suggests that IgA antibodies may serve an important role in conferring passive immunity on the human neonate.

Although IgA antibodies do not activate complement, there is evidence that they are capable of exerting anti-microbial activity in some other way, as yet not understood. There is some evidence that IgA antibodies alone are able to neutralise certain viruses, but their anti-bacterial activity may depend on the presence of additional factors in the secretions (other than complement). More data is clearly needed to establish the mechanisms of antimicrobial activity by IgA antibody.

Transmucosal exposure to antigens usually stimulates the local production of secretory IgA antibodies,

* *i.e., antibodies found in faeces. These are believed to be important defense mechanisms against potentially- or frankly-pathogenic gut flora.*

which appear in high titre in local mucous secretions. Eventually, however, serum IgA antibodies may appear in the circulation as well.

<u>IgD Antibodies</u>: Until recently, no antibody activity had been associated with the IgD class immunoglobulins. However, antinuclear antibodies of the IgD class have been reported in 40-50% of patients with disseminated lupus erythematosus, and 20% of patients with rheumatoid disease. IgD antibodies to diphtheria toxoid were noted in one subject following repeated immunisation with this antigen. An IgD anti-thyroid antibody was described in 1 of 26 patients with Hashimoto's thyroiditis. Three patients who were sensitive to cow's milk demonstrated IgD antibodies to bovine gamma globulin (BGG), and two of these patients also demonstrated IgD antibodies to bovine serum albumin (BSA). (It may be noted that both BSA and BGG are constituents of cow's milk). IgD antibodies to insulin and to penicillin have been reported.

Since all of the patients who demonstrated IgD antibodies also produced antibodies of several other classes to the same antigen*, no specific biological role can yet be assigned to antibodies of the IgD class. Experimental studies have been limited by failure to demonstrate IgD immunoglobulins in any experimental animal; this class of immunoglobulins thus far appears confined to man.

<u>IgE Antibodies</u>: IgE antibodies are of great clinical importance as mediators of atopic (allergic) reactions and atopic diseases. Serum IgE is usually elevated in patients with allergic asthma, allergic rhinitis, atopic dermatitis and parasitic infestations of many types. IgE antibodies are cytophilic for mast cells, blood basophiles, and blood neutrophiles; the affinity for cell membrane receptors resides in the *Fc*-portion of the IgE molecule. When specific antigens (allergens) react with IgE antibodies attached to mast-cell or leucocyte membrane receptors, the reaction results in degranulation of mast cells or leucocytes, liberation of histamine, and other biologically-active effective molecules, and the development of inflammatory changes *in situ (vide infra*, Chapter 11). IgE antibodies, then, are important as mediators of pathologic reactions.

Recently, however, it has been suggested that IgE antibodies may play some role in the body's defenses.

* *The patient in whom IgD antibodies to diphtheria toxoid were demonstrated developed antibodies of all five immunoglobulin classes to this antigen. One of the milk-sensitive patients similarly developed antibodies to BGG which belonged to all five immunoglobulin classes.*

IgE antibodies have been identified in plasma-cells within the *lamina propria* of the gastrointestinal tract, and in plasma-cells within pharyngeal lymphoid tissue. Moreover, it has been noted that two patients with isolated deficiency of IgE (and normal levels of other classes of immunoglobulins) suffered from chronic sinopulmonary infections, which could not be modified appreciably by treatment with pooled human gamma-globulin. (Pooled human gamma-globulin does not provide significant amounts of IgE).

It is as yet too early to make definitive statements about the role of IgE in the body's defense system; better understanding of the functions of IgE must await further studies of IgE antibodies and monoclonal IgE proteins. However, it would not be surprising if IgE antibodies were capable of acting both as defense mechanism and pathogenetic mechanisms under different circumstances, since most immunological reactions can be shown to exhibit this dual potential.

Figure 9 presents a summary of the more important properties of immunoglobulins and antibodies, most of which have been discussed above.

Fig. 9 BIOLOGICAL, IMMUNOCHEMICAL, AND PHYSICO-CHEMICAL PROPERTIES OF THE IMMUNOGLOBULINS OF MAN

Ig Class	*Established Antibody Activity*	*Sedimentation Value*	*Where Found In Highest Concentration*	*Valence in Antigen Binding*	*Complement Fixation*	*Cross Placenta*
IgG	+	7S	Serum	2	+	+
IgA	+	7S - 11S	Seromucous Secretions	$2^{2} - 4^{3}$	-	-
IgM	+	19S	Serum	5-(10)[5]	+	-
IgD	+	7S	Interstitial Connective Tissue	?	-	-
IgE	+	8.2S	Skin and Epithelium	2	-	-
Ig Class	*Molecular Weight*	*Carbohydrate*	*Operational Categories*	*Antigenic Types*	*Serum Conc. (Mg.%)*	*Known Subclasses*
IgG	140,000	2.9%	Opsonin, Lysin, Precipitin, Agglutinin	K,L (γ)[4]	800-1680	4
IgA	170,000[2] 400,000[3]	7.5%	Principal Secretory Globulin Coproantibody, Colostral-antibody	K,L (α)[4]	140-420	2
IgM	900,000	11.8%	Opsonin, Lysin, Precipitin, Agglutinin	K,L (μ)[4]	50-190	2
IgD	200,000	14.8%	No Known Biological Function	L,K (δ)[4][1]	0.3-40	-
IgE	200,000	10.7%	Reagins (mediating atopic states)	K,L (ε)[4]	0.1-0.7 μgm/ml[6] (in normal patients)	-

1 Conversely to the other classes, which have a preponderance of K-types, IgD has a predominance of L-types

2 Serum IgA

3 Secretory IgA

4 The antigenic type of the H-chain for each class is included in parentheses ()

5 Although 1 IgM molecule (19S) contains 10 antigen binding sites, only 5 are available. The other 5 are "blocked".

6 Note change in unitage for IgE. Average normal serum IgE ≃ *0.33* μgm/ml. Significantly higher concentrations occur in the serum of most atopic patients.

Chapter 6

ANTIGEN-ANTIBODY REACTIONS

It is appropriate at this point to examine the mechanisms of certain antigen-antibody reactions, which are of interest as *in vitro* clinical laboratory methods or which serve as mechanisms of pathogenesis or defense *in vivo*.

Antibodies are often designated as haemolytic, agglutinating, precipitating, or complement-fixing. These are largely operational terms, which merely indicate the method used to demonstrate or measure the activity of antibodies. It is therefore evident that antibodies may be measured in a variety of ways. Generally speaking, one chooses the method that best reflects the particular parameters or properties of the antibodies in which the investigator is interested. Since many antibodies are capable of mediating a variety of reactions under different circumstances, they can be measured in any of several ways. Other antibodies are less versatile, however, and may require one particular technique to be employed for their measurement.

A partial list of antigen-antibody reactions of medical interest are provided in Table 1.

Table 1 NOMENCLATURE OF ANTIGEN-ANTIBODY REACTIONS OF MEDICAL INTEREST

Type of Reaction	*Trivial Name (Antigens)*	*Trivial Name (Antibodies)*	*Immunoglobulin Classes Involved in Reactions*
Agglutination	Agglutinogens	Agglutinins	IgG, IgM, IgA, (IgE ?)
Precipitation	Preciptinogens	Precipitins	IgG, IgM, IgA, (IgE ?)
Opsonisation	Opsinogens	Opsonins	IgG, IgM, (IgA ?, IgE ?)
Lysis[1]	(Membrane Antigens)	Lysins	IgG (except $\gamma 4$), IgM
Complement Fixation[1]	--	Complement-Fixing Antibodies	IgG (except $\gamma 4$), IgM
Cytotoxicity[1]	(Membrane Antigens)	Cytotoxic Antibodies	IgG (except $\gamma 4$), IgM
Enzyme Inactivation	Enzymes	Antienzymes	IgG, Igm, (IgA ?)
Virus Neutralisation	Cell Receptors of Viruses	Neutralising Antibodies	IgG, IgM, (IgA ?)
Atopic Reactions[2]	Allergens	Reagins	IgE, (IgG ?, IgM ?)

[1] - These Reactions Involve the Complement System

[2] - Certain "Allergic Reactions" (*i.e.*, anaphylaxis, complement-dependent histamine release) may involve the complement system, and IgG and IgM antibodies capable of activating it. All of these are of doubtful significance in human disease states.

Precipitation Reactions

Antibody molecules have multiple (at least 2/ molecule) antigen-binding sites, and most antigen molecules are large enough to have multiple antigenic determinants on them. Thus, when one mixes a solution of soluble antigen with antibodies directed against that antigen, an opportunity is presented for extensive cross-linking of antigen and antibody to occur. The ultimate result is the formation of a three-dimensional lattice-work of antigen and antibody, which precipitates out of solution.

The proportion of antigen-to-antibody molecules that is present in the mixture determines the extent of the cross-linking, and consequently the precipitation, that ultimately occurs. When an optimal proportion of antigen-to-antibody is present, cross-linkage is extensive, and large, insoluble complexes are formed, which are recognised as a visible precipitate. Where the antigen-to-antibody ratio is such that all antigen and antibody are bound into insoluble complexes and co-precipitated out of solution, the antigen and antibody are said to be "at equivalence". However, where the ratio of antigen-to-antibody is altered so that either antigen or antibody are in excess (*i.e.*, above or below the point of equivalence), the solution will contain at least some soluble complexes which are of sufficiently small particle size to allow them to remain in colloidal suspension*. Conditions of antigen-excess are particularly conducive to the development and maintenance of soluble complexes, for reasons not entirely understood. Soluble complexes are small antigen-antibody aggregates each containing only a few molecules. These are formed when all of the antigen-binding sites of an antibody are occupied by individual antigen molecules (as in antigen-excess) or, conversely, when all available antigenic determinants are bound by individual antibody molecules (as occurs in antibody-excess). No significant cross-linking occurs under such conditions. Consequently, the complexes do not become large enough to precipitate from solution. The foregoing can be illustrated in the following example:

> A series of test-tubes is prepared, each containing the same amount of antibody. The antigen, however, is varied serially, so that an increasing amount is added to each tube in the series (*e.g.*: 1 mg./ml. to the first tube, 2 mg./ml. to the second tube, 3 mg./ml. to the third tube, etc.). After mixing the fixed-amounts of antibody with the serially-increasing

* *Vide infra, discussion on reversibility of antigen-antibody reactions.*

amounts of antigen, the tubes are incubated at 37°C for 30 minutes to allow the reaction to proceed to completion, and the amount of precipitate in each tube is determined.

The precipitation curve obtained in such an experiment is represented in Figure 1, and the immune complexes characteristic of such reactions are illustrated in Figure 2.

Fig. 1 THE PRECIPITATION CURVE

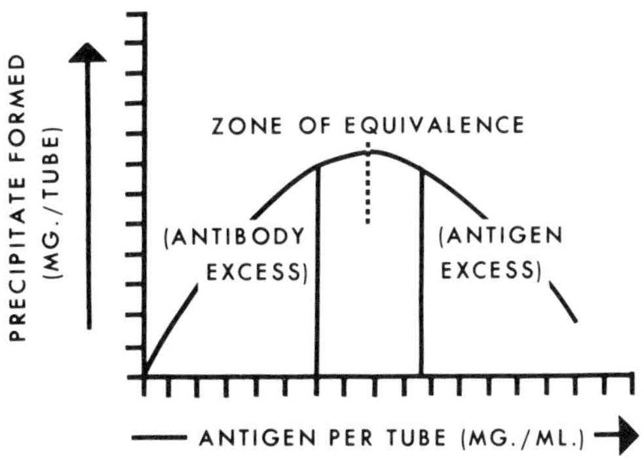

Increasing amounts of antigen are added to a constant amount of antibody. At the equivalence zone the precipitate is maximal and no unreacted antigen or antibody is left in solution. Soluble complexes occur on either side of the equivalence zone.

Fig. 2 IMMUNE COMPLEXES FORMED IN ANTIBODY EXCESS (A), EQUIVALENCE (B) AND ANTIGEN EXCESS (C). NOTICE THAT VERY LARGE LATTICE STRUCTURES CAN OCCUR AT EQUIVALENCE; THESE ARE RESPONSIBLE FOR PRECIPITATION REACTIONS

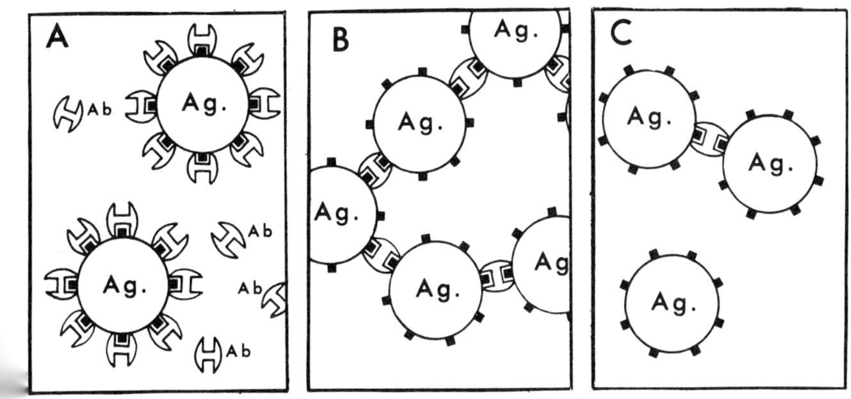

It will presently be seen that soluble complexes which form in the circulating blood are important in the pathogenesis of several types of immune vasculitides which occur as human diseases (*vide infra*, Chapter 14).

In the clinical and research laboratories, precipitation reactions have found a great variety of uses, since they are simple to perform, do not usually require costly equipment, are reproducible, accurate, and capable of providing useful information.

Precipitation reactions can be employed to measure the titre of antibody in a patient's serum. For example:

> In this instance, blood is drawn, and allowed to clot. Serum is prepared, and inactivated at 56°C for 30 minutes, to destroy complement activity (*vide infra*, Chapter 7). The serum is then diluted serially into a series of test tubes, mixed with a fixed amount of antigen, and incubated at 37°C for 30 minutes to allow reaction to occur. The tubes are then inspected to determine the serum dilution that produces maximal precipitation, since this will occur at the zone of equivalence. The dilution at equivalence is chosen for assay of the precipitate, since all of the antibody in the tube should be in the precipitate at equivalence. The amount of protein in the washed precipitate is determined, and the protein content of the antigen subtracted from the total precipitated protein, to yield a figure representing the antibody protein in that tube. When multiplied by the dilution factor of the serum in the tube, the total antibody protein of the patient's serum is obtained.

The molar ratio of antigen-to-antibody at equivalence varies with the valence of the antibody and the number of antigenic determinants per molecule of the antigen. For example, large molecular weight antigens can be expected in general to bind many antibody molecules, whilst small molecular weight antigens would bind fewer antibodies.

Precipitation reactions are widely employed in the clinical laboratory in the form of agar diffusion techniques for detection and measurement of serum proteins. These are described below:

Agar Diffusion Techniques

Because of their simplicity and sensitivity, techniques of studying antigen-antibody reactions in agar have become widely used. There are three methods (*i.e.*, single diffusion in agar, double diffusion in agar, and immunoelectrophoresis) all of which depend on precipitation reactions between antigen and antibody, and can therefore only be applied to systems that form precipitates. The antigen must be in a dissolved or colloidal state so that it is able to diffuse through an agar gel to react with its antibody.

(1) Single Diffusion in Agar: A glass slide is covered with a layer of agar containing antibody specific for the antigen. A hole is punched in the agar and this is filled with antigen. After twenty-four hours, the antigen will have diffused into the agar, and a ring of precipitate will have formed around the hole, indicating where the antigen and antibody have reacted at equivalence, as illustrated in Figure 3 and 4.

The diameter of this ring will be proportional to the concentration of antigen in the well, and the concentration of antibody in the agar. By setting up suitable standards, fairly accurate figures can be obtained for either antibody or antigen concentration. This has become a widely-used method for determining the concentrations of immunoglobulins in human serum. Prepared agar plates are available commercially for this purpose.

Fig. 3 SINGLE DIFFUSION IN AGAR

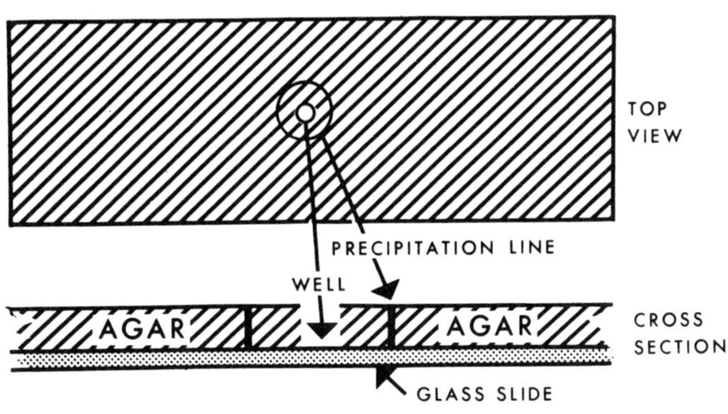

The agar contains specific antibody and buffer. A ring of precipitate has formed around the well which has been filled 24 hours previously with antigen. The diameter of the ring will be proportional to the concentration of antigen.

Fig. 4 ANALYSIS OF SINGLE DIFFUSION IN AGAR

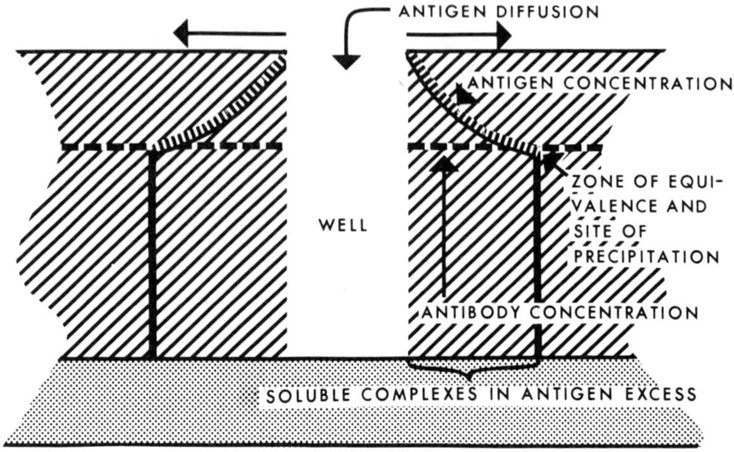

The position of the line of precipitation indicates that antigen and antibody are reacting at equivalence. Between this and the well, no precipitation is seen because of antigen excess. The precipitation ring moves outwards with time because antigen diffuses outwards and dissolves the inner side of the precipitate, while a new zone of equivalence is formed at the outer surface.

(2) Double Diffusion in Agar: In double diffusion precipitation reactions, the antigen is placed in one well cut in an agar gel overlying a glass slide or plate, and the antiserum is placed in another well. Both antigen and antibody diffuse toward each other, and form precipitate lines where they meet at equivalence. In a double diffusion system, one line of precipitate will form for each antigen-antibody system that is present. Double diffusion systems can be employed to determine the number of antigens or antibodies present in an unknown system, to identify these antigens or antibodies, and to determine their relationships to each other by direct comparison. This is illustrated in Figure 5.

Figure 5 is a diagram of the type of double diffusion system devised by Orjan Ouchterlony, and hence referred to as the Ouchterlony double diffusion test. The figure represents the following experiment:

> A substance is prepared from the plasma of a patient with a particular disease. This substance is denoted as Z. An antiserum to Z is prepared by injecting the substance repeatedly into a rabbit. This antiserum is denoted as anti-Z. Substances are similarly prepared from three other patients, suspected of having a disease similar to that of the patient from whom

Fig. 5 DOUBLE DIFFUSION IN AGAR

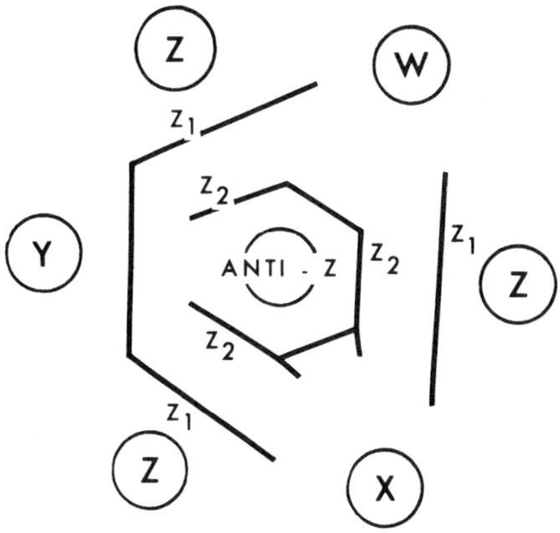

(1) Substance "Z" contains two separate antigenic components, denoted by the precipitate lines "Z_1", and "Z_2".

(2) "Y" contains a component that appears antigenically identical to component "Z_1"; *i.e.*, "Y" shows a "reaction of identity" with "Z_1".

(3) "W" contains a component that appears antigenically identical to component "Z_2"; *i.e.*, "W" shows a "reaction of identity" with "Z_2".

(4) "X" contains a component that shares at least one antigenic determinant with component "Z_2", but "Z_2" contains at least one antigenic determinant which is non-identical to "X". The evidence for the partial identity of "X" and "Z_2" is the merging of the "X" line with the "Z_2" line, but the "Z_2" line has a *spur* which overlaps the "X" line.

Z was prepared. These substances are denoted as W, X, and Y. An Ouchterlony plate is prepared by coating a glass slide with a thin layer of agar gel, and punching out a pattern of wells, in which six antigen wells are radially arranged around a single antibody well. The anti-Z antibody is placed in the centre well, whilst antigen-preparations, W, X, Y, and Z are arranged in the antigen-wells as indicated.

As the antigens and antibodies diffuse toward each other, a series of precipitate lines form, and the location of these is indicated in the figure.

Analysis of these lines enables one to draw several conclusions about the antigens under investigation, which are outlined beneath the diagram.

Electrophoresis and Immunoelectrophoresis

The separation of serum proteins by an electric

field (electrophoresis) depends on the net charge of the protein molecules and (to a lesser extent) their size. Most proteins have a net negative charge at pH 8 and migrate toward the anode at this pH. The rate at which proteins migrate in an electric field is also affected by the ionic strength of the electrolyte-buffer and the nature of the material used for support. Some materials (such as agar or cellulose acetate) have large net negative charges which fix positive buffer ions, resulting in a flow of buffer towards the cathode. This is called electroendosmosis and causes some plasma proteins (such as IgG) to migrate towards the cathode when electrophoresis is performed on these media at pH 8. In contrast, other support media (like agarose) do not produce electroendosmosis. In consequence, all of the plasma proteins migrate toward the anode (at pH 8) when electrophoresis is performed on agarose medium.

Other support media in common use for electrophoresis include paper, starch gel, plastic beads, and polyacrilamide gel.

Fig. 6

CELLULOSE ACETATE ELECTROPHEROGRAM
OF NORMAL HUMAN SERUM

(The protein bands are stained with Amido - Schwartz)

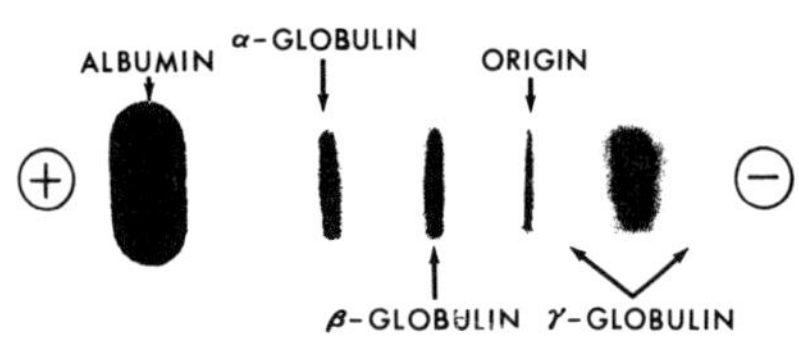

0.05 Barbital Buffer, pH 8.2
250 Volts - 20 min. (Constant voltage)

In immunoelectrophoresis, the techniques of electrophoresis and double-diffusion precipitation are combined, as is illustrated in Figure 7, 8 and 9:

> A glass slide is covered with an agar gel, which contains an electrolyte solution buffered at pH 8.8

Fig. 7

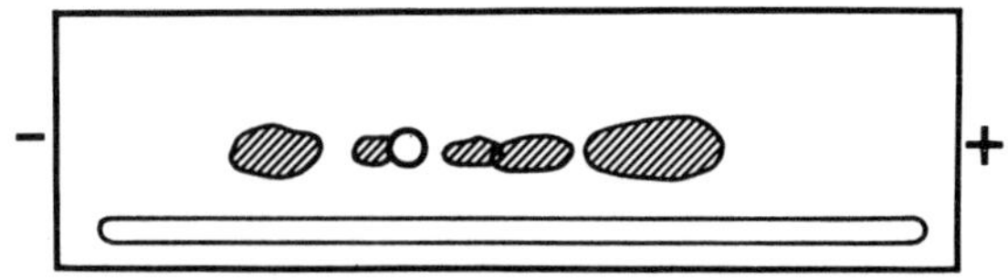

(1) Serum is placed into a well cut in the agar. The serum proteins are separated electrophoretically. The albumin migrates toward the anode, but the IgG migrates toward the cathode in agar support medium, due to electroendosmosis. (The electrophoretically-separated serum proteins are not visible at this stage, unless they are stained).

Fig. 8

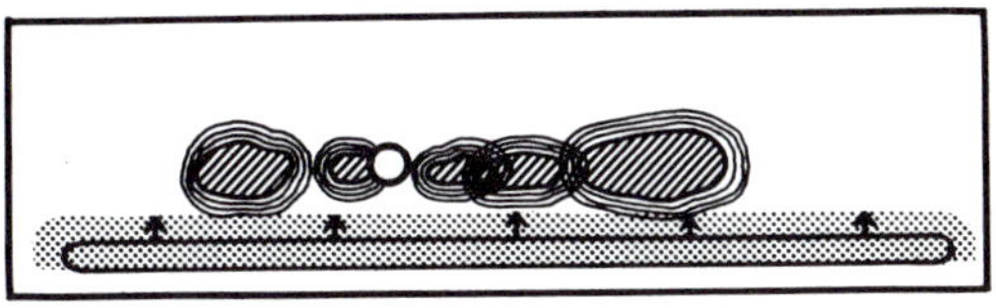

(2) A trough is cut in the agar parallel to the axis of electrophoretic separation of the proteins. This trough is filled with an antiserum made against whole serum. The antiserum and the separated serum proteins diffuse toward each other through the agar gel. Where antigen and antibody meet at equivalence, lines of precipitate will form. These precipitate lines delineate each antigenically-definable protein in the serum.

Fig. 9

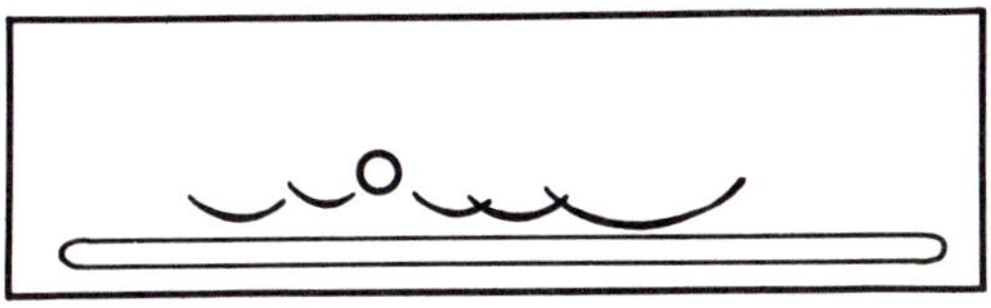

Immunoelectrophoresis, a technique depending on both electrophoretic mobility and double diffusion in agar gel, enables high resolution of antigenic components from complex mixtures of antigens (*e.g.*, human plasma-proteins). It was the development of immunoelectrophoresis, in fact, that first provided evidence that human immunoglobulins were divisible into classes (*e.g.*, IgG, IgM, IgA).

Figure 10 illustrates immunoelectropherograms which show the whole spectrum of serum proteins and each major class of immunoglobulin individually.

Fig. 10
IMMUNOELECTROPHEROGRAM OF NORMAL HUMAN SERUM
(The precipitin lines are stained with Amido - Schwartz)

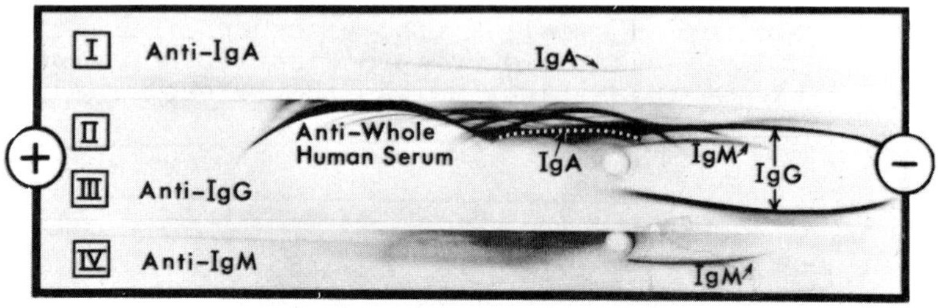

The serum is obtained from the same patient as the serum in Figure 6. The principal classes of immunoglobulins are pointed out in Part II of the figure which represents Human Serum vs. Goat Anti-Whole Human Serum. A separate immunoelectrophoretogram is shown for each class of immunoglobulin using sera directed against IgG, IgM, and IgA (Parts III, IV, & I, respectively). These sera are also of goat origin and are directed against the antigenically distinctive H-chains of each immunoglobulin class; i.e.,....γ-chains (IgG), μ-chains (IgM), and α-chains (IgA).

Agglutination Reactions

Antigens are often associated with particles which are too large to form solutions or colloidal suspensions in aqueous media. Such particles (e.g., bacteria, erythrocytes, latex particles, etc.) can be suspended in saline, and mixed with specific antiserum. When mixture of particulate antigens with specific antisera results in aggregation of the antigenic particles, the phenomenon is referred to as an agglutination reaction. Agglutination usually is visible to the naked eye, but in some instances, may require microscopic examination of the test preparation.

Antibodies of different immunoglobulin classes differ in their ability to mediate agglutination reactions. These differences are largely a matter of the antigen-binding valence of different classes of antibody. It is not surprising, therefore, that IgM antibodies (with 5 effective antigen-binding sites per 19S molecule) have higher agglutinating activity than IgG antibodies (with 2 antigen-binding sites per molecule) directed against the same antigen. In other words, a low concentration of IgM antibodies will produce an agglutination reaction of equal intensity to the agglutination reaction produced by a high concentration of IgG antibodies.

The mechanism of an agglutination reaction is similar to that of a precipitation reaction; both are produced by multivalent antibodies which cross-link antigen particles into complexes of antigen and antibody. The only difference between a precipitation reaction and an agglutination reaction is that precipitating antigens are of molecular size whilst agglutinating antigens are associated with larger particles. Like precipitation reactions, agglutination tests require proper pH and molarity of saline buffers (so that the antigen-antibody complexes formed will be stable) and proper ratio of antigen-to-antibody should be present (so that optimal cross-linking of antigen with antibody can occur). When antibody concentration is sufficiently excessive to allow all of the antigenic sites on the particles to be occupied by single antibody molecules, cross-links will not form between particles, and a falsely-negative agglutination test will result. This inhibition of agglutination in antibody-excess is known as the prozone phenomenon, because it appears before the zone of agglutination when constant amounts of particulate antigens are tested against serial dilutions of an antiserum. Figure 11 illustrates the results of an agglutination test using the serum of a patient who has had a past transfusion of improperly-matched blood with washed red cells from the blood donor as the antigen.

Agglutination tests have many uses in the clinical laboratory, both for measuring antigens and for assessing antibody titres. Agglutinating antibody titre is defined as the highest dilution of antiserum that will agglutinate the test antigen under the conditions employed in the test. In general, agglutination tests are operationally simple, quite reproducible, and highly sensitive. Indeed, such tests are usually capable of detecting 0.1 μgm/ml. of serum.

In cases where soluble antigens are to be tested, they can usually be coated onto particles like sheep erythrocytes or latex particles, which then can be utilised in agglutination tests. Both types of particles can be easily coated with a wide variety of antigens, by the use of several standard techniques.

Agglutination tests are employed routinely in the cross-matching of blood, prior to giving transfusions. This will be discussed in a later chapter in some detail, because of its medical importance (*vide infra*, Chapter 16). The example given in Figure 11 below is an example of a direct agglutination test used in this way.

When a patient develops antibodies to antigens present on the red cells of a previous blood donor, demonstration of these antibodies requires mixing red cells of the previous donor with recipient serum. If

Fig. 11 AN AGGLUTINATION TEST FOR BLOOD GROUP MISMATCH

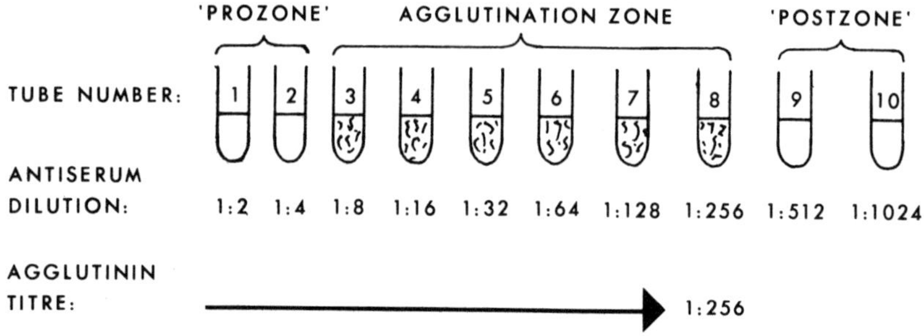

(NOTE THAT CONCENTRATION OF ANTIGEN PARTICLES IS CONSTANT)

Blood is drawn from the transfusion donor in anticoagulant solution, and the specimen centrifuged to separate the cells. The red cell fraction is washed several times and standardized to a 2% suspension of the cells in buffered saline solution. One ml. of the red cell suspension is added into each of ten tubes containing one ml. of a serial dilution of serum from the transfusion recipient. The serum was prepared from clotted blood, and inactivated at 56° C for 30 minutes prior to serial dilution and use in the test (to destroy the complement activity of the serum).

a prospective new donor's red cells share red cell antigen(s) with the previous donor against which the patient has made antibodies, an agglutination reaction may occur upon mixing, as is usual in mismatches relating to ABO blood group antigens. However, this method of mixing donor red cells directly with recipient serum (and *vice versa*) is not sufficient to detect many potential transfusion mismatches, especially where there is a mismatch in antigens belonging to the *Rh* system.

Therefore, an additional test is employed routinely. This test utilises rabbit antiserum specific for human immunoglobulins (Coombs' serum). The test described above is the indirect Coombs' test; it serves as an example of an agglutination reaction employed in the clinical laboratory as an amplifier, to increase the detection of potential blood group mismatches. The indirect Coombs' test uses the rabbit antiserum to human immunoglobulins to detect the presence of recipient antibodies coating the surfaces of donor erythrocytes. The antibodies bound to antigens on the red cell membranes which require the indirect Coombs' test for demonstration, do not of themselves agglutinate the red cells in saline suspension. In most cases these antibodies are of the IgG type, and the reason for their failure to agglutinate the red cells to which they are bound is not known with certainty. It is thought, however, that conditions of extreme antigen-excess result in both antigen-binding sites on each antibody molecule being bound to the same red cell, so that cross-links between adjacent erythrocytes do not form. In other words, relatively low concentrations of antibody might result in a postzone phenomenon similar to that shown in Figure 11, in which no free combining sites on antibody molecules are present to form cross-links between red cells.

Whatever the reason for the failure of these antibodies to agglutinate the red cells to which they are bound, their presence on red cells can be detected by the indirect Coombs' test.

Moreover, a similar principle may be employed in the diagnosis of autoimmune haemolytic anaemias (*vide infra*, Chapter 19), in which patients develop antibodies to their own erythrocyte membranes. Since the erythrocytes of such patients become coated with antibodies in the circulation, direct addition of rabbit anti-human globulin serum (Coombs' serum) to a suspension of washed erythrocytes from these patients will result in agglutination of the antibody-coated erythrocytes. This is referred to as the direct Coombs' test for autoimmune haemolytic anaemias.

Fig. 12. THE COOMBS' TESTS

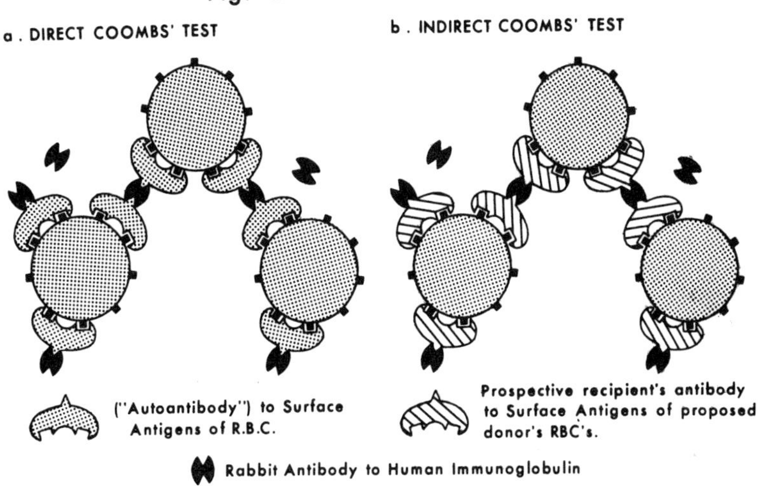

(a). The direct Coombs' test is a test for autoimmune haemolytic anaemia. Both red cells and the antibodies to them are from a single individual.

(b). The indirect Coombs' test is a test for potential blood transfusion mismatch Red cells from a prospective donor are mixed with serum (containing antibody to donor red cell antigens) from the proposed recipient.

The addition of rabbit antiserum to human immunoglobulins (Coombs' Serum) enables positive tests in both situations to be recognised in the clinical laboratory as agglutination reactions — even when both antigen binding sites of single (human) anti-red cell antibodies have combined with two antigenic determinants on single red cells.

In performing the direct Coombs' test, a sample of blood is drawn from the patient suspected of having non-agglutinating antibodies on his red cells in an anticoagulant, and centrifuged to sediment the red cells. The red cells are washed several times in saline to remove non-specifically bound immunoglobulins, and resuspended in saline as a 2% suspension. Rabbit antiserum to human immunoglobulin (Coombs' serum) is added to the suspension of red cells. Where the red cells contain specific non-agglutinating antibodies on their membranes, visible agglutination will be provoked by the addition of Coombs' serum, as indicated in Figure 12. Where no such antibodies are present, no agglutination of the patient's red cells occurs.

The direct Coombs' test differs from the indirect only in that Coombs' serum is added directly to a washed erythrocyte suspension in the former, whilst the latter requires the addition of serum from one individual (*e.g.*, the prospective transfusion recipient) to a washed erythrocyte suspension from another individual (*e.g.*, the prospective transfusion donor) before the addition of Coombs' serum to the system.

The Paul-Bunnell test is a clinical agglutination test which is based on the fact that patients with infectious mononucleosis develop heterophile antibodies, which cross-react with an antigen on sheep erythrocytes. The reason for the development of such antibodies in infectious mononucleosis is still poorly understood.

Blood is drawn from a patient suspected of having infectious mononucleosis, and allowed to clot. The serum is separated, and inactivated at 56°C for 30 minutes to destroy complement activity. It is diluted serially into a series of tubes, and mixed with a 2% suspension of washed sheep erythrocytes in each tube. A positive reaction is judged by the appearance of agglutination at serum dilution of 1:32 or greater.

The Widal test makes use of the fact that patients infected with certain gram-negative bacteria develop antibodies in their sera which agglutinate suspensions of the infecting organisms.

Serum from such a patient is mixed with suspensions of killed *Salmonella typhi*, *Salmonella paratyphi A*, *Salmonella paratyphi B*, *and Brucella abortus*. A rising titre of agglutinins specific for one of the above organisms during a severe febrile illness may help to confirm the clinical impression of an enteric fever.

The rheumatoid factor test (latex test) is another example of a clinically-employed agglutination reaction. Patients with rheumatoid arthritis (and certain other mesenchymal diseases) often, in the course of their illness, develop an IgM antibody which reacts with *Fc*-determinants of human IgG molecules. By coating latex particles with human IgG, and exposing the coated particles to serum from a rheumatoid patient, one can confirm the presence and estimate the titre of this peculiar antibody, known as rheumatoid factor. Rheumatoid factor is alleged to occur in about 70% of adult patients who meet the diagnostic criteria for rheumatoid arthritis established by the American Rheumatism Association.

The immunological pregnancy tests are also examples of clinically-useful agglutination tests, which will be considered next.

Human chorionic gonadotrophin (HCG) is a protein hormone produced by the developing foetal trophoblast, which is antigenic to the rabbit. HCG is excreted in the urine of pregnant women, and can be purified from such urine as a source of immunising antigen. Rabbit antibodies to HCG are employed to detect HCG in the patient's urine, as follows:

- A standard purified preparation of HCG is absorbed onto latex particles (or onto specially-prepared sheep red cells).

- These HCG-coated particles are mixed with serial dilutions of rabbit anti-HCG, and the highest dilution at which agglutination occurs is noted.

- A fixed amount of the anti-HCG, is then mixed with the patient's urine. If the urine contains HCG, it will react with the antibodies and inhibit these antibodies from agglutinating HCG-coated particles, if these are subsequently allowed to react with such particles. Thus, a positive agglutination-inhibition test would mean that the patient's urine lowers the agglutinating titre of the anti-HCG serum. In a negative test, the agglutinating titre of the rabbit anti-HCG serum would be unchanged by first mixing it with the patient's urine. When the urine does not contain HCG, it cannot bind antibodies to HCG.

This test is illustrated in Figure 13.

Fig. 13

POSITIVE AND NEGATIVE IMMUNOLOGICAL TESTS FOR PREGNANCY (by agglutination inhibition)

POSITIVE TEST							
ANTISERUM DILUTION:	1:2	1:4	1:8	1:16	1:32	1:64	1:128
RESULTS W/O URINE	±	+	+	+	+	+	—
RESULTS WITH URINE	+	+	+	—	—	—	—

NEGATIVE TEST							
ANTISERUM DILUTION:	1:2	1:4	1:8	1:16	1:32	1:64	1:128
RESULTS W/O URINE	±	+	+	+	+	+	—
RESULTS WITH URINE	±	+	+	+	+	+	—

\+ AGGLUTINATION OBSERVED IN TUBE

— AGGLUTINATION NOT OBSERVED

Immunofluorescent Staining

The fluorescent dye, fluorescein isothiocyanate, can be coupled onto antibody molecules by allowing the isothiocyanate group to react with free amino-groups present on the antibody molecule. This coupling reaction, if properly performed, does not interfere with the antibody's ability to bind antigen. The fluorescent group attached to the antibody serves as a label which enables the antibody to fluoresce *in situ* when it is exposed to light of the appropriate wave length. When fluorescent antibodies react with their antigen, the resultant complex is rendered fluorescent. When the antigen is associated with cells (or other microscopic structures such as nuclei), the structure containing the antigen bound to the fluorescent antibody will consequently fluoresce when it is observed with a fluorescence microscope. Because immunofluorescent staining reflects the serological specificity of the antibody employed, it is a highly specific histochemical tool.

Two methods of immunofluorescent staining are commonly employed:

(1) Direct Immunofluorescence: This method employs a fluorescent antibody that reacts directly with the antigen under study, and is commonly employed in the diagnostic laboratory to identify bacteria in tissue sections, blood, C.S.F., urine, faeces or other clinical specimens. Figure 14 shows an example of

direct immunofluorescent identification of *Salmonella typhi* from the blood of a patient in the bacteraemic phase of thyphoid fever.

Fig. 14

DIRECT IMMUNOFLUORESCENCE TEST IN DIAGNOSTIC BACTERIOLOGY

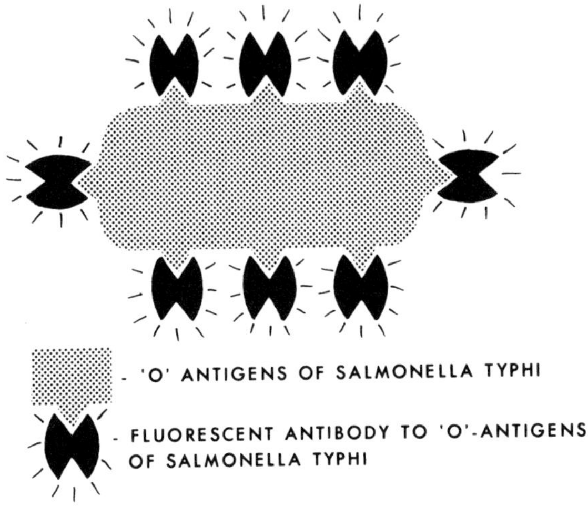

In this instance, a blood film is made from the patient, fixed in 95% ethanol for five minutes, and then allowed to dry. The slide is then overlaid with fluorescent antibody (made by immunising rabbits with the "O"-antigen of *Salmonella typhi*) and incubated for 30 minutes at 37°C. After incubation with fluorescent antibody, the slide is washed exhaustively to remove all antibody that is not bound specifically to antigen, and then examined with a fluorescence microscope.

Positive preparations are recognised by observing fluorescent bacteria on the slide, either free or within phagocytic cells.

(2) Indirect Immunofluorescence: This is a method commonly employed for detection of antibodies in serum. It is employed in many situations, but will be illustrated here by the anti-nuclear factor (A.N.F.) test. The mechanism of the A.N.F. test is presented diagrammatically in Figure 15.

A preparation of buffy-coat leucocytes is prepared from a normal human donor. These are washed several times to remove any non-specifically absorbed immunoglobulins. A suspension of these washed leucocytes is then used to prepare a series of slides, which are air-dried and fixed in 95% ethanol. After fixation and drying, these slides may be stored for long periods at -10°C prior to use in A.N.F. tests.

The A.N.F. test is then performed as follows:

Blood is drawn from a patient suspected of having A.N.F. This is allowed to clot, and the serum is removed and inactivated at 56°C for 30 minutes, to destroy complement activity. A leucocyte slide is overlaid with this serum and incubated at 37°C for 30 minutes. Following incubation, the slide is then overlaid with fluorescent anti-human immunoglobulin serum prepared in a rabbit, and again incubated for 30 minutes at 37°C. The slides are again washed exhaustively, and examined with a fluorescence microscope.

The test is positive when the nuclei of the leucocytes are fluorescent.

Fig. 15
THE INDIRECT IMMUNOFLUORESCENCE TEST FOR ANTI-NUCLEAR FACTOR (A.N.F.)

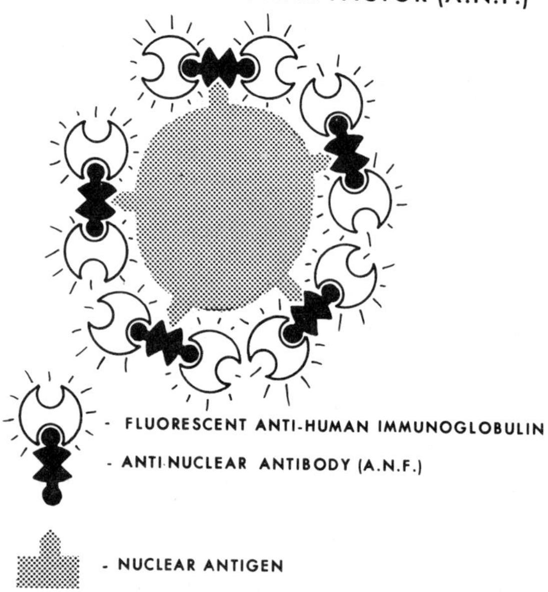

- Anti-nuclear Factor is an immunoglobulin with antibody activity against nucleoproteins. It binds these specifically, and in doing so, coats the nucleus of the cell. When fluorescent antibody against human immunoglobulin is added, the nuclei become fluorescent, and the test is considered positive for A.N.F.

The clinical significance of anti-nuclear factors is discussed more fully in Chapter 19 (*vide infra*). They occur in mesenchymal diseases like disseminated lupus erythematosus, and in certain rheumatic diseases such as rheumatoid arthritis.

Immuno-autoradiography

Fluorescent dyes are not the only method for labelling an antibody. Radioactive iodine (I^{125} and I^{131}) can also be used for this purpose, since it can be attached to tyrosyl residues on antibody molecules. If the antibody is not saturated with radioactive iodine, labelling can be accomplished without interfering appreciably with the labelled antibody's capacity to bind antigen. Cells (or other structures) to which such labelled antibodies are bound can be identified by the method of autoradiography on conventionally-stained preparations. Radioactive iodine can be used to label either antibodies or protein antigens containing tyrosine. However, the reader is cautioned that *saturation* labelling of antigens or antibodies with radioactive iodine will interfere with antigen-antibody reactions (*vide supra*, Chapter 4).

For example, I^{131}-labelled antigen was employed in autoradiographic experiments to demonstrate specific antibodies within the cytoplasm of plasma-cells as early as 1953.

> After immunising an animal with specific antigen, the animal was sacrificed and impression-slides were prepared which contained a variety of cell-types from lymph-nodes and spleens. After fixing in 95% ethanol, these slides were soaked in a solution of I^{131}-conjugated antigen. After allowing ample time for antigen-binding, the impression slides were dipped in photographic emulsion, and incubated for a suitable period in the dark. The slides were then developed in the same manner as photographic film, following which, they were stained with a standard Romanowski stain (*e.g.*, Giemsa's, Wright's, or Leishman's).

The decay of the radio-isotope attached to the bound antigen was visualised by counting photographic emulsion grains over the cells that contain labelled antibody; moreover, the cytology of antibody-containing cells could be clearly recognised, because they appeared exactly like Romanowski-stained cells in the clinical laboratory.

Virus Neutralisation

Most viruses are covered with an antigenic protein coat, wherein resides the ability of the virus to attach itself to, and to penetrate potential host cells. The region of the viral protein coat responsible for host cell recognition and attachment, and the complementary region on the cell membrane of the host cell, are known as specific receptor sites of virus and host cell, respectively.

Antibodies to viral protein coat often have the property of binding antigenic determinants on the viral specific receptor site which prevent the viral receptor from combining effectively with the complementary sites on susceptible cells; these antibodies therefore prevent the attachment of virus to host cell, and render the virus non-infective. Viral neutralisation by antibody is believed to play an important role in acquired resistance to viral infections. However, such antibodies do not affect the course of events within a cell once a viral infection has occurred.

It may be noted that some viruses (including certain bacteriophages) may be inactivated or neutralised by a single antibody molecule per infective unit. This extraordinary sensitivity of virus to the action of antibody has been utilised in the research laboratory to study antibody synthesis by single cells *in vitro*.

In the diagnostic laboratory, neutralisation tests are routinely employed in the serological typing of many viruses. The following example describes a method employed to type polioviruses:

> Clinical specimens (*e.g.*, C.S.F. or faeces) are obtained from patients suspected of poliovirus infections. These are treated to kill or eliminate all organisms other than viruses; following which, they are inoculated into monkey kidney cell cultures. The inoculated cultures are then incubated at 37°C for several days and observed periodically for the appearance of cytopathogenic effects (CPE). When characteristic CPE's are noted, the culture fluids are collected and divided into four aliquots. The first aliquot serves as a control, while each of the others is mixed with a fixed titre of antiserum of known specificity for one of the three serotypes of poliovirus. Each of the aliquots is then diluted serially, and each dilution inoculated into fresh tissue cultures. The particular antiserum which neutralises the isolated poliovirus identifies its serotype.

Bacterial Toxin Neutralisation, Antitoxins

Several types of bacteria are able to produce severe disease in man by virtue of their ability to synthesise and secrete potent exotoxins. These substances are protein in nature, and usually strongly antigenic. Some toxins exert their pathogenic effects by interfering with the physiological functions of certain target tissues of the infected host. Examples of these toxins are diphtheria toxin (which blocks protein synthesis in a wide variety of target tissues), tetanospasmin (or tetanus toxin - which blocks post-synaptically the action of inhibitory neurones on motoneurones of the anterior horn of the spinal cord, and consequently produces tetanic spasms of skeletal muscles), and anthrax toxin (which results in profound, irreversible systemic shock, with haemoconcentration, electrolyte imbalance, and acute renal failure).

Other bacterial exotoxins, such as botulin (botulinus toxin), are released into the external environment when the organism grows in contaminated food. (The toxic effects in this case are produced following ingestion of the toxin, which blocks acetylcholine release by the motor end plates of anterior horn motoneurones).

All of the bacterial toxins mentioned above are antigenic; moreover, most or all are capable of stimulating the production of antibodies which neutralise their toxic effects - *i.e.*, antitoxins. It is thus possible to prevent these toxins from causing disease by providing antitoxic antibodies to persons at risk. One may immunise actively or passively, as circumstances dictate. The decision in this regard is based on evaluation of the nature of the risk to the patient, the amount of time elapsed subsequent to exposure, the likelihood of recurring risk, the materials available for immunisation, etc. For example:

Tetanospasmin and diphtheria toxin are both readily obtainable in unlimited amounts by growing the toxigenic bacteria on simple broth culture media. The broth in which the bacteria are grown contain the toxins, which are easily purified from culture filtrates. Moreover, both tetanospasmin and diphtheria toxin can be detoxified chemically by treatment with formalin. Formalin-treated toxin (toxoid), although rendered non-toxic by the treatment, retains the antigenicity of the intact toxin. Thus, toxoids of diphtheria or tetanus toxins can be used as non-toxic antigens to induce long-lived active immunity in man. Since *Clostridium tetani* and *Corynebacterium diphtheriae* are both endemic organisms, it is advisable to immunise the entire population with these agents in coördinated health programmes. However, when an individual is at high immediate risk (*e.g.*, from exposure to a known case of diphtheria or from a soil-contaminated traumatic injury where tetanus infection is probable) it may be desirable to immunise such patients passively as well. Both animal and human antitoxin preparations are available for this purpose. The human antitoxins are the agents of choice. Animal antitoxins today have no legitimate use in prophylaxis of either tetanus or diphtheria, because the risk of anaphylactic reactions or serum sickness consequent to their use is not balanced by any therapeutic advantage. Where human antitoxin is not readily available, a combination of active immunisation with toxoid plus chemoprophylaxis (*e.g.*, with penicillin) should be used. The chemoprophylactic agent will suppress the growth of toxigenic bacteria until the level of antitoxic antibodies stimulated by the toxoid is sufficient to prevent the disease.

Since the risks of anthrax and botulism are extremely low for most people, toxoids are not usually available for active immunisation. Botulin presents an additional problem in that it occurs in five antigenically-distinct serotypes, each requiring type-specific antitoxin for positive prophylactic or therapeutic effect. Moreover, even type-specific antitoxins are effective only before the toxin is fixed to (susceptible) motor end plates. Once sufficient toxin is fixed, antitoxin has no effect on the course of this disease. Persons suspected of having ingested food containing botulin should be treated immediately with polyvalent antitoxin (of equine origin) containing antibodies to the three most common antigenic types of botulin.

Persons exposed to anthrax, however, are best treated by short-term chemoprophylaxis (with penicillin, erythromycin, tetracycline, streptomycin, or chloramphenicol), which ensures that infection will be prevented or suppressed before the toxin accumulates in sufficient amount to cause serious illness. Recently, a toxoid prepared from alum-precipitated anthrax toxin has been developed, which is safe for human use. This toxoid, where available, can be used to immunise actively certain persons who are chronically at high risk to this disease (*e.g.*: wool-carders, hide-processors, wool-shearers, etc.).

Finally, mention should be made of one toxin-antitoxin reaction that is clinically-useful in the assessment of immunity to diphtheria toxin - *i.e.*, the Schick test. A small amount of purified diphtheria toxin is injected intradermally into the volar surface of the forearm. If the patient has circulating antitoxin antibodies (and is therefore refractory to the effects of this toxin and clinically immune to diphtheria), the toxin will be neutralised *in situ* and no reaction will occur. This is denoted as a negative Schick test. However, patients lacking such antibodies develop a local zone of erythema and necrosis at the site of injection, which is due to the local effect of the toxin. This is designated as a positive Schick test*.

Enzyme Neutralisation: Anti-Enzymes

Since enzymes are proteins, the enzymes of one species are frequently antigenic to vertebrates of other species. Antibodies to enzyme antigens may inhibit the catalytic action of the enzyme. However, inhibition is not an invariable consequence of reaction with an antibody. Antibodies that possess the ability to inhibit enzymatic activity are called antienzymes. Usually, antienzyme activity is specific for the species from which the enzyme was derived. However, since enzyme evolution is usually highly conservative in the region of the catalytic site, it would therefore be predicted that antibodies directed against antigenic determinants within the catalytic site region of the molecule would cross-react with the homologous enzymes of species distantly-related to the animal from which the enzyme-antigen was derived. Nonetheless, observed fact differs from theoretical prediction in this case. For this reason, it is generally believed that antibodies with anti-enzyme activity are directed against regions of the molecule other than the catalytic site, but upon reacting with non-catalytic regions of enzyme molecules, antibodies could exert antienzyme activity by altering the conformation of the entire enzyme molecule, including the catalytic site (*i.e.*, allosteric inhibition).

Alternatively, antienzyme antibodies could induce mechanical blockade of catalytic sites (*i.e.*, steric hindrance), which would inhibit access of substrate to the catalytic site of the enzyme.

Antienzyme antibodies to enzymes of infecting parasites may interfere with parasite physiology, thus promoting eradication of the infection. In this situation, antienzyme antibodies would serve as a host defense mechanism. Some evidence exists that antienzymes do, in fact, have adaptive value in resisting certain helminthic infections.

* *Appropriate control inoculations are employed to differentiate sensitivity reactions to non-toxin components of the Schick test antigens from the effects of the toxin itself; i.e., to distinguish positives from false-positives.*

Hormone Neutralisation: Antihormones

Polypeptide hormones from foreign species are frequently antigenic to vertebrates. In many cases, reaction of hormones with antibodies directed against them results in a loss of hormonal activity. Antibodies which neutralise hormonal activity are denoted as antihormones. These are believed to be the basis of acquired insulin resistance, an infrequent complication following the long-term treatment of diabetic patients with animal insulins.

The Reversibility of Antigen-Antibody Reactions

The binding of antigen and antibody into a complex is a reversible phenomenon, as represented in the following equation:

$$Ag + Ab \leftrightarrow Ag \cdot Ab$$

Under physiological conditions, this reaction proceeds strongly to the right, whilst in acid solution (pH∿3), complete dissociation of the antigen-antibody complex occurs. However, some interchange between antibody in solution and antibody bound with antigen into complex occurs - even under neutral conditions.

Chapter 7

ANTIGEN-ANTIBODY REACTIONS INVOLVING COMPLEMENT

Most antibodies of the IgG and IgM types are capable of activating a complex system of serum β-globulins called complement (denoted as *C*). Complement plays an important role in several types of immune reactions (*e.g.*, haemolysis, cytotoxicity, immobilisation, opsonisation, and others). Although the end results observed differ in each of these reactions, an initial antigen-antibody reaction stimulates a similar sequence of biochemical reactions, involving the complement system, in all of them. The complement system may be regarded as a biological amplifier of the actions of antibodies. Complement is known to have a number of different physiologic functions, many of which are influenced by the nature of both the antigen and the experimental system employed to detect the action of complement. For example, antibodies to erythrocyte membrane antigens usually promote a haemolytic reaction when they are added to a suspension of red cells in the presence of complement, whilst antibodies to membrane antigens of nucleated mammalian cells usually promote a cytotoxicity reaction, wherein cell death occurs usually without cytolysis upon addition of antibodies and complement to the cell suspension. The identical sequence of reactions involving the complement system occurs in both situations resulting in similar lesions of the plasma membranes of the target cells. However, erythrocytes seem more prone to undergo lysis following membrane damage or destruction than do nucleated cells; thus the differences in end results observed in this case are due almost entirely to differences in target cell structure.

Similarly, differences in microbial cell antigens may lead to a variety of end reactions involving antibodies and complement. For example, antibodies to certain surface antigens of Gram-negative bacteria frequently promote lysis of the bacteria in the presence of complement, but similar antibodies to Gram-positive bacteria usually do not. Antibodies to surface antigens of *Treponema*, on the other hand, result in loss of motility by these spirochaetes in the presence of complement. This reaction is used frequently to detect antibodies in the serum of patients in whom luetic infection is suspected (*i.e.*, the *Treponema pallidum* immobilisation (TPI) test). Finally, antibodies to the type-specific capsular antigens of *Diplococcus pneumoniae* promote the phagocytosis of encapsulated *Pneumococcal* organisms in the presence of complement (opsonisation).

All of the above reactions activate the complement system in a similar way (denoted the *classical* pathway of complement activation). Differences in visible final reactions are due largely or entirely to differences in the structure of target cells or organisms. A second pathway of activation, termed the alternate pathway or *properdin* pathway can be independent of antibody under certain circumstances.

The Nature of Complement

Complement is a complex of eleven distinct protein components, most of which are associated with the β-globulin fraction of plasma. Complement can be activated and bound by IgM and (most) IgG antibodies upon reaction with antigen. Complement-binding represents a sequence of enzymatic reactions always occurring in a specified, stereotyped order. Certain of these reactions require the presence of Ca^{++} and Mg^{++} to occur; all of them proceed maximally at 37°C. The individual components of the complement system have been designated as C1, C2, C3, C4, C5, C6, C7, C8 and C9. C1 has been identified as a complex of three proteins (designated C1q, C1r, and C1s) held together by a Ca^{++} ligand. Certain components of the complement system are highly thermolabile; for example, C1, C2, C5, C8 and C9 are inactivated by heating sera to 56°C for 30 minutes.

The sequence in which the complement system is activated in both the classical and the alternate (*properdin*) pathways is given in Figure 1. In this figure, it may be noted that certain functions of complement (*e.g.*, opsonisation) do not require the sequence of reactions to proceed to completion, whilst others (*e.g.*, haemolysis) do require activation of all components. Most of the complement components have now been purified, and the reaction studied by sequential addition of each component in the test tube. If an intermediate component is omitted, subsequent components of the complement system fail to react.

Mechanisms of complement action are still imperfectly understood at the molecular level. In a haemolytic system, no evidence of damage to the red cell membrane appears until the last component of the system (*i.e.*, C9) is bound. An area of focal membrane dissolution has been noted (in electron micrographs) at the site of reaction immediately upon completion of the full reaction sequence.

The Classical Pathway

Not all antibodies are capable of binding comple-

Fig. I REACTIONS OF THE COMPLEMENT SYSTEM (simplified)

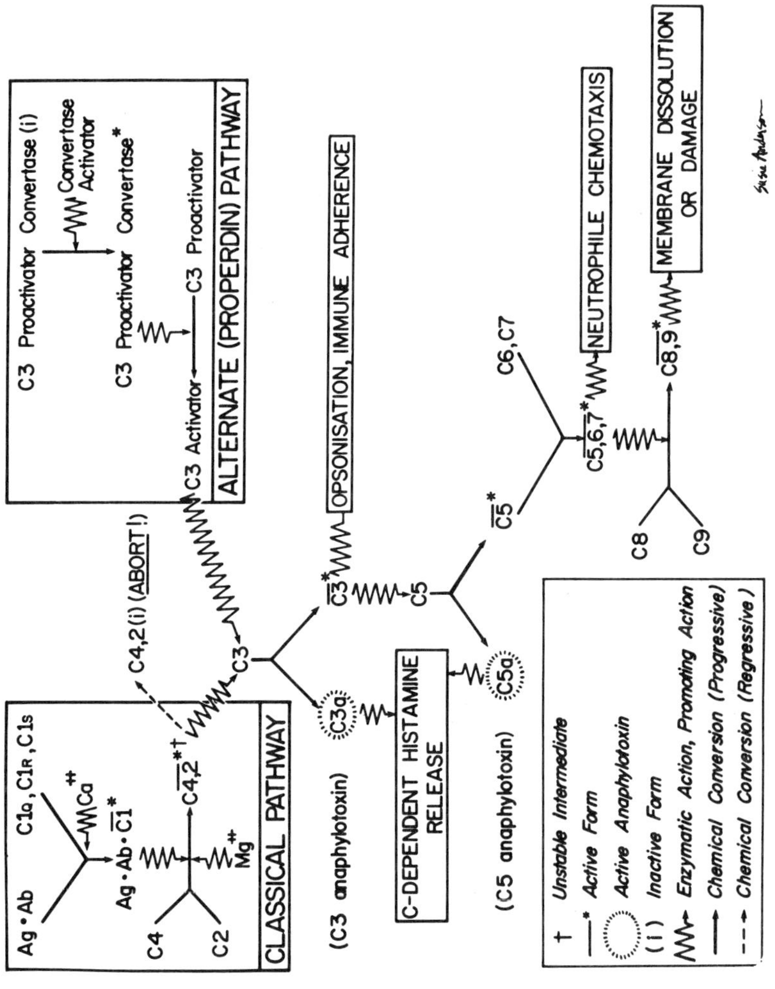

ment. Ability to activate complement via the classical pathway appears to be restricted to IgM antibodies and IgG antibodies (exclusive of the γ4 subclass). Complement-binding is a function of the *Fc*-region of the antibody molecule. The sequence is initiated by conformational changes in that region following reaction of the *Fab*-regions of the antibody molecule with antigen ("allosteric activation").

When a complement-binding antibody reacts with an antigen, the *Fab*-regions undergo changes in conformation. Allosteric changes in the *Fab*-regions alter the conformation of the entire molecule, including the *Fc*-region. Conformational changes occurring within the *Fc*-region enable the antibody molecule to bind C1. Bound C1 acquires esterase activity, preparing the site of antigen-antibody reaction for the subsequent binding of C4 and C2. From this point, reaction may proceed either to completion or decay via an "abort" sequence.

The Alternate Pathway

Many substances have been shown to be effective activators of the alternate (properdin) pathway. These include various types of immunoglobulin aggregates, polysaccharides such as inulin, agar, endotoxin, and yeast cell walls, as well as other substances, such as a protein factor derived from the venom of the common cobra (*Naja naja*) and the enzymes trypsin and plasmin.

Complement as a Homeostatic Mechanism in Vertebrates

Since the complement system can serve both as an important defense mechanism and as a powerful pathogenetic mechanism under different circumstances, it must be subject to precise control at all times. Thus, the system can be activated under circumstances where it may function in a defensive capacity, but deactivated where it would be likely to serve a pathogenetic role. It is thought that the multiple steps in complement activation afford maximal opportunity for precise control of this system, particularly where intermediate complexes are short-lived. The presence of short-lived intermediates allows the activation sequence to abort whenever the next component of the sequence is not activated and bound within a very short period (*vide supra*, Figure 1). Multiple enzymatic steps also provide maximal amplifying ability of the whole system.

The complement system is widely distributed amongst

the vertebrates. Despite wide variation in complement activity amongst vertebrate species, nearly all of these possess some complement.

With respect to the distribution of complement amongst the vertebrates, its multifactorial nature, and its ability to serve as an important defense mechanism or a powerful pathogenetic mechanism under different circumstances, the complement system is analogous to the blood-clotting system and the fibrinolysis system. Each of these systems requires precise control mechanisms to prevent inappropriate activation and excessive reaction, whilst permitting the system to function as a valuable homeostatic mechanism where circumstances require.

Clinical Assay of the Complement System

Because the complement system is involved in many types of human disease, it is sometimes desirable to assess the activity of this system in the clinical laboratory. Laboratory assessment is performed in two ways at present.

The routine determination of serum complement represents a direct immunoassay for component C3 (β1C globulin) using a commercially-available single-diffusion precipitin test in which C3-specific serum is incorporated into an agar plate (*vide supra*, Chapter 6). Single-diffusion plates for assay of component C2 are also commercially available at present, but this determination is not commonly performed as a routine clinical laboratory procedure. If demand for routine assay of other components of the complement system becomes evident, additional commercial assay kits will undoubtedly become available in the future. At present, however, such assays represent research tools primarily. Table 1 expresses the normal levels for all components of the complement system in man, with a summary of their physico-chemical properties.

Direct immunoassay of C3 (and occasionally C2) is a quick and operationally-simple procedure, but the results do not necessarily reflect the biologic activity of the whole complement system. For example, deficiencies of other components, not assayed in this test, may interfere with the integrated function of the system. Furthermore, the antisera used to prepare the C3-assay plates do not distinguish between biologically-active C3 and inactive C3. Thus, even when the serum-C3 is normal by immunodiffusion test, one cannot assume that the C3 measured by the immunodiffusion method is biologically-active.

Table 1 SERUM CONCENTRATIONS OF COMPONENTS OF THE COMPLEMENT SYSTEM IN MAN

C-Component	*Serum Concentration*	*Sedimentation Coefficient (S)*	*Molecular Weight*	*ELφ*	*(CH₂O)*	*Reactive Sulfhydryl*
$C1_q$	190 μgm/ml.	11.1	400,000	γ2	15%	-
$C1_r$	-	7.0	-	β	-	-
$C1_s$	22 μgm/ml.	4.0	79,000	α2	-	-
C2	20-40 "	5.5	117,000	β2	-	2(?)
C3	1200 "	9.5	185,000	β1	2.7%	1-2
C4	430 "	10.0	240,000	β1	14%	-
C5	75 "	8.7	-	β1	19%	-
C6	-	5-6	-	β2	-	-
C7	-	5-6	-	β2	-	-
C8	<10 μgm/ml.	8.0	150,000	γ1	-	-
C9	<10 "	4.5	79,000	α	-	-

For these reasons, it is sometimes necessary to assess the physiologic activity of the entire complement system. This is done by a bio-assay which requires all of the components of the system to be active - *i.e.,* by measurement of complement-dependent haemolysis. Since this assay tests the overall activity of the complement system, it can only indicate general reductions or increments in complement activity, without pinpointing which components are responsible.

This test employs an antiserum against sheep red blood cells made in the rabbit:

Washed sheep erythrocytes are mixed with heat-inactivated antiserum to allow the cells to become sensitised (*i.e.,* coated with the antibody). The sensitised erythrocytes are suspended in isotonic buffered saline containing Ca++ and Mg++, and dispensed into a series of tubes, containing serial dilutions of serum prepared from the freshly-drawn blood of the patient to be tested. After mixing the serum with the sensitised cells, the tubes are incubated at 37°C for 30 minutes, in order to allow complement-binding to occur.

The complement titre is read as the highest dilution of serum which will allow 50% haemolysis of the sensitised erythrocytes (expressed as CH_{50}-titre) to occur.

The Complement-Fixation Test

Complement-fixation tests are employed to determine the presence (or titre) of complement-fixing antibodies. They depend on the fact that appropriate types of antibodies combining with antigen will consume complement. Thus, by adding a known amount of complement to a mixture of antigen and serum suspected of containing antibody to the antigen, one can detect the presence of reaction by determining the amount of complement that has been consumed (or fixed) by the reaction. This can be done by adding haemolysin-sensitised sheep erythrocytes to the mixture, after allowing time for the fixation of complement to occur in the antigen-antibody reaction under test. Thus, we have the unknown antigen-antibody reaction occurring, which fixes the complement. This is followed by the addition of sensitised sheep erythrocytes to serve as an indicator of complement activity remaining after the test system has reacted.

The procedures used for complement-fixation tests vary somewhat in detail, but the principle will be illustrated by the following example:

(1) The Test System: Fresh guinea-pig serum is prepared as a source of complement, and diluted serially. Each dilution is mixed with a standardised suspension of sensitised erythrocytes and incubated at 37°C for 30 minutes in order to determine the dilution at which 50% haemolysis occurs - *i.e.*, the CH_{50}-titre. (A typical CH_{50} determination on fresh guinea -pig serum might yield a CH_{50}-titre of 1:1024).

Blood is drawn from the patient under test, allowed to clot and the serum removed. The serum complement is inactivated at 56°C for 30 minutes, and mixed with a standardised fixed amount of antigen. An equal volume of the titred guinea-pig serum is added to the tube, so that the contents represent a 1:2 dilution of this serum. The tube is incubated with shaking at 37°C for 30 minutes to allow complement-binding to occur.

(2) The Indicator System: The test tube is removed from the incubator, and the contents are diluted serially into a series of fresh test tubes. Each dilution is again mixed with a standard preparation of haemolysin-sensitised sheep red cells, and incubated once more for 30 minutes at 37°C. The CH_{50}-titre of the guinea-pig serum is again determined (corrected for the 1:2 dilution in which it is present in the test mixture).

If the test is positive (*i.e.*, if the complement has been fixed) the CH_{50}-titre will decrease. For example, in a typical positive test where the original CH_{50}-titre was 1:1024, the CH_{50}-titre after incubation of the test system might be 1:32. In a negative test, the CH_{50}-titre would still approximate 1:1024.

In spite of the apparent complexity of complement-fixation tests, they are clinically-useful in a variety of situations. Screening tests for syphilis, like the Wassermann test and the Kolmer test, are examples of clinically-useful complement-fixation tests. The test system consists of the patient's inactivated serum mixed with a bovine heart extract called cardiolipin, which represents the test antigen. These tests are empirical screening tests, based on the fact that syphilitic patients produce an antibody that reacts with cardiolipin, a substance unrelated to the aetiologic agent of the disease. Antigens like cardiolipin are designated generically as heterophile antigens. Heterophile screening tests for syphilis, although quite useful, may be falsely-positive in a number of other diseases (*e.g.*, yaws, leprosy, malaria, infectious mononucleosis, primary atypical pneumonia, vaccinia, disseminated lupus erythematosus, relapsing fever, rat-bite fever, lymphocytic choriomeningitis, and other diseases). For this reason, the highly-specific *Treponema pallidum* immobilisation (T.P.I.) test is preferred to the heterophile tests when syphilis is suspected clinically.

Complement is fixed in many antigen-antibody reactions in which it plays no evident role. In some cases, complement may, in fact, obscure or inhibit a desired reaction. For example, the presence of complement in a haemagglutination system may convert an agglutinating antiserum into a haemolytic one. Moreover, the haemolysing titre of the antiserum may differ from the haemagglutinating titre of the same serum, since certain classes of antibody molecules may serve as agglutinins, but cannot bind complement or serve as lysins. For these reasons, antisera to be used for antigen-antibody reactions not requiring complement (such as agglutination or precipitation reactions) are usually inactivated prior to use (by heating them for 30 minutes at 56°C).

Opsonisation

Opsonisation is derived from the Greek οψων, meaning dressing or relish. Opsonisation reactions are defined as immunologic reactions which alter the surface properties of pathogenic microörganisms in such a way as to render them susceptible to phagocytosis.

Specific opsonins are antibodies directed against surface-antigens on bacteria, which promote phagocytosis by coating the bacterial cells. The action of specific opsonins is greatly enhanced by certain components of complement, although appropriate antibodies alone are capable of exerting slight opsonising activity. Completion of the entire complement activation sequence is not necessary to provide maximal opsonic activity *in vitro*; components Clq, r & s, C4, C2 & C3 (in the presence of Ca++, Mg++, and specific antibody) will promote phagocytosis of encapsulated bacteria as effectively as will the complete complement system.

Opsonic activity of an antiserum is assessed *in vitro* by a test called the *opsonocytophagic index*, in which the phagocytosis of bacteria is compared after additions of normal and immune sera.

Opsonins are important defense mechanisms against infections by encapsulated *Pneumococci*. Although the polysaccharide capsular antigens of these bacteria are themselves non-toxic to the host, they act as virulence factors because they inhibit the phagocytosis of those bacteria whose surfaces they coat. Encapsulated *pneumococci* are thus not ingested or destroyed by phagocytic cells. Consequently, they are able to multiply within sites of infection until the level of opsonin is sufficient to allow phagocytic cells of the host to engulf and destroy the microbial invaders.

Miscellaneous Functions of Complement

Components of the complement system are able to:

(a) stimulate the production of an *anaphylotoxins** (substances which may produce an anaphylactic shock state when they circulate in the plasma and promote systemic histamine release),

(b) stimulate the *immune adherence* of certain microörganisms to platelets and other non-phagocytic cells, and

(c) serve as *chemotactic stimuli* to neutrophiles, causing these cells to migrate into foci of immunologic activity.

* *Two anaphylotoxins have been recognised in the human complement system. One is derived from component C3 and is denoted C3a, whilst the second is derived from component C5 and is denoted C5a. The two anaphylotoxins exert similar effects on smooth muscle, but probably react with different tissue receptors, since smooth muscle rendered unresponsive to C3a by repeated applications of it retains full responsiveness to C5a, and vice versa. Both, however, are inactivated by the same inhibitor in human plasma.*

(All of these functions are noted in Figure 1 above).

Many of the observations and concepts described in this chapter were developed by Dr. H. J. Müller-Eberhard and his colleagues of La Jolla, California.

Chapter 8

FORMATION OF ANTIBODIES IN HUMORAL RESPONSES

Parenteral injections of antigens and systemic bacterial or viral infections usually stimulate the production of IgM and IgG antibodies in a combined response, wherein most of the antibodies are of the IgG type.

When antigens are introduced to the body via mucous membranes (*e.g.*, as in local respiratory tract infections, gastrointestinal tract infections, or inhalation of pollens) the antigens may also initiate a combined IgM/IgG response. Perhaps more importantly, however, transmucosal exposure to antigen stimulates the production of IgA antibodies and/or IgE antibodies *in situ*. Locally-produced IgA antibodies may thus appear in high titre in mucous secretions, or IgE antibodies (attached to the membranes of submucosal mast-cells) may appear in connective tissue underlying mucosal epithelium. Eventually, IgA and IgE antibodies may be detected in circulating plasma.

Any of the above events may occur alone or in virtually any combination, depending on circumstances. The presence of one type of antibody does not usually preclude the simultaneous presence of others, although one type of antibody may block some or all of the biological functions of another (and ultimately favour its disappearance from the circulation).

The remaining discussion is restricted to the combined IgM/IgG responses that usually follow (non-transmucosal) exposure to antigens.

The Kinetics of Humoral Responses

The Primary Response

When an immunologically-competent vertebrate is exposed to an antigen for the first time, a primary response will occur.

During the 24-48 hours following first antigenic stimulation, no antibody is detectable. Thereafter (depending on the sensitivity of the detection method employed) antibodies begin to appear in the plasma.

Antibodies are usually readily detected by the fourth or fifth day after antigenic exposure; initially they consist entirely of IgM.

By the sixth or seventh day, IgG antibodies are usually detectable; these reach much higher titres than the IgM antibodies. The IgM titre usually begins to wane before the IgG peak is reached (usually around the fourteenth or fifteenth day). After the IgG titre peaks, the total antibody titre begins to decline, and may become virtually undetectable within 30-40 days after a single antigenic exposure.

The events of a primary response as outlined above are summarised in Figure 1.

Fig. 1 THE PRIMARY RESPONSE

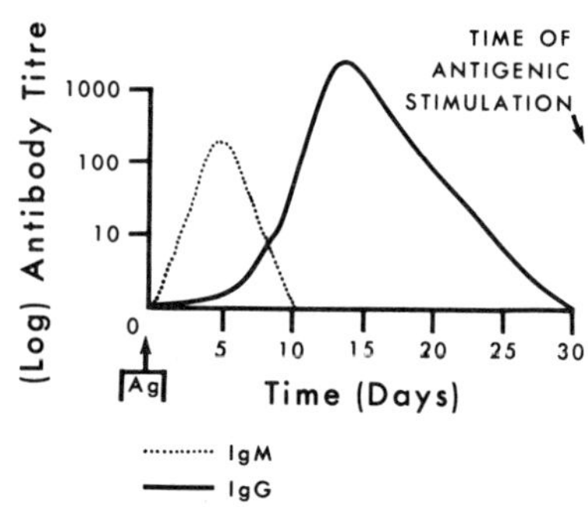

The Secondary Response

A second (or booster) exposure to the same antigen will result in the development of a secondary response.

Initially, a flurry of IgM production occurs - but without apparent lag. The IgM phase of the secondary response is accelerated in its course when compared with the IgM production observed during the primary response.

The IgG component of the secondary response is also accelerated; the titre climbs to a much higher value, and remains elevated much longer than during the primary response.

Because the lymphoid system seems to "remember" its first contact with the antigen, the accelerated and intensified secondary response may be called alternatively the *anamnestic** response.

* *Amnesia = a state of "forgetfulness"*
Anamnesia = a state of "remembrance"

The primary and secondary responses are compared in Figure 2 and 3. Figure 2 illustrates the events for IgG and IgM separately, whilst Figure 3 indicates the total antibody titres only.

Fig. 2 PRODUCTION OF IgM AND IgG IN PRIMARY AND SECONDARY RESPONSES

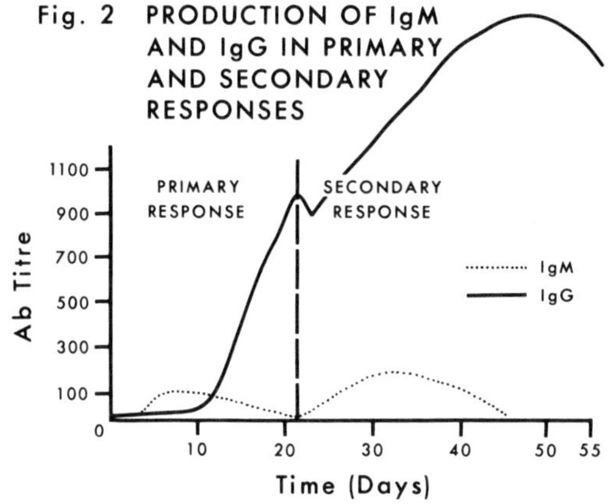

Fig. 3 PRODUCTION OF ANTIBODIES (BOTH IgM AND IgG) IN PRIMARY AND SECONDARY RESPONSES

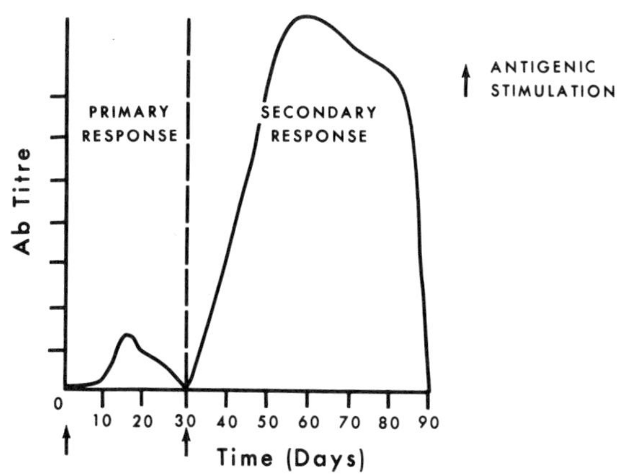

Secondary (or anamnestic) responses demonstrate a most important feature of immune responses - *i.e.*, immunological memory. Even where primary exposure to an antigen has occurred in the remote past, a second exposure to that antigen can be expected to elicit an anamnestic response. Anamnestic responses provide the rationale for employing multiple doses of antigen in certain clinical immunisation programmes (*e.g.*, Salk poliomyelitis vaccine, diphtheria and tetanus toxoid, etc.).

Adjuvants

Certain compounds or mixtures are capable of stimulating enhanced titres of antibody when they are mixed with antigenic substances. These preparations, termed adjuvants, need not themselves be antigenic. Many unrelated substances have been found to enhance immune responsiveness to antigens (and thus to have adjuvant activity). The mechanism(s) whereby these substances act is not understood. Generally, adjuvants decrease the solubility of antigen, slow the absorption of antigen from deposition sites, and/or promote infiltration of inflammatory cells —such as macrophages— into the tissues surrounding the antigen. Some example of adjuvants:

(1) Freund's Complete Adjuvant: Mineral oil + killed *Mycobacteria* emulsified with the antigen in aqueous base.

(2) Freund's Incomplete Adjuvant: Above but without *Mycobacteria*. Generally less efficient than the complete adjuvant.

(3) Calcium Alginate Adjuvant (Algivant®): 6% sodium alginate is mixed with antigen and injected into the desired depot. This is followed by injection of Ca++ (usually as calcium gluconate) into the site of antigen deposition, resulting in the immediate precipitation of the antigen within a matrix of insoluble calcium alginate gel.

(4) Alum Precipitates: Soluble antigens are mixed with an aqueous solution of alum. The pH is then adjusted to flocculate the antigen maximally. The flocculated (precipitated) antigen is then injected.

In many cases, a single dose of antigen, when injected as an antigen-adjuvant mixture, is capable of eliciting both a primary and a secondary response, whilst the same dose of antigen, administered alone, can elicit only a primary response.

(5) Laevo-Tetramisole (Laevamisole, Decaris®): The laevo-isomer of tetramisole* is an anthelminthic agent effective against most nematode infections of man and domestic animals. Recently, this drug has been found to possess marked ability to stimulate the reticulo-endothelial system, as well as both divisions of the lymphoid system. It thus may be considered as a new type of chemical adjuvant, which is capable of

* *(1) - 2, 3, 5, 6 - tetrahydro-6-phenyl-imidazo-2, (1b) thiazole HCl*

stimulating increased production of antibodies and sensitised lymphocytes to concurrently-administered antigens. Moreover, it differs from other adjuvants in that it does not exert maximum effects when injected together with the antigen, but rather when administered orally as a short course of drug concurrent with parenteral administration of antigen. Its mechanism(s) of action are not understood presently, but have nonetheless stimulated great interest in many centres throughout the world.

Cellular Aspects of Humoral Responses

The principal cells responsible for antibody and immunoglobulin synthesis are morphologically members of the plasmacytic series. However, it has been demonstrated conclusively that some cells which would be assigned to the lymphocytic series on the basis of their appearance alone are also able to synthesise immunoglobulins. These cells have been termed lymphoblasts, lymphocytes, or B-immunocytes by different authors. However, because they synthesise immunoglobulins, these cells must be considered functionally as members of the B-cell division of the lymphoid system (*e.g.*, as B-lymphocytes).

Unfortunately, no general agreement exists as to precise definition of "lymphocytes", because these cells lack specific histochemical and ultrastructural markers. All too often, the term "lymphocyte" is used as a "catch-all" category for non-phagocytic mononuclear leucocytes of variable sizes with large nonlobed nuclei. Electron-micrographic studies have not as yet provided final answers to lymphocyte definition and classification as to T- or B-origin. However, recent electron-micrographic studies appear to have made important strides in this direction. If these preliminary observations are confirmed, it may be possible to assign lymphocytes to the T-cell and B-cell series without ambiguity on the basis of their ultrastructure. At present, however, the term "lymphocyte" as used in the immunological literature refers to a functionally-heterogeneous group of cells, some of which are thymus-dependent ("T-cells") and others of which are members of the B-cell series.

No universally-accepted morphological criteria have yet unambiguously distinguished "lymphocytoid" or T-lymphocytes *en masse* from "plasmacytoid" or B-lymphocytes. That is why, in this text, the author has not attempted to define lymphoid cells morphologically-preferring, wherever possible, to define these cells in terms of function. Thus, lymphoid cells involved in the expression of cellular immunity are T-cells, whilst those synthesising and secreting humoral antibody are B-cells —by definition— irrespective of their morphological characteristics.

Primary Responses

Let us now consider some of the cells involved in primary immune responses (when exposure to an antigen is not via the transmucosal or intravenous route).

The antigen may be phagocytosed at the site of deposition and carried intracellularly to the regional lymph-nodes via the afferent lymphatics.

Alternatively, antigen may traverse the same route in a non-phagocytosed state.

Where the latter occurs, the antigen will be phagocytosed by macrophages within the medulla of the regional lymph-node, upon arrival.

Medium-to-large lymphocytes* (and/or plasmacytes) then appear in the medulla; cell proliferation and *DNA* synthesis can be demonstrated at this time. These proliferating immunocytes appear initially within the medulla of the node, but in later stages of primary responses, occur within the follicles of the cortex as well.

Small lymphocytes also accumulate within the medulla of antigen-stimulated lymph-nodes in the early phases of primary responses. These are derived primarily from a recirculating pool of lymphocytes, the members of which wander through the tissues of the body, collect in the afferent lymphatics and migrate through these lymphatics to the lymph-nodes. These lymphocytes percolate through the medulla and around the efferent lymphatics. Eventually, these cells gain access to the circulation via the thoracic duct. After circulating through the blood stream for a variable period of time, they emigrate through capillary walls and begin the cycle anew. In contrast, another population of lymphocytes, which appears later in the antigen-stimulated node, are thought to be derived from the medium-to-large lymphocytes of the lymph-node itself. These cells are thought to be carriers of immunologic memory.

Antibody-production in primary responses is usually most intense initially within the regional lymph-nodes draining the site of antigen deposition.

* *or lymphoblasts*

However, this activity usually spreads to distant sites in the course of time. Dissemination of antibody production occurs as a result of the proliferation of immunocytes accompanying local antibody synthesis. Antibody-forming cells escape from the regional nodes via the efferent lymphatics, eventually reaching the blood stream via the thoracic duct. Having gained access to the circulation, they again emigrate through the walls of capillaries to reach the tissue spaces, and, eventually, distant lymph-nodes as well.

Antibody-synthesising B-cells initially produce IgM antibodies, somewhat later shifting over primarily to the production of IgG antibodies. The precise mechanism by which this switch from IgM to IgG production is accomplished is only partially understood at present, but T-cells appear to be necessary to allow the change to occur (*vide infra*).

Secondary Responses

A second exposure to an antigen results in cellular events which differ from those accompanying a primary exposure to the antigen. In secondary responses, antigen localises rapidly - both in macrophages at the site of deposition, and on the surface of dendritic reticular cells* located throughout the cortex of regional lymph-nodes. These dendritic cells attract the antigen specifically by means of cytophilic antibody - developed during the primary response - which is attached to surfaces of their dendrites. The antibody-coated dendritic processes, in close contact with the lymphoid cells of the germinal follicle, represent an efficient method of concentrating antigen at the cellular sites at which it acts to stimulate antibody synthesis. The dendritic cells may also serve to initiate the development of germinal follicles. Cells derived from the recirculating lymphocyte pool percolate through the network of dendritic processes of lymph-nodes in the course of their extravascular migrations. Some of these lymphocytes are believed to represent immunologic memory cells, capable of being stimulated by contact with antigen. Primed lymphoid cells of this type contact the antigen bound to the cytophilic antibody on the surfaces of the dendritic processes, and transform into *immunoblasts*. Immunoblasts are large pyroninophilic** cells which prolifer-

* *also referred to by some authors as dendritic macrophages*

** *"pyroninophilic" means that these cells have an affinity for the dye "pyronine", as a result of their high concentration of intracytoplasmic RNA.*

ate *in situ*, giving rise to a developing germinal centre at the periphery of the dendritic cells.

Coöperation of T-cells, B-cells, and Macrophages in Humoral Immune Responses

It will be recalled from Chapter 2 (*vide supra*) that at least three types of cells are involved in humoral immune responses. These include:

(1) T-cells: These are lymphocytes which have developed and differentiated under the influence of the thymus. These represent the cells responsible for cell-mediated immune responses; however, they also participate in the development of many humoral immune responses, despite the fact that they do not themselves secrete antibodies that appear in the circulation.

(2) B-cells: These include plasmacytes and lymphocytes of bone marrow origin, which have differentiated and developed under the influence of the Bursa of Fabricius in birds or its (as yet undefined) analogue in mammals. Ultimately, B-cells differentiate into immunocytes which synthesise and actively secrete humoral antibodies.

(3) Macrophages: These phagocytic cells do not synthesise or secrete antibodies; however, they are thought to be important components of humoral immune responses by serving to present antigens to T-cells and B-cells in a form suitable to initiate specific immune responses.

The necessity for coöperation between macrophages, T-cells and B-cells in some humoral immune responses has been known for some time, though the actual mechanisms involved in these cellular interactions is only now becoming clarified. The methods employed to elucidate these mechanisms have included the transfer of certain populations of lymphoid cells from immunocompetent donor animals to irradiated (and therefore immunoincompetent) recipient animals. Such transfer is designated as "*adoptive immunity*". *In vitro* experiments have also served to elucidate cellular coöperation in humoral immune responses.

In order to better understand the nature of cellular coöperation in these circumstances, let us consider the "carrier effect". If we consider the case of immunogens made up of carrier moieties attached to haptenic determinants, the nature of the carrier moieties in addition to the nature of the haptenic determinants appears to be of great importance in the formation of antibodies. For example, the antibody response to a single hapten is generally better when the carrier itself is a strong immunogen. Moreover, carrier specificity can be demonstrated clearly by the frequent observation that secondary responses to a hapten are better when the hapten is attached to the same carrier as was used in initiating the primary response. Furthermore, induction of immunologic unresponsiveness to a given carrier results in a reduced antibody response to the hapten conjugated to the carrier to which the immunised individual has been rendered unresponsive (*vide infra*, Chapter 9).

T-cells recognise the carrier in those humoral responses wherein T-cell/B-cell coöperation occurs - *i.e.*, in T-dependent B-cell responses. In this way, T-cells serve a "helper" role in antibody formation by B-cells with certain antigens.

In order to develop a model for this cellular coöperation, we must first consider antibody responses to those antigens which are independent of T-cells. All T-cell independent antigens appear to be polymers having a large number of repeating identical determinants. Such antigens include *Pneumococcal* polysaccharides, endotoxic lipopolysaccharides, leavans, polyvinylpyrrolidone (*PVP*), and polymerised flagellin. Some of these show loss of immunogenicity when their molecular size falls below a critical number of polymeric units. These antigens are capable of stimulating B-cells directly; however, they appear to primarily stimulate the synthesis of IgM antibodies.

Several models have been proposed to account for the mechanisms of T-cell/B-cell interaction in humoral responses to T-cell dependent antigens. The simplest and earliest hypothesis of this type has been termed "antigen focusing"; in this theory the helper T-cells are thought to bind antigen and to present it to antibody-forming B-cells. Such a totally passive role for the T-cell, however, now appears unlikely in light of present evidence. Concentration of antigen by T-cells appears to require an active differentiation process; moreover, it appears that T-cells exert a regulatory influence on B-cells. For example, the switch from production of IgM antibodies to IgG antibodies by B-cells seems to require the regulatory influence of T-cells, since T-cell independent antigens elicit the production of IgM antibodies primarily (*vide supra*). Evidence has also been presented recently for T-cells having a regulatory influence on the binding affinity of antibodies produced by B-cells.

Recent experiments have suggested that soluble factors with biological and immunological activities are released from activated T-cells, which account for many of the observed phenomena following T-cell/B-cell interaction. For example, two major activities have been associated with soluble factors present in supernatant fluids of antigen-stimulated T-cell cultures.

(1) B-cells become activated *non-specifically* to synthesise immunoglobulins in general, and to undergo mitosis. These functions are mediated by lymphokines (*vide supra,* Chapter 3).

(2) Antigen-primed B-cells become activated *specifically* to produce antibodies specific for the antigen which stimulated the T-cells under study. Moreover, the carrier specificity alluded to earlier in this discussion (*vide supra*) may be abrogated by supernatant fluid from these antigen-primed T-cells. Thus, if a hapten "*H*" attached to carrier "*A*" (immunogen "*H-A*") is presented to previously-primed T-cells in tissue culture, these T-cells will be induced to produce a soluble factor which is capable of stimulating a culture of B-cells previously activated with the same hapten-carrier ("*H-A*") conjugate to produce antibodies to the hapten "*H*", even when it is attached to an entirely different carrier "*B*", as "*H-B*". In other words, a pure culture of B-cells stimulated by the immunogen "*H-A*" in a primary response, will yield a poor secondary response if subsequently exposed to the same hapten attached to another carrier, *e.g.,* as "*H-B*". However, if the same culture of B-cells is exposed to soluble factors from T-cells activated by "*H-A*" in addition to the second conjugate "*H-B*", the "*H-B*" conjugate will now stimulate the B-cells to yield a strong secondary response to the hapten "*H*".

Both *specific* and *non-specific* activation of B-cells by soluble factors from antigen-primed helper T-cells are favoured by the mitogenic activity of a soluble lymphokine on the B-cells. This mitogenic activity serves to increase the number of B-cells interacting with the helper T-cells (*i.e.,* initiates B-cells amplification). However, mitogenic activity alone cannot account for all of the observed phenomena in T-cell/B-cell coöperation. Evidence presently favours the existance of both a non-specific lymphokine and another soluble substance specific for the antigen in question.

Recently, an *in vitro* model was developed to study T-cell/B-cell coöperation in more detail. Populations of B-cells and T-cells were purified and separated from each other by a porous membrane permeable to molecules but impermeable to passage of the cells themselves. The T-cells were activated by an antigen, following which they released soluble factors into the medium which diffused across the membrane. In the presence of macrophages, these soluble factors induced the B-cells on the other side of the membrane to respond specifically to hapten determinants present on the antigen molecule. Moreover, the soluble factors were able to stimulate both T-cells and B-cells to respond *specifically* to the immunogen. Accordingly, antigen-activated T-cell populations were shown to release IgM monomers of molecular weight 180,000, with antibody activity for the antigen and with cytophilic affinity for the membranes of macrophages. These observations suggest that T-cell antigen-binding specificity resides in monomeric IgM receptors, released upon activation of the T-cells by antigen. These IgM monomers do not circulate to an appreciable extent, but exert their activity locally.

Antigen is thought to become bound to the membranes of macrophages and dendritic reticular cells (*vide supra*) by means of cytophilic antibodies categorised as IgM monomers. The cytophilic properties of the IgM monomers produced by the helper T-cells resides in the *Fc* region of the molecule. The spacing of the receptors for IgM monomers on the surface of the macrophages appears to permit the formation of an immunogenic lattice of antigen - *i.e.*, a matrix of repeating antigenic determinants is thus formed, wherein the surface configuration resembles that of the linear repeating antigenic units characteristic of T-cell independent antigens (*vide supra*). Thus, by virtue of the cytophilic antibody receptor arrangement on the membranes of macrophages, the antigenic determinants of T-cell dependent antigens are presented to the responding B-cells in a manner similar to that of (T-cell independent) polymerised antigens composed of linear repeating polymeric units. Thus, it is not surprising, for example, that an anti-*DNP* response requires the presence of macrophages when the *DNP* hapten is conjugated to a polymeric (T-cell dependent) carrier,whilst macrophages are *not* required, and B-cells are stimulated directly, when the *DNP* hapten is conjugated to a T-cell independent carrier. These findings imply a single mechanism of B-cell activation by T-cell dependent and T-cell independent antigens (*vide infra*, Figure 4). An observation related to activation of B-cells by linking their immunoglobulin receptors by linear series of repeating antigenic determinants, is the finding that immunoglobulin molecules on the surfaces of B-cells are capable of moving among these surfaces, and becoming aggregated at one pole of the cell following reaction with specific anti-immunoglobulin antibody, thus forming a "cap". Following formation of a cap, these molecules of membrane-bound immunoglobulin then become interiorised, thus forming intracellular vesicles. The "capping" phenomenon depends upon linear

Fig. 4

T-CELL / B-CELL COÖPERATION IN HUMORAL IMMUNE RESPONSES (DIAGRAMMATIC)

(Modified from Basten & Howard)

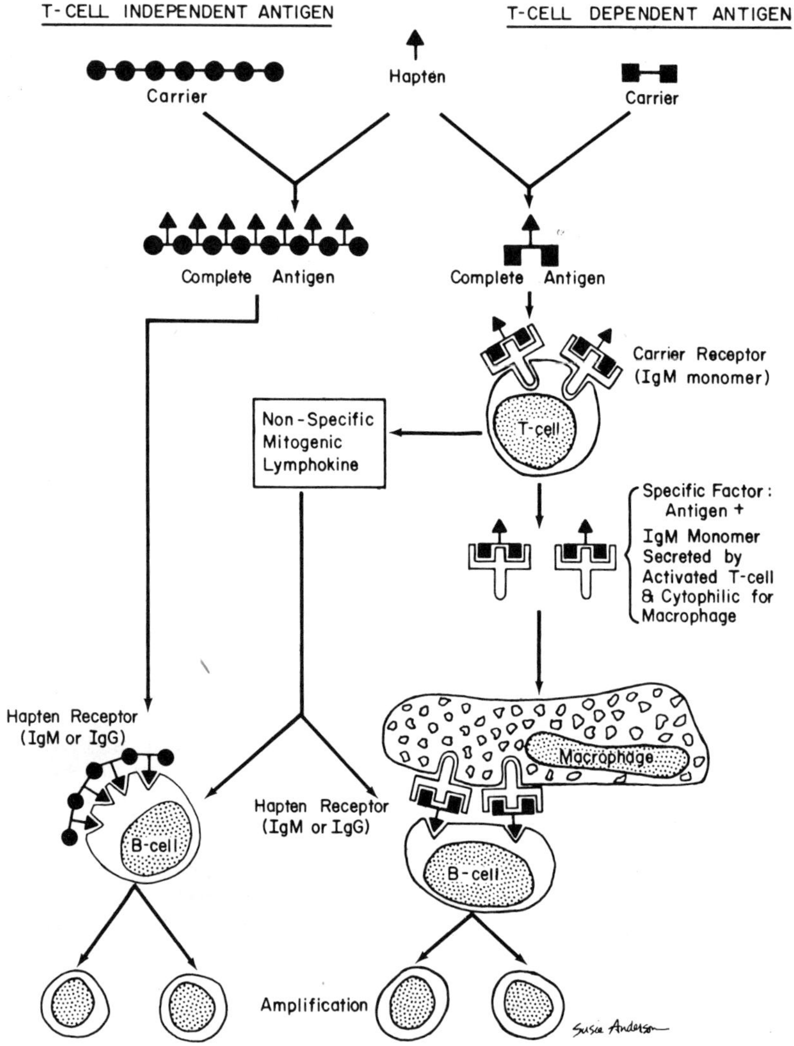

linkage of immunoglobulin receptors, and will not occur if the B-cells are treated with univalent anti-immunoglobulin *Fab* fragments, which prevent linkage of adjacent immunoglobulin molecules (and consequently their receptors) from occurring.

Chapter 9

THE RECOGNITION OF "SELF"

In general, antigenic substances are foreign to the individual responding to them. Normal, healthy individuals do not respond immunologically to their own tissues. It is self-evident that immune responses against one's own tissues could be detrimental to bodily function, since damage or destruction to tissue might be expected to result from such responses. Paul Ehrlich considered this problem many years ago, coining the Latin neologism "*horror autotoxicus*" to refer to conditions where immunologic responses to one's own tissues occur. A wide variety of clinical "*autoimmune*" diseases have been recognised, and are discussed more fully in Chapter 19. For purposes of the present discussion, these are diverse clinical entities, wherein a break in the body's ability to discriminate *self* from *non-self* appears to occur, which results in immune reactions developing against some constituent of the body, and leads to clinical disease. Where similar reactions occur in the absence of frank clinical disease, they are referred to as *autoimmune phenomena*. Since autoimmune phenomena do not ordinarily develop in normal individuals, some physiological mechanisms probably enable immunocompetent individuals to distinguish the components of *self* from the many *non-self* constituents encountered constantly throughout life.

Immune Tolerance

How, then, might such an extraordinary ability for self-recognition arise? Abundant evidence suggests that this capacity is acquired during embryonic development, although the mechanisms by which it occurs remain enigmatic. Sir F.M. Burnet suggested some years ago that autologous antigens become marked as "*self*" *in utero* during the period of embryogenesis. He conjectured that any antigen presented to a developing vertebrate embryo during this period might also become categorised falsely as *self*. In other words, Burnet predicted that exposure to any antigen during a certain period of immaturity of the lymphoid system might result in a state of *immunologic tolerance* to that antigen. Thus, exposure to that antigen after birth would fail to elicit an immune response in an individual rendered *tolerant* to it by previous exposure *in utero*.

Burnet's theory has been somewhat substantiated by experimental work in which immune tolerance states were produced by exposing certain animals to foreign antigens during foetal or early neonatal life. However, certain antigens induce tolerance better than others (*i.e.*, are better *tolerogens*), and the duration of tolerance is also variable with different antigens. Initiation and maintenance of tolerance to self-antigens (*intrinsic antigens*) is believed to require direct exposure of the immature lymphoid system to these substances; however, it is not yet known whether the exposure must be continuous in order to allow the tolerant state to persist. Such direct exposure does not always occur during development. For example, certain potentially-antigenic substances occurring in tissue are sequestered in such a way as to be inaccessible to cells of the lymphoid system. As long as structural integrity of the tissue is maintained, these substances remain sequestered.

Lymphoid cells cannot be stimulated by such occult antigens unless disruption of tissue integrity occurs, exposing the antigens to contact with immunocompetent lymphoid cells after maturation of the lymphoid system has occurred. Since direct exposure to these occult antigens did not occur *in utero*, tolerance could not have developed, and subsequent contact could therefore be expected to elicit an immunologic response to the antigen. A pathogenetic mechanism of this type has been postulated in certain autoimmune diseases - often without direct proof - as will be seen in Chapter 19.

Naturally-occurring immune tolerance to foreign antigens appears to be extremely rare. Even congenitally-acquired infections do not usually result in a state of immune tolerance to the infecting organism. For example, foetal infections with rubella virus stimulate an antibody response that appears to persist throughout infancy, childhood, and even throughout life. Neonates with congenital rubella develop serum antibody titres comparable to the titres present in their mothers. Both IgM and IgG antibodies to the rubella virus are present at birth. Moreover, the total plasma IgM is elevated at birth in infants with congenital rubella. In all of these respects, infants with congenitally-acquired rubella differ from normal infants, whose anti-rubella antibodies are maternally-acquired and all of the IgG type, whose anti-rubella antibody titres become undetectable by six months of age, and whose serum IgM is absent or negligible at birth*.

* *The effect of congenitally-acquired rubella infections on the cellular immune response is still controversial. Conflicting reports appear in the literature regarding deficiency and/or tolerance in this system.*

Neither the mechanism whereby an antigen induces tolerance or the mechanism whereby tolerance to an antigen is lost are adequately understood at present. Since this is an extremely important area of immunology, it is under intensive investigation at many centres. Hopefully, major advancement in our understanding will soon be forthcoming (*vide infra*, Chapter 17).

Immunologic Competence of the Neonate

The maturity of the lymphoid system at birth differs widely amongst various animal species. Human neonates are endowed with varying degrees of immunologic competence, correlating to some extent with gestational age and maturity in other systems. Most full-term human babies are able to form appreciable quantities of IgM antibodies upon antigenic stimulation at time of birth. IgA antibodies begin to appear about three weeks post-natally. IgG antibodies are produced in significant amounts usually only after the fourth postnatal week. Antibody responses of premature infants are usually less well developed than are antibody responses of full-term infants.

In spite of the relative immaturity of the human lymphoid system at birth, there is little danger of antigens to which babies are exposed in early postnatal life inducing immunologic tolerance. Thus, for example, early vaccination of newborns is considered relatively safe though probably less than optimally effective in preventing variola.

As a general rule, development of the lymphoid system precedes the development of immunologic competence. The human neonate at term possesses a complete lymphoid system, although germinal follicles are usually absent or poorly-developed. Immunoglobulins initially circulating in the plasma of normal full-term human neonates are almost entirely maternally-derived IgG, as this is the only major class of immunoglobulin capable of transplacental transport. However, IgM synthesis begins at birth and the level of IgM in the plasma rises rapidly. The rise in plasma IgM contrasts with an initial fall in circulating IgG*. This decline in plasma IgG continues steadily during the first three to four weeks of life. At the third week of age, however, developing competence to form IgG enables the infant to replenish its dwindling stores of maternal

* *This is not surprising since all of the IgG is maternally-derived.*

immunoglobulin. The plasma IgG level rises as new antigenic stimuli continue to stimulate the increasingly-competent IgG-forming cells of the infant.

Maternal colostrum contains significant levels of IgA antibodies. These antibodies are believed to represent an important mechanism for resisting infection of the intestinal tract by providing passive protection against the infant's constantly-developing and expanding intestinal flora. Little, if any, colostral IgA is absorbed systemically by human neonates. In this respect, the neonatal human stands in marked contradistinction to neonates of certain other species of mammals, in which significant colostral antibody is absorbed systemically.

SECTION II

CLINICAL IMMUNOLOGY AND IMMUNOPATHOLOGY

INTRODUCTION

This section, dealing with clinical immunology and immunopathology, is of greatest concern to the medical student and physician. However, its importance to the basic scientist should not be underestimated either - and an understanding at least of the principles of immunopathology is essential to understand immunobiology in general.

The system of Gell and Coombs for classifying immunologic mechanisms of disease has gained great favour in recent years, and will be presented here as an overview of the subject. These authors divide such mechanisms into four categories, as follows:

Type I Reactions: These reactions include all immunologic phenomena involving *atopy*. They are mediated by antibodies of the IgE class, denoted as *reagins*, which become passively attached to tissue mast-cells, blood basophiles, and blood neutrophiles. Upon contact with allergen, such reagin-sensitised cells undergo rupture, with consequent release of pharmacologic mediator substances such as *histamine* and *SRS-A*. These reactions are considered in detail in Chapter 11 (*vide infra*).

Type II Reactions: These reactions include all immunologic phenomena mediated by *cytotoxic antibodies* and *complement*. These are discussed in detail in Chapter 15, with special aspects being dealt with in Chapter 7, and Chapters 16, 17 and 19 (*vide supra et infra*).

Type III Reactions: These include all reactions mediated by *immune complexes - i.e.*, those conditions in which *free circulating antigen* forms complexes with *circulating antibodies* and *complement*. These reactions are discussed in detail in Chapter 10 (*vide infra*).

Type IV Reactions: These include all cell-mediated immune reactions leading to tissue damage. These reactions are mediated by the thymus-dependent division of the lymphoid system, and are considered as a group in Chapter 12. Special aspects of these reactions are also dealt with in Chapter 4 and in Chapters 17, 18 and 19 (*vide supra et infra*).

Chapter 10

IMMUNE INJURY DUE TO ANTIGEN-ANTIBODY COMPLEXES

The Arthus Phenomenon: An Experimental Model for Immune Complex Injury

If a rabbit is given small doses of an innocuous protein, such as bovine serum albumin (BSA), by weekly subcutaneous injections, a gradually-increasing reaction at the site of injection will be observed. The first one or two injections elicit no visible response, but the third or fourth injections will initiate the development of local reddening and swelling at the injection site within a few hours. Subsequent injections will elicit progressively more violent responses, and ultimately, the injection sites develop extensive haemorrhage and necrosis. This sequence of events is known as the Arthus reaction, after its discoverer, Maurice Arthus.

The initial stage in the pathogenesis of the Arthus reactions is the primary response provoked by the first injection of the antigen (BSA). Each subsequent injection of BSA provokes secondary responses so that rising titres of serum antibody to BSA develop. These antibodies circulate in the blood and, on subsequent subcutaneous injections of BSA, react with the antigen *in situ*. Initially, the Ag-Ab reaction occurs within the lumina of small blood vessels, injured by the trauma of injection. The Ag-Ab complexes thus formed, fix to themselves the components of complement (C)*. The Ag-Ab-C complexes, due to the properties of the complement system initiate a sequence of pathological events, *i.e.*, agglutination of platelets, degranulation of mast-cells, and chemotaxis of leucocytes. The agglutinated platelets and degranulated mast-cells release vasoactive substances (*e.g.*, histamine, serotonin, kinins, etc.) which alter the permeability of blood vessels and favour the transudation of additional antibody molecules and components of the complement system through the vessel walls. This efflux of antibody and complement promotes further formation of Ag-Ab-C complexes, both within the vessel walls and in the extracellular spaces. The accumulation of polymorphonuclear leucocytes within the site of immune complex deposition contributes to the increasing inflammation through release of lysosomal enzymes by living and dead leucocytes. The consequence of these events is the development of vasculitis, which is the characteristic lesion of the Arthus reaction.

* *Vide supra, Chapter 7.*

Proof that the mechanism of the Arthus reaction is as described may be derived from several sources.

The histology of the Arthus lesion is that of an acute inflammation with conspicuous involvement of blood vessels, *i.e.*, vasculitis with haemorrhage and thrombosis.

Direct immunofluorescence studies using fluorescent antisera directed against initiating antigen, antibody or complement demonstrates Ag-Ab-C complexes in the walls of affected blood vessels, as well as in surrounding tissues.

In animals depleted of complement or polymorphonuclear leucocytes, the Arthus reaction cannot develop.

Substances which block the action of vasoactive substances released from platelets, mast-cells and polymorphonuclear leucocytes inhibit the Arthus reaction.

Arthus reactions occur in humans as well as other species of vertebrates possessing the necessary components (*i.e.*, antibody, complement and polymorphonuclear neutrophiles); however, it is likely that certain minor details of mechanism vary from one species to another.

Arthus reactions are not of great clinical importance, since strongly antigenic substances are not usually administered as repeated subcutaneous injections. The great importance of the Arthus reaction is that it can be elicited reproducibly in animals, and thus has served as a major experimental model for unravelling the mechanisms of tissue injury by antigen-antibody complexes in certain human diseases.

Human Disorders Due to Immune Complexes

Serum Sickness

When an individual is injected with ~10 ml. of a foreign serum, a characteristic illness usually results. Six to ten days after the injection, the patient may develop fever, arthritis, lymphadenopathy, splenomegaly, urticaria, and haematuria. A severe acute glomerulonephritis may occur. In past years, when serotherapy was common, this condition usually arose after the injection of horse serum used for passive immunisations against (or immunotherapy of) an infectious disease. At present, horse anti-lymphocyte serum is a potential offender, and occasionally, certain slowly-excreted drugs (*e.g.*, benzathine penicillin) may initiate an identical disorder.

The injected foreign serum acts as an antigen and initiates an immune response. Antibodies produced in consequence of the antigenic stimulation provided by foreign serum antigens are released into the circulation in ever-increasing titres, where they meet these antigens - still circulating in significant titres - usually between the sixth to the tenth day following injection of serum. Complexes between antigen and antibody thus form within the vascular bed. These are soluble initially, because they form under conditions of antigen excess (*vide supra*, Chapter 6). The complexes deposit in vessel walls, particularly within the vessels of the renal glomeruli. Penetration of complexes into vascular walls is favoured by increased permeability resulting from the release of vasoactive substances from platelets and neutrophiles. Fixation of complement within the Ag-Ab complexes results in an inflammatory sequence similar to that in the Arthus reaction. Acute vasculitis and acute glomerulonephritis result. The location of the vasculitis determines the nature and distribution of symptoms; arthritis and urticaria are often the predominating manifestations.

In animals, experimental serum sickness can be produced by mixing antigen and antibody in a test tube and injecting the mixture, if the Ag-Ab complexes are formed in antigen-excess. Under these circumstances, soluble complexes are formed which initiate development of serum sickness readily. Under conditions of antibody-excess or at equivalence, larger complexes form, which are cleared rapidly by the reticulo-endothelial system before they provoke inflammation or initiate serum sickness. (*Vide supra*, Chapter 6).

Immune Vasculitis (Allergic Vasculitis)

Not uncommonly, patients develop symptoms and signs attributable to inflammatory lesions occurring in blood vessels, usually pyrexia associated with localised disturbances of function explainable on the basis of obstruction of arterial blood flow. Occasionally, patients with localised vasculitis will demonstrate local tenderness and pain related to the particular vessel involved. Biopsy of the involved vessel will show intramural inflammation. Fluorescein-labelled rabbit anti-human gamma globulin, or fluorescent anti-human C3, applied to frozen sections of the arterial lesions, may indicate the presence of immune complexes. It is now thought that the pathogenesis of most immune vasculitis is through the inflammatory effects of these immune complexes. Certain drugs (*e.g.*, sulfonamides, thioureas, diphenylhydantoin, iodides, penicillin, and others) are not infrequently implicated as initiators of immune vasculitis; thus, patients in whom this condition develops should be queried specifically about a drug history.

Polyarteritis Nodosa

Polyarteritis nodosa is a disease which can occur at any age; it is characterised by segmental inflammation and necrosis of small arteries and arterioles, and may affect almost any organ in the body. Whereas the more acute immune vasculitides usually demonstrate spontaneous improvement over the course of a few weeks, polyarteritis nodosa tends to be recurrent and progressive, and leads to serious consequences from organ damage due to arterial insufficiency. Because of the great similarity of the vascular lesions to those seen in immune vasculitis and serum sickness, it would appear reasonable for these diseases to have similar pathogenetic mechanisms (*i.e.*, circulating immune complexes). Nonetheless, the pathogenetic mechanism of polyarteritis nodosa has not been proven; it is best for the time being to regard the pathogenesis of this condition as still unsolved, whilst continuing to search for a possible mechanism.

Glomerulonephritis

There are many forms of glomerulonephritis, with varied primary aetiology. Pathogenetic mechanisms, however, are frequently similar, the common denominator being the ability of Ag-Ab-C complexes to initiate foci of inflammation at deposition sites within glomerular capillaries.

There are two main types of pathological lesions:

(A) In the commonest type, Ag-Ab-C complexes form "lumpy-bumpy" deposits on the glomerular basement membranes, which are well-seen in the electron microscope (*e.g.*, post-Streptococcal glomerulonephritis).

(B) In the less common type, the glomerular basement membrane itself appears to be both the antigen and the site of localisation of antibody and complement.

Post-Streptococcal Glomerulonephritis: This is an acute inflammation of the glomerulus which develops about 10 days after an upper respiratory infection with Lancefield Group A haemolytic Streptococci, especially types 4, 12, 21 and (rarely) other types as well. Clinically, there is haematuria, proteinuria, oedema, hypertension, and, in severe cases, renal failure. Grossly, the kidneys appear swollen and demonstrate petechial haemorrhages; microscopically, the glomeruli are swollen and hypercellular. In children, the vast majority of cases recover completely, but in adults, chronic renal disease is a relatively common sequela.

Whilst there are still some gaps in our understanding of the pathogenesis of this condition, the following outline indicates the most probable sequence of events. Streptococcal infection elicits formation of antibodies to this organism, which react with circulating Streptococcal antigens, yielding soluble complexes. These complexes are filtered out by the renal glomeruli and deposited on the Bowman's space aspect of capillary basement membranes. Complement, bound by the complexes, initiates an acute inflammatory response within the glomerulus, with increased glomerular permeability resulting in leakage of proteins and cells into the urine. Immunofluorescent techniques demonstrate deposition of IgG and complement in a characteristic "lumpy" pattern on the outside surfaces of the glomerular basement membranes, as in Figure 1.

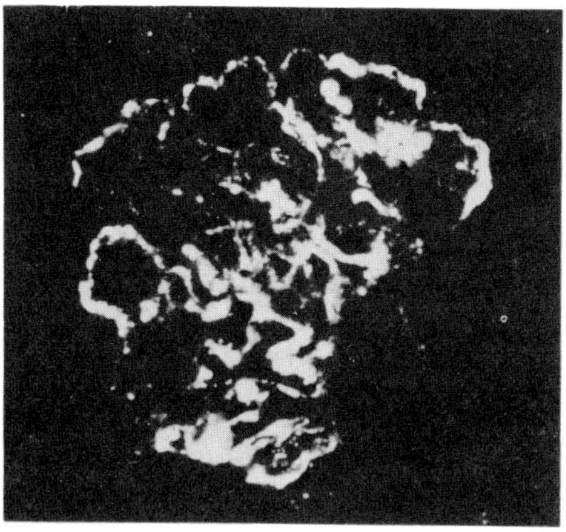

Fig. 1 Immunofluorescent staining of a Renal Biopsy from a patient with Post Streptococcal Glomerulonephritis showing 'lumpy' deposits on outer surface of Glomerular Basement Membrane. (Fluorescein-labelled anti-human immunoglobulin, prepared in a goat, is employed.)

The "lumpy-bumpy" deposits are readily demonstrable by electron micrography (Figure 2). Streptococcal antigens can also be demonstrated in the capillary walls by immunofluorescence.

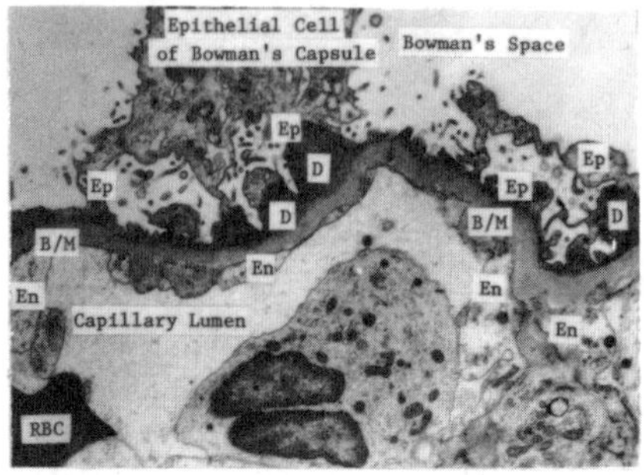

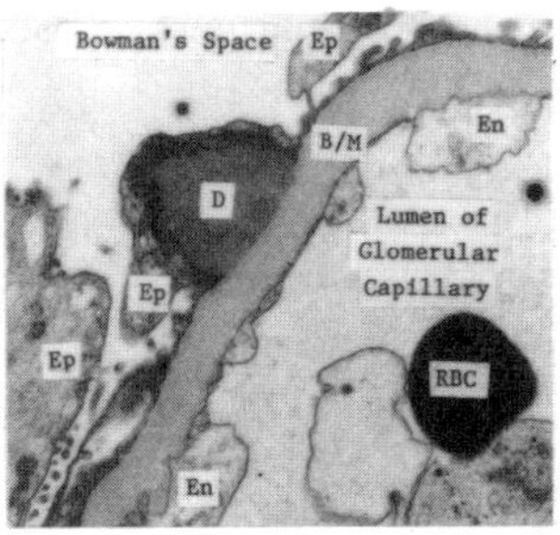

D - Deposit

Ep - Epithelial Cell Layer

En - Endothelial Cell Layer

RBC - Red Blood Cell

B/M - Basement Membrane

Fig. 2 Electron micrographs of a Renal Biopsy from a patient with Post Streptococcal Glomerulonephritis showing 'lumpy' deposits on outer surface of Basement Membrane. (Fluorescein-labelled anti-human immunoglobulin, prepared in a goat, is employed.)

Experimental glomerulonephritis, very similar to naturally-occurring human post-Streptococcal glomerulonephritis, can be induced in rabbits by repeated intravenous injections of foreign protein, thus allowing circulating soluble immune complexes to form. Repeated intravenous injections of nephritogenic Streptococci will also produce glomerular injury in rabbits; however, the reason why certain strains of Streptococcus are more apt to cause the disease than others remains obscure.

Other Diseases with Glomerulonephritis Histologically Similar to Post-Streptococcal Glomerulonephritis:

In several other diseases, glomerulonephritis with similar pathologic appearance may occur. That is, electron microscopy of the glomeruli will show "lumpy" deposits on the Bowman's space aspect of the glomerular basement membrane as seen in Figure 2 above.

For example, in *disseminated lupus erythematosus (DLE)*, a variety of glomerular lesions, including the type just described (*vide infra*, Chapter 19) may be seen. In this disease, the Ag-Ab-C complexes are thought to consist, at least in part, of nuclear antigen, antinuclear antibody, and complement.

Moreover, the glomerulonephritis occurring in serum sickness, as well as that associated with immune vasculitis, is attributed to circulating immune complexes.

Idiopathic Membranous Glomerulonephritis: This is a distinctive disease, seen mainly in adults, and marked by insidious onset of the nephrotic syndrome.* Renal biopsy demonstrates diffusely thickened glomerular capillary walls, with little evidence of hypercellularity or inflammation. Electron microscopy reveals extensive amorphous "lumpy" deposits on the outer surface of glomerular basement membranes, and immunofluorescent stains show "lumpy" deposits of IgG and complement. The disease is slowly progressive over a period of many years, ultimately ending in renal failure.

The features of idiopathic membranous glomerulonephritis discussed above strongly suggest that it, too, is due to immune complexes. However, there is usually no history of antecedent infection, so the provoking antigen remains unknown.

A similar experimental disease can be produced in rats by immunisation with a renal tubular antigen. However, until the significance of this rather unexpected observation is worked out, it is best to regard the aetiology of the human disease as still unsolved.

Autoimmune Glomerulonephritis: Glomerular basement membranes are relatively antigenic; thus, a rabbit immunised to rat kidney will produce antibodies which will bind to rat glomerular basement membranes. If the rabbit anti-rat kidney serum is injected into the rat, an acute glomerulonephritis is produced, which binds complement and involves polymorphonuclear neutrophiles similarly to the Arthus reaction. This experimental model is called Masugi nephritis, after the man who

* *The nephrotic syndrome is a clinical entity characterised by massive proteinuria, hypoproteinaemia (particularly hypoalbuminaemia), hyperlipidaemia, lipiduria, and oedema.*

first developed the experimental system. Immunofluorescent staining shows IgG and complement bound to glomeruli in a "linear" pattern, quite different in appearance from the "lumpy-bumpy" pattern seen in glomerulonephritis due to immune complexes. The linear pattern is due to the binding of anti-basement membrane antibodies to the surfaces of glomerular basement membranes.

In certain cases of human glomerulonephritis, an identical linear pattern of fluorescence is seen using fluorescein-conjugate anti-IgG or anti-C3, as illustrated in Figure 3. This suggests that antibodies to glomerular basement membrane are present. Indeed, such antibodies have been detected in acid eluates of affected kidneys.

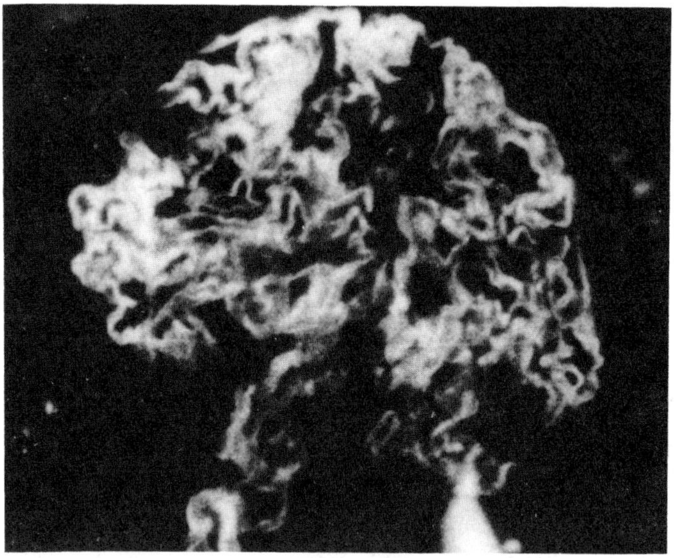

Fig. 3 Immunofluorescent staining of Renal Biopsy from a patient with Goodpasture's Syndrome, showing linear pattern of Immunofluorescence. (Fluorescein-labelled anti-human immunoglobulin, prepared in a goat, is employed.)

The linear type of glomerulonephritis, although less understood than the post-Streptococcal form may represent an example of an "autoimmune disease" (*vide infra*, Chapter 19) in that the patient appears to produce antibodies directed against an autologous antigen which are capable of initiating a disease state.

This type of glomerulonephritis occurs characteristically in a rare disease called Goodpasture's Syndrome, in which nephritis is associated with pulmonary lesions.

Also, certain patients who develop progressive post-Streptococcal glomerulonephritis show both a linear and a "lumpy-bumpy" pattern of immunofluorescence. These patients may develop circulating anti-kidney antibodies in the course of their disease which may not be detectable in serum except following nephrectomy prior to renal transplantation.

Linear immunofluorescence has also been described in certain cases of glomerulonephritis associated with DLE.

Many of the observations and concepts described in this chapter were developed by Dr. Frank Dixon and his colleagues in La Jolla, California.

Chapter 11

IgE-MEDIATED IMMUNE INJURY (ALLERGY, ATOPY, IMMEDIATE HYPERSENSITIVITY)

Certain individuals are genetically predisposed to react in an abnormal way to contact with certain antigens termed "allergens", which are not harmful to normal people. When these antigens contact mucosal surfaces of such individuals, they respond by producing antibodies of the IgE class. IgE antibodies, termed "reagins", mediate "allergic" or "atopic" states. Patients with an atopic diathesis are referred to as "atopic" individuals.

Atopic individuals are susceptible to a number of clinical disorders, the stigmata of which depend upon many factors- *e.g.*, the route of exposure to allergen and the distribution of sensitised tissues within the body (*i.e.*,"Shock organs"). Thus, an atopic individual may exhibit any of the following reactions, alone or in combination:

(1) *Anaphylactic Shock* - this consists of a sudden profound vasomotor collapse leading to shock, which occurs when the sensitised patient is given the offending antigen. Paroxysmal bronchoconstriction usually occurs as well. Typically, the inciting dose is given intravenously, but anaphylactic reactions can occur after oral, subcutaneous or intramuscular administration. Death may occur in a matter of minutes, if prompt treatment is not undertaken.

(2) *Allergic (Extrinsic) Asthma* - this consists of paroxysmal bronchospasm, usually with excessive viscid bronchial mucus secretion. Attacks are usually precipitated by inhalation of the specific offending "allergen". The condition occurs typically in children and young adults, although it may often persist into middle and late life.

(3) *Allergic Rhinitis (Hay-Fever)* - exposure of the nasal mucous membranes to allergen causes a profuse watery nasal discharge with sneezing. Frequently, the nasal symptoms are accompanied by a similar reaction in the conjunctiva, resulting in redness, irritation and watering of the eyes.

(4) *Urticaria (Hives)* - although the aetiology of urticaria is not always atopic, allergic urticaria may occur following exposure to allergens, usually by ingesting them. Wheals and erythematous areas in the skin cause intense pruritis and discomfort. Considerable local oedema, known as "angio-oedema", may accom-

pany urticaria, and this may be life-threatening when it affects the mucosa of the pharynx or larynx, resulting in severe acute respiratory obstruction.

(5) *Atopic dermatitis (infantile eczema, atopic eczema)* - This condition arises most commonly in infants and young children with a familial history of allergic disorders. It is commonly the first indication of an atopic diathesis in an infant, presenting clinically as a persistent, pruritic dermatitis, which may be versicular, papular, exudative or lichenified, and involves the head, neck and flexor aspects of the trunk and extremities most commonly (*e.g.*, the antecubital fossae, popliteal fossae, wrists, hands, face, and neck). Although in many cases the provoking allergen cannot be identified, a large number of patients with this disease react to animal products such as wool and other epidermal allergens (hair and danders), or to foods in the diet, such as milk, wheat, eggs, pork, shellfish, citrus, tomatoes, strawberries, or chocolate.

The Prausnitz-Küstner Reaction

Historically, serum from atopic individuals was found to contain a hitherto-unidentified category of antibody called reagin which could transfer sensitivity to specific allergens from allergic patients into the skin of normal (non-atopic) people. Thus, if reagin-containing serum from an atopic individual is injected into the skin of a normal (non-allergic) person, the passively-sensitised skin will react to a subsequent injection of offending allergen with development of a wheal and erythema; *i.e.*, non-atopic recipients of atopic serum respond to intradermal injections of allergens in a similar manner to the atopic serum donors. This test, evolved by Prausnitz and Küstner, is known as the Prausnitz-Küstner (P-K) reaction. Reagins may thus be referred to as P-K antibodies, as well as skin-sensitising antibodies.

The recent discovery of the IgE class of immunoglobulins and its association with reaginic activity by the Ishizakas represents a major advance in our understanding of the atopic diseases.

Further information, however, is needed to clarify many aspects of atopic diseases that are still poorly-understood.

Relationships of Atopic Diseases to IgE

IgE (*vide supra*, Chapter 5) will be discussed here only in the context of its relationship to (atopic) allergy. Human IgE will "fix" itself to human skin; fixation being due to a cytophilic affinity of this immunoglobulin for the plasma membranes of mast-cells within the dermis. This cytophilic affinity resides in the Fc region of the ε-chain. IgE antibodies bind allergens specifically - each (8S) IgE molecule containing 2 antigen-binding sites. Reaginic antibodies are not capable of activating the complement system, and there is little evidence that complement is involved in true atopic diseases.

IgE levels in serum are extremely low (*i.e.*, 10-70μg.%) - this immunoglobulin thus comprising only ∿0.002% of the total serum immunoglobulin. Although atopic patients frequently have elevated serum IgE titres, the degree of elevation is often not great.

IgE antibodies have cytophilic affinity for the plasma membranes of tissue mast-cells, blood neutrophiles and blood basophiles, and can sensitise these cells to allergens. Such reagin-sensitised cells will rupture and undergo degranulation immediately on contact with allergen, the result of which is the release of vasoactive mediator substances, or their precursors from the cells undergoing degranulation. Vasoactive substances, released in consequence of the contact of these cells sensitised by cytophilic IgE antibodies with provoking allergen, represent the "deputy messengers", which produce the signs and symptoms characteristic of atopic conditions. To some extent, these signs and symptoms depend on the location where the reagin-sensitised cells contact the allergen and release chemical mediators in the body.

Nature of the Atopic Response

The release of histamine and other pharmacologic mediator substances by reagin-sensitised cells on contact with allergen is the initiating stimulus for a variety of subsequent reactions.

The pharmacological actions of histamine on the vascular system include the dilation of capillaries, small arterioles and venules. Thus, systemic histamine release produces a rapid fall in blood pressure. On the other hand, local histamine release produces congestion of small blood vessels adjacent to the site. Intradermal injection of pure histamine will produce a wheal and erythema similar to that observed when atopic patients are given intradermal injections of allergens to which they are sensitised.

Histamine directly stimulates bronchiolar smooth muscle to contract. It may be responsible for some of the bronchospasm seen in allergic asthmatics. However, although atopic asthma (*vide infra*, this Chapter) shares a number of features with known IgE-histamine-mediated reactions, antihistamines are usually of no therapeutic value, because mediators other than histamine are primarily involved in extrinsic asthma.

Histamine can also stimulate certain exocrine glands, possibly, in part, through vagal stimulation. This may account for some of the bronchial hyper-secretion seen in asthma and the nasal hyper-secretion seen in hay-fever.

Contact of reagin-coated mast-cells with offending allergens will also liberate pharmacologically-active mediator substances other than histamine. One such substance, thought to be of primary importance in atopic asthma, has been designated "slow-reacting substance of anaphylaxis", or "SRS-A". SRS-A, as its name suggests, acts more slowly than histamine. Over a course of time 6 to 12 hours long, it exerts several pharmacologic activities similar to those of histamine. For example, SRS-A is able to induce bronchiolar smooth muscle to contract; however, SRS-A induced bronchospasm is not alleviated by antihistamines.

A third class of pharmacologically-active substances may be liberated by allergen-reagin reactions. These reactions are capable of activating the kallikrein system of proteolytic enzymes, which eventually results in release of bradykinin. Bradykinin is able to exert marked vasoactive and bronchospastic activities.

At this time, the eosinophilia which is so characteristic of atopic states is inadequately understood. It is known, however, that eosinophilia increases with increased contact with the allergen. Eosinophilia is favoured by release of Eosinophile-Chemotactic Factor (ECF) from degranulating mast-cells.

Peculiarities of the Allergic Individual

There is a strong hereditary predisposition to the development of allergic manifestations; usually parents or siblings of allergic patients will also have a history of allergies. The reasons for this are not yet understood. It has been suggested that atopic individuals manufacture more IgE than normal, possibly of variant type. Overproduction of IgE antibodies by atopic individuals may be particularly stimulated when the antigen is introduced by the transmucosal route. The higher serum levels of IgE found in allergic subjects supports this view but does not rule out another possibility - that reagin-coated mast-cells of allergic individuals may degranulate and release histamine and other mediators more readily than do mast-cells from non-atopic subjects upon contact with allergen. Furthermore, some allergic subjects may even be more sensitive to the pharmacologic effects of histamine than are non-atopic individuals. In fact, all three suggestions could represent additive peculiarities which might function alone or in combination, in different individual patients.

Recognition of Offending Allergens in the Clinic

The patient's historical account of the precipitating causes of his allergic manifestation often incriminates the offending allergens. For example, symptoms may arise only when the patient is exposed to one particular pollen, dust, food or drug. A trial exposure to the suspected antigen may confirm its aetiological role, by inducing a typical attack. Quite often, however, the history is imprecise, or the diagnostic induction of an attack by challenge with a suspected allergen is not safe, convenient, or practical. In these circumstances, skin-tests provide valuable diagnostic assistance. For example, if a patient complains of seasonal hay-fever or asthma, the physician may test his skin reactivity to scratch tests or intradermal injections of appropriate potential allergens, such as pollens. The offending antigen will produce a wheal- and erythema response at the site of injection. The skin provides a large area for testing multiple antigens; thus, complex situations involving possible sensitivities to several antigens can be evaluated. Unfortunately, a positive skin reaction to a given allergen does not constitute *ipso facto* proof that a patient's symptoms of hay-fever or asthma are related to that antigen. In fact, the allergic individual may frequently demonstrate positive skin tests to allergens which are not related to his clinical symptoms. Moreover, the skin of certain allergic individuals may react to the non-specific minor trauma of the intradermal injection or scratch with a spurious wheal-and erythema response, which can easily confuse the interpretation of skin testing. Thus, interpretation of skin tests is best attempted only by clinically-competent allergists.

Atopic Disorders of Uncertain Status

Anaphylaxis

The types and mechanisms of anaphylaxis in different animal species are varied and complex. Some of the main differences between animal species are as follows:

(a) *Clinical Features of Anaphylaxis:* In the guinea pig, intense bronchospasm is the dominant feature of anaphylaxis. In the rabbit, however, pulmonary artery constriction and heart failure are pronounced, whilst in the dog, the splanchnic circulation is affected maximally.

(b) *Immunologic Mediators of Anaphylaxis ("Primary Messengers"):* In man, anaphylaxis appears to be mediated primarily by IgE antibodies. However, anaphylactic responses in certain animals can be mediated by IgG antibodies, and a possible role for some IgG and IgM antibodies as activators of C3a and C5a anaphylotoxins from the complement system (*Vide supra*, Chapter 7) has not been excluded in man. Once liberated, C3a and C5a actively promote the release of pharmacologic mediators from the granules of nearby mast-cells.

(c) *Pharmacologic Mediators of Anaphylaxis ("Deputy Messengers"):* The chemical mediators responsible for anaphylactic reactions also vary between species. For example, serotonin appears to be the major pharmacologic mediator of anaphylaxis in the mouse and the rat, whilst histamine serves the same role in guinea pigs and in man.

Intrinsic Asthma

Intrinsic asthma arises most commonly in later life, is usually associated with chronic bronchial infection, and tends to be persistent, rather than occurring in short attacks, as does atopic asthma. The aetiology and pathogenesis of intrinsic asthma remain obscure; anti-histamines and immunologic desensitisation attempts have no therapeutic value. Patients who have had atopic asthma in early life may subsequently develop intrinsic asthma, but this progression is by no means invariant.

Atopic Eczema

Atopic eczema is a poorly-understood condition wherein it is frequently impossible to demonstrate skin sensitivity to allergens by means of scratch tests or intracutaneous tests. Occasionally foods may be incriminated as allergens, and the condition may resolve entirely when these foods are eliminated from the diet. Histamine appears to play no role in eczema, and antihistamines have no effect on this condition. However, most patients with this condition develop other stigmata of an atopic diathesis sooner or later, and eosinophilia is almost a constant feature of this disease.

Therapeutic Principles in Managing Atopic Diseases

Immunologic Desensitisation

Allergic patients may be desensitised to an offending allergen by repeated injections of it. Initially, extremely minute amounts are given to minimise the risk of anaphylaxis. The dose is gradually increased, and a course of injections usually extends over a period of months. Such treatment is usually effective, if the antigens are, in fact, the ones responsible for the allergic manifestations. However, appropriate selection of antigens for this type of treatment is difficult, for it requires a knowledge of local atmospheric conditions, assessment of skin tests and evaluation of the patient's history. Furthermore, injection of the extracts may be dangerous, since it can precipitate rapid untoward systemic reactions. Thus, immunologic desensitisation therapy is best initiated under the direction of an adequately-trained allergist; it can not be considered a part of routine general practise.

The desensitisation process is believed to stimulate the production of IgG antibodies to the antigen. These antibodies will be available subsequently to react with the antigen before it is bound by reaginic antibodies of the IgE class. Because these IgG antibodies "block" the action of reagins they have been called "blocking antibodies". The IgE may be blocked - not only because the therapeutically-induced antibodies are present in greater abundance - but also because the IgG has a greater affinity (avidity) for the sensitising antigen. Thus, serum IgE levels usually fall over the course of time as a result of desensitisation therapy, probably because the stimulus to continued production of IgE antibodies is removed before it can act.

Antihistamine Therapy

As expected, antihistaminic drugs are effective agents in the treatment of histamine-mediated allergic states. Indeed, antihistamines are the mainstay of treatment for allergic rhinitis and urticaria. Because mediators other than histamine are important in asthma and atopic eczema, however, antihistamines are usually totally ineffective in these conditions. All of these drugs act as competitive inhibitors of histamine for receptor sites within the shock organs (*e.g.*, the nasal vasculature). There are no particular advantages or disadvantages to one antihistamine over another; all have similar side-effects (*e.g.*, drowsiness) in therapeutic doses. These drugs are best administered orally under most circumstances. Examples including chlorpheniramine (Chlor-Trimeton , Chlor-Tripolon), brompheniramine (Dimetane), triprolidine (Actidil), tripelennamine (Pyrabenzamine), diphenhydramine (Benadryl), etc.

Topical and Systemic Vasoconstrictors

Both topical and systemic α-adrenergic agents are employed in the treatment of atopic rhinitis to constrict the widely-dilated sub-mucosal blood vessels, and thus physiologically reverse the action of histamine and other vasoactive mediators on the vasculature of the nose, following their local release in nasal mucosa.

The systemic decongestants, thus, all raise systemic blood pressure, since their vasoconstricting action is not specific for nasal mucosal vasculature. For this reason, systemic agents of this type are contraindicated in hypertensive patients.

Topical vasoconstrictors, however, instilled intranasally (as nose drops) are highly effective in shrinking the nasal mucosa without appreciable systemic absorption; they may be employed therefore in hypertensive patients to relieve symptoms of rhinitis without deleterious effects on hypertension.

Topical vasoconstrictors have two adverse effects worth considering; firstly, all are potentially habituating to some degree, and patients using them for chronic problems thus tend to develop a dependency on them; secondly, nearly all such drugs are capable of producing a rebound phenomenon, wherein initial vasoconstriction is followed by delayed vasodilation, resulting ultimately in a similar mucosal swelling to that for which the drug was administered. Commonly employed topical vasoconstrictors include xylometazoline (Otrivin®), naphazoline (Privine®), phenylephrine (Neo-Synephrine®), and 1% ephedrine solution. Commonly employed systemic vasoconstrictors include phenylephrine (Neo-Synephrine®), pseudoephedrine (Sudafed®), and phenylpropanolamine. Many proprietary formulae are available wherein a systemic, vasoconstrictor is combined in fixed - ratio with an antihistamine, *e.g.*, Actifed®, Triaminic®, Dimetapp®, Novahistine®, etc. There is no particular advantage to any of these fixed-ratio mixtures.

Bronchodilators in Asthma

For many years, systemic (both oral and parenteral) and inhalant bronchodilators have been the mainstay of therapy for the acute asthmatic attack. In general, two types of agents have been employed as bronchodilators:

(1) *Methylated xanthines (e.g.*, theophylline and aminophylline) may be employed in acute asthma for re-

Fig. I

THE PHARMACODYNAMICS OF ATOPIC ASTHMA

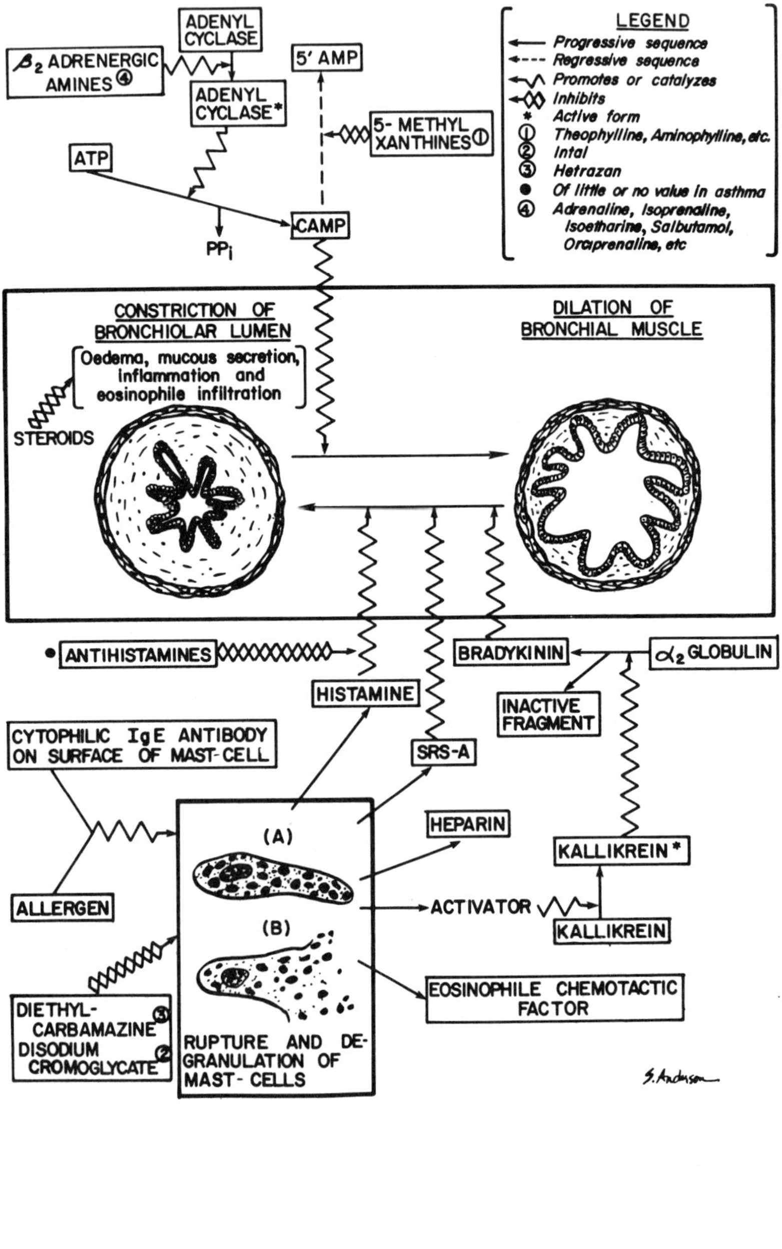

lief of bronchospasm. This class of agents acts by inhibiting reversibly the enzyme phosphodiesterase in smooth muscle fibres. Phosphodiesterase splits 3', 5' cyclic adenosine monophosphate (cAMP) to 5' adenosine monophosphate (AMP). cAMP is an intracellular mediator of physiologic relaxation of the smooth muscle fibres of the bronchi, whilst AMP is inactive in this regard. Thus, by inhibiting the degradation of cAMP, physiologic relaxation of the muscle, with consequent dilation of the lumen is sustained by this type of drug (*vide supra*, Figure 1). Methylxanthines are frequently employed in oral anti-asthmatic formulae in fixed ratio with a β-adrenergic amine (*vide infra*). The two classes of agents employed together act synergistically for reasons that will become clear. Therapeutic doses of methylxanthines alone are therefore necessarily higher than when the two types of drugs are used together. Therapeutic doses of these methylxanthine compounds are often poorly tolerated by the oral route because they are quite irritating to the gastric mucosa. However, aminophylline administered by I.V. route, and in adequate doses by slow injection is highly effective in aborting acute asthmatic attacks. Aminophylline is also available as rectal suppositories, but these are frequently unsatisfactory because of their tendency to produce irritative proctitis and also because they are often absorbed inadequately through the rectal mucosa.

(2) Let us turn, then, to the second class of bronchodilator drugs employed in treating asthmatics - *i.e.*, the β-adrenergic amines. These are the drugs most commonly employed for relief of acute bronchospasm. They act in the following manner:

Bronchial smooth muscle fibres have adrenergic receptors on their surface membranes. These receptors are of the β-type, and can be further subclassified as β_2-receptors, since agents have been synthesised which can differentiate between the β-receptors of the heart (β_1-receptors) and the β-receptors of the bronchial musculature (β_2-receptors). Attachment of a β-adrenergic amine to the membrane receptor of the muscle activates the enzyme adenyl cyclase (*vide supra*, Figure 1), which catalyses the hydrolysis of ATP to cAMP. As we have just seen, cAMP is an intracellular mediator of bronchial muscle relaxation; thus, these drugs induce bronchodilation. Since these drugs initiate formation of cAMP and the methylxanthines inhibit its degradation, the reason for the observed synergism of these two classes of drugs becomes readily apparent - the combination favours the development of high concentrations of mediator (cAMP) intracellularly.

Let us then consider the various types of β-adrenergic agents useful as bronchodilators in the clinic.

(a) *Ephedrine:* This agent has both α- and β-adrenergic activity, but is nonetheless useful in the treatment of asthma. It is administered orally, where it requires about 20 minutes to exert a therapeutic effect. The drug is occasionally administered by itself, but more commonly in combination with a methylxanthine and a barbiturate - the latter being employed as a sedative to counteract the CNS and cardiovascular stimulant effects of ephedrine. Tedral and Amesec are examples of fixed-ratio combinations frequently encountered in clinical practise.

(b) *Epinephrine (Adrenaline):* This drug is commonly employed as subcutaneous injections (in dilution of 1:1000) for relief of acute asthma. When used in this manner, a relative risk of life-threatening cardiac arrythmias must always be borne in mind. Moreover, the therapeutic and toxic doses of adrenaline are dangerously close to each other when administered by injection. If possible, therefore, this route is best avoided except in acute emergencies. Although ineffective when administered orally, adrenaline can be administered by inhalation, where it usually effects immediate relief of acute bronchospasm. If used repeatedly over a short time, however, it loses its effect rapidly - and this must always be kept in mind. Since adrenaline inhalers can be purchased over the counter in the United States and Canada, patients frequently overmedicate themselves with these, and become refractory to further treatment (*i.e.,* "adrenaline-fast"). When such patients present themselves in acute distress, the physicians must attempt to elicit a history of self-medication by inhaler. If the patient denies use of an inhaler, a small dose of adrenaline may be injected subcutaneously and the effect observed. If no effect is evident, it is generally better to employ another drug, such as aminophylline.

(c) *Other β-adrenergic amines:* Isoprenaline or isoproterenol (Isuprel , Medihaler-Iso® and others) is a more selective β-adrenergic agent than is adrenaline. However, it is not selective for β_1 receptors of the heart or for β_2 receptors of the bronchus - it stimulates both subclasses of β-receptors equally. Because of this, the drug is very liable to induce cardiac tachyarrhythmias on repeated use - even when administered as an aerosol for direct inhalation. This liability is further increased by its brief duration of action, which causes many patients to repeat the drug more frequently than recommended. Moreover, the β-receptors in the bronchus become "isoprenaline-fast" on repeated use, and prodigious doses of the drug are consumed without giving relief. High doses of the drug, particularly in a hypercapnic hypoxaemic patient renders the heart particularly susceptible to dangerous tachyarrhythmias such as ventricular tachycardia and ventricular fibrillation. A large number of documented fatalities by this mechanism consequent to isoprenaline abuse have occurred during the past two decades.

Another β-adrenergic amine which acts on both cardiac and bronchial β-receptors is a newer agent called **orciprenaline** or **metaproterenol** (Alupent®). This drug has one advantage over isoprenaline in that it has a much longer duration of action on bronchial musculature, and thus has slightly less **potential** for patient abuse. Nonetheless, it can be overused, and, if it is, is capable of inducing dangerous **tachyarrhythmias** as well.

At least two adrenergic amines have been developed which have some selectivity for the β_2-receptors of the bronchi. Thus, these agents are far less likely to initiate **tachyarrhythmias** in effective bronchodilatory doses than are the less selective agents mentioned above. These β_2 agents are isoetharine (Bronkometer®) and salbutamol (Ventolin®). Isoetharine is a short-acting drug (like isoprenaline), and therefore has a relatively high potential for abuse when self-administered. Its selectivity, moreover, is only relative - and some β_1 stimulation does occur, especially when the drug is administered repeatedly over a short time. Thus, **tachyarrhythmias** can occur with isoetharine, although the frequency is less than with isoprenaline. Salbutamol, on the other hand, is almost entirely devoid of β_1 activity in therapeutic doses, and, moreover is long-acting, and therefore less subject to patient abuse during self-administration. Salbutamol thus appears to be one of the safest and best bronchodilators yet developed with the least potential for initiating cardiac tachyarrhythmias. (Salbutamol not yet released by USFDA.)

The most common form of administration of all these β-adrenergic amines mentioned is as aerosol nebulisers for direct inhalation.

Adrenal Corticosteroids in Asthma

In asthma, corticosteroid therapy is often highly effective, though not curative. Possible benefits of such therapy must always be weighed against the real dangers of toxicity from prolonged use of these potent anti-inflammatory agents. Therefore, these drugs are usually reserved for the treatment of patients refractory to all other forms of therapy, and in whom the disability is severe, or for patients with acute severe manifestations, like status asthmaticus, where corticosteroids may be employed to terminate a single severe attack, after which they are immediately withdrawn. None of the many steroid preparations available have any advantages over prednisone for oral use and prednisolone for I.V. use.*

Disodium Cromoglycate or Cromolyn Sodium (Intal®, Aarane)

Disodium cromoglycate represents a major advance in the prophylaxis and treatment of atopic asthma. This drug is a highly effective agent in preventing the occurrance of asthmatic attacks. It is administered by inhalation of the dry powder through a rather ingenious inhaler called a Spinhaler®.

Cromolyn acts to stabilise the membranes of reagin-sensitised mast-cells and leucocytes, thus preventing the rupture of these cells with consequent release of mediator substances upon contact with allergen (*vide supra*, Figure 1).

Although by itself of little use in the acute attack, therapy can be initiated with Intal®and bronchodilators, which may both terminate the acute attack and prevent recurrence of symptoms following its termination. Intal® exerts a powerful prophylactic effect, which frequently allows severe, otherwise intractable asthmatics, formerly requiring long-term maintenance on corticosteroids, to be withdrawn from these agents. It thus is said to have a "steroid sparing effect"; yet available data indicate that unlike steroids, it has virtually no intrinsic toxic properties when used in the recommended therapeutic dose range.†

Diethylcarbamazine (Hetrazan®)

Diethylcarbamazine is an anthelminthic that has long been in use in the treatment of filarial infections. Recently, it was noted that when administered to asthmatic subjects, it reduced the frequency and severity of attacks. Its mode of action is essentially identical to that of disodium cromoglycate - it stabilises mast-cell membranes and prevents the rupture and degranulation of these cells on contact with allergen. However, it differs from cromolyn in that it is much more toxic; therefore, it has little if any clinical use in the routine treatment of asthma (*vide supra*, Figure 1).

* *In addition to their use in asthma, adrenal corticosteroids are often of great value applied topically in the treatment of chronic atopic eczema.*

† *Recently, this drug has been released for intranasal inhalation in the U.K., under the proprietary name of Rynacrom for the prophylaxis of allergic rhinitis in atopic individuals prone to this condition and (unavoidably) exposed to allergens.*

Chapter 12

CLINICAL ASSOCIATIONS OF DELAYED HYPERSENSITIVITY

Cell-mediated immune reactions have been considered in some detail in Chapter 3. The purpose of the present chapter is to emphasise the clinical importance of cell-mediated responses, rather than their underlying mechanisms, with which familiarity is assumed.

Diagnostic Skin Tests

Because of the frequency of cell-mediated hypersensitivity reactions to infecting organisms, and because of the exquisite specificity of these reactions, these hypersensitivity reactions have been employed frequently as aids to specific diagnosis. In many cases, clinical appearance, definitive history, and positive skin test may be sufficient to establish the aetiology of a patient's illness, but one must always be wary of any diagnosis based on the results of a skin test alone.

The tuberculin reaction, representing by far the commonest diagnostic skin test employed today in North America or Europe, has already been discussed in some detail (*vide supra*, Chapter 3). Many adaptations of this test have been developed, but the Mantoux test (*i.e.*, intradermal injection of PPD into the volar surface of the forearm) is still most widely used. The reaction is read at 48 hours, at which time an area of induration >0.5 cm. in diameter is considered positive.

Similar tests are employed for many other parasitic organisms; a partial list of which is presented in Table 1.

As is obvious from Table 1, many different types of organisms elicit cell-mediated hypersensitivity reactions.

Amongst the bacteria, delayed hypersensitivity reactions accompany infections with *Streptococcus sp.*, *Staphylococcus aureus*, *Diplococcus pneumoniae*, *Salmonella typhosa*, *Brucella sp.*, *Haemophilus ducreyi*, *Bordetella pertussis*, *Pasteurella tularense*, *Mycobacterium sp.*, and many others.

Cellular hypersensitivity is likewise characteristic of *Chlamydia (Bedsonia)* infections, occurring regularly in *lymphogranuloma venereum, psittacosis, trachoma*, and *inclusion conjunctivitis*.

Table 1

Some Examples of Diagnostic Tests Involving Cellular Immunity

Name of Test	Disease Tested for	Test Material
Lepromin Test	Leprosy	Cell-free extract of skin from patient with leprosy
Brucellergen Test	Brucellosis	Nucleoprotein extract of *Brucella sp.*
Histoplasmin Test	Histoplasmosis	Culture filtrate of *Histoplasma capsulatum*
Coccidioidin Test	Coccidioidomycosis	Culture filtrate of *Coccidioides immitis*
Casoni Test	Hydatid Disease	Cyst fluid from *Echinococcus granulosus*
Frei Test	Lymphogranuloma Venereum	Yolk-sac extract from egg on which LGV-agent has been grown

Viruses also characteristically induce delayed hypersensitivity. Such reactions accompany infections by *measles, mumps, influenza, herpes simplex, vaccinia, variola*, and other viruses.

Mycotic infections likewise elicit cell-mediated sensitivity reactions. Examples: *Coccidioides immitis, Blastomyces sp., Aspergillusniger, the dermatophytes, Histoplasma capsulatum, Candida (Monilia) albicans, Cryptococcus neoformans*, and others.

Protozoal infections, *e.g., Leishmaniasis*, can elicit delayed hypersensitivity, particularly where the parasite occurs intracellularly.

A metazoan infestation, *i.e.*, hydatid disease, is almost invariably accompanied by delayed hypersensitivity to cyst fluid from *Echinococcus granulosus*, the aetiological agent of this disease. Other helminthic infections have been said to elicit delayed reactions, but atopic sensitivity usually dominates the clinical picture.

Finally, delayed hypersensitivity to insect bites has been frequently described, but is of lesser importance than atopic hypersensitivity to insect bites, which, when severe, may represent a real medical emergency leading to rapid death from anaphylactic shock.

Delayed Hypersensitivity as a Cause of Pathological Lesions

Many parasitic organisms, of which the tubercle bacillus is an excellent example, are not directly toxic to cells or tissues of the body. However, these organisms actively provoke cell-mediated hypersensitivity reactions, which may result ultimately in a great deal of tissue damage or necrosis. Thus, an agent of this type may do little or no damage when introduced into the non-sensitised body for the first time. Histological sections through infected tissues may reveal the presence of the infectious agent, but usually also reveal adjacent host tissues and cells to be undamaged; *i.e.*, host and parasite appear to coexist in an atmosphere of relative symbiosis with each other.

However, over the course of time, the situation begins to change as the host develops cell-mediated hypersensitivity to antigens of the parasite. Inflammatory reactions develop around the parasites, in which macrophages and lymphocytes are seen to occur prominently. These reactions are consequences of developing cellular hypersensitivity to antigens of the parasites, and usually serve to assist the host in limiting, and ultimately destroying the infection. In part, these reactions tend to alter the balance between host and parasite in favour of the host by concentrating phagocytic cells and cytotoxic factors at the site of infection.

Nevertheless, under certain circumstances, the inflammatory reactions following the development of cellular hypersensitivity may result in harmful, rather than beneficial effects to the host. For example, delayed hypersensitivity to *M. tuberculosis* contributes to the tissue necrosis resulting in pulmonary cavitation. (*Vide supra*, Chapter 3).

Contact Dermatitis (Dermatitis Venenata)

Dermatitis venenata, an acute or chronic skin lesion following direct contact of skin with chemical substances, may occur in two ways.

Firstly, the chemical substance may have direct irritant properties; in such instances, immunological phenomena are not involved.

Alternatively, the chemical substance may be non-irritating *per se*, but may act as an antigen or hapten and provoke cell-mediated hypersensitivity reactions on prolonged or repeated contact with the skin. Such cases are examples of true immunological reactions, and the resultant contact sensitivity shows exceedingly fine immunological specificity for the sensitising antigen or hapten.

Many non-irritating chemical agents can serve as contact allergens. The pathogenesis of the contact dermatitis following exposure to these agents frequently depends on attachment of the chemical to structural proteins of skin, whereupon the chemical functions as a hapten and leads to alteration results in stimulation of the T-cell division of the lymphoid system and the development of a lymphocyte population which has become sensitised to the hapten. An inflammatory reaction thus ensues, the stigmata of which may include pruritis, burning or stinging sensation, erythematous macules, papules, vesicles, exudation and crusting.

Some examples of common contact allergens follow:

(a) Nickel is a contact allergen responsible for a great number of cases of industrially-acquired contact dermatitis.

(b) The *Rhus* antigen is a simple phenolic compound which acts as a powerful hapten. It occurs in plants of the genus *Rhus*, including poison ivy, poison oak, and poison sumac.

(c) Picroyl Chloride and Dinitrochlorobenzene (DNCB) are examples of simple organic chemicals which are able to serve as powerful haptens in both humans and experimental animals, and have been employed frequently in laboratory studies of cellular hypersensitivity.

(d) Various dermatological medicaments, applied topically, can elicit contact dermatitis (*Dermatitis Medicamentosa*); amongst the most common of these are antihistamines, local anaesthetics, and topical antimicrobial agents.

Allograft Rejection - The principal mechanism by which tissues transplanted into immunologically-competent recipients are rejected is by cell-mediated immune reactions. This is covered in some detail with the discussion of transplantation (*vide infra*, Chapter 17) and is mentioned here merely for the sake of completeness. This clinical association of cellular immunity is assuming far greater importance than it has in the past because of the rapidly expanding frontiers of surgical technology. It is perhaps unfortunate at this moment that surgical techniques are far advanced over clinically-available means of immuno-suppression, since it is ultimately the failure to inhibit effectively the cell-mediated immune response to transplanted tissue or to develop a practical means of initiating and maintaining a state of specific tolerance to transplantation antigens that has led to the failure of many organ transplantation programmes throughout the world.

Chapter 13

NATURE'S EXPERIMENTS IN IMMUNITY: IMMUNE DEFICIENCY DISEASES OF MAN

It was noted in Chapter 2 (*vide supra*) that our present concepts of the organisation of the lymphoid system were derived from combined studies of clinical diseases and laboratory experimentation. Careful study of human diseases as "Nature's Experiments" provides a most valuable tool for understanding basic biological mechanisms; disordered function (pathophysiology) provides the key for understanding normal physiology.

Although successful studies of this type can be illustrated from many branches of medical and scientific endeavour, nowhere has this aphorism proven more true than in the study of immunologic diseases in man.

Not only has this approach provided the concept of semi-autonomous B-cell and T-cell divisions of the human lymphoid system, but it has also indicated the adaptive values of different types of immune responses. For example, patients with immune deficiency diseases may be subject to repeated infections, and the type of infections occurring in patients with particular deficiencies will reflect the adaptive functions of that part of the immune system which is deficient or absent. Thus, a patient with Bruton's Agammaglobulinaemia will often present clinically with recurrent infections caused by extracellular pyogenic bacteria, whilst a patient with Di George's Syndrome will present clinically with repeated viral, mycotic, or *Pneumocystis carinii* infections (in addition to the anatomical and endocrinological anomalies accompanying failure of the IIIrd and IVth pharyngeal pouches to develop).

The following discussion will attempt to consider some of the more important immune deficiency diseases of man, to illustrate how they have influenced our current concepts of immunobiology, and to discuss the recent concept of immunologic reconstitution (*i.e.*, correction of immunologic defects by tissue grafts of immunologically-competent lymphoid tissue from other individuals).

Bruton's Agammaglobulinaemia

In 1952, Col. Ogden Bruton described an 8-year-old boy under treatment at the Walter Reed Army Hospital in Washington, D. C., for severe,recurrent, life-threatening, pyogenic bacterial infections. In the course of investigating this child, serum electrophoresis was performed, revealing an absence of detectable gamma globulins. Human gamma globulin was administered to the patient in attempt to ameliorate his infections, which responded dramatically to this treatment. This patient has subsequently received large doses of gamma globulin at 2-3 week intervals, and consequently, has grown normally, remained well, and has been able to lead a normal life, provided that the injections are continued regularly.

It is a matter of conjecture at present whether the patient originally described by Bruton, and referred to above, suffers from an acquired form of agammaglobulinaemia or from the congenital sex-linked recessive disease now known as Bruton's Agammaglobulinaemia.

Bruton's Agammaglobulinaemia is a congenital sex-linked disease that becomes manifest in infancy, usually as a virtually endless succession of infections caused by extracellular pyogenic bacteria - such as *Pneumococcus, Streptococcus, Haemophilus, Staphylococcus, Pseudomonas, Meningococcus* or *Coliforms* - beginning about the sixth month of age. The serum of patients with this disease contains virtually no immunoglobulins of any class. These patients are unable entirely to respond to bacterial or viral infection (or other antigenic stimulation) with the synthesis of humoral antibody, but in striking contrast to this deficit, develop normal cellular immunity as evidenced by delayed hypersensitivity and allograft rejection (*vide supra et infra,* Chapters 3, 12, 17).

If one examines lymphoid tissue from these patients histologically, an absence of germinal follicles in lymph-nodes and spleen, and an absence of plasma-cells in bone-marrow, connective tissue, lymph-nodes, and spleen will be noted. Tonsils and Peyer's Patches may be totally absent or hypoplastic and devoid of follicular architecture. Circulating lymphocytes, in contrast, are present in normal or near-normal numbers, as are the lymphocytes of the thymus and the thymus-dependent regions of the lymph-nodes and spleen.

Although these patients resist pyogenic bacterial infections poorly, they recover well from most viral infections and resist reinfection by the same viruses normally. Moreover, the immunity to viral infections developed by these patients appears to be long-lasting, although little or no antibody to viral antigens is demonstrable. A notable exception to this rule, however, is the virus of *infectious hepatitis;* infection by this agent usually leads to *acute fulminant hepatitis* or to *chronic active hepatitis* progressing to total destruction of the liver and death of the patient from liver failure.

Resistance to tuberculosis, mycotic infections, and certain other pathogens appears to be normal, reflecting the fact that resistance to these agents is primarily cell-mediated and thymus dependent.

Patients with this disease inexplicably are very prone to develop *arthritis*, *vasculitis*, *dermatomyositis*, and other mesenchymal diseases. These patients also have a high incidence of neoplasms, especially malignant lymphomas and gastrointestinal tumours.

Chronic administration of gamma globulin whilst greatly ameliorating the severity of this disease, does not control it completely. Thus, these patients are prone to develop persistent respiratory tract diseases (such as *bronchiectasis*, *chronic bronchitis*, and *pulmonary fibrosis*) which may proceed ultimately to respiratory failure and death. Good and his colleagues feel that the respiratory sequelae of Bruton's Agammaglobulinaemia result from absence of local IgA and IgE production in these patients (*vide supra*, Chapter 5).

As noted in Chapter 2 (*vide supra*), Bruton's Agammaglobulinaemia shares many features with an experimental disease of birds produced by neonatal extirpation of the bursa of Fabricius. Both diseases represent selective deficits of the B-cell division of the lymphoid system, with normal or near-normal function of the T-cell division. Thus, humoral immunity cannot be expressed, whilst cellular immunity remains virtually unimpaired.

Class-Specific Dysgammaglobulinaemias

These are isolated deficiencies of certain classes of immunoglobulins, in which the remaining immunoglobulin classes are represented in normal or increased amounts. For example:

An isolated deficiency of IgA has been described repeatedly in the medical literature. This is a relatively common condition, occurring in more than 1 in 1,000 persons. In many of these, it is an "orphan dyscrasia"; the patient is clinically-well and apparently suffers no ill effects from the absence of IgA. However, many such patients suffer from recurrent gastrointestinal infections and a sprue-like syndrome. Recurrent respiratory infections in these patients are unusual, unless other immunological defects are also present. Some of these patients suffer from mesenchymal diseases like *rheumatoid arthritis*, *disseminated lupus erythematosus (DLE)*, and *tenosynovitis*, but the relationship of these diseases to the deficiency of IgA is not understood.

Fig. 1 ELECTROPHEROGRAM OF PATIENT WITH AGAMMAGLOBULINAEMIA

NORMAL HUMAN
ELECTROPHEROGRAM

+ 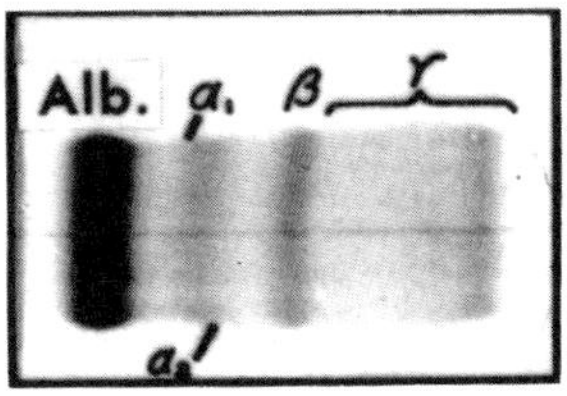

−

IgG = 1000 mg% (700-1500)
IgA = 300 mg% (125-425)
IgM = 125 mg% (50-150)

AGAMMAGLOBULINAEMIA

+ 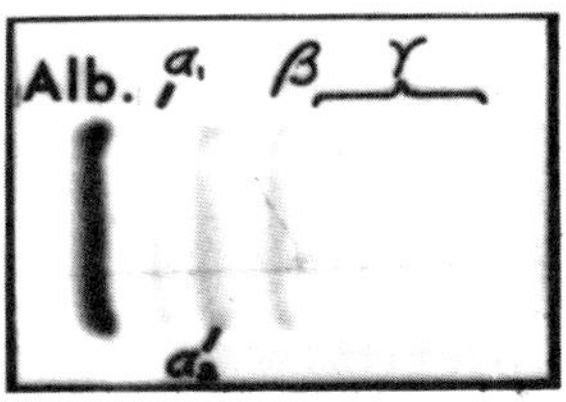

−

IgG<50 mg%
IgA Not detectable
IgM Not detectable

Current constant at 2 mA/strip
Voltage ~ 80 V.
Time = 30-40 min.
Buffer = TRIS-BARBITAL, pH = 8.8, μ = 0.05
Stained with Ponceau-S

Courtesy of Dr. John Griffiths
Mrs. J. Kozier and Miss A. Kyriakidis
Dep't. of Clinical Chemistry, Vancouver General Hospital

Two patients have been described recently with isolated deficiencies of IgE and histories of recurrent sino-pulmonary infections, as was noted in Chapter 5 (*vide supra*).

A number of patients have been described with a combined deficiency of IgA and IgE. These patients tend to suffer from recurrent sino-pulmonary infections, which resemble those seen in both patients with isolated IgE deficiencies.

Late-Occurring (Acquired) Dysgammaglobulinaemias

A poorly-understood group of immunologic deficiency diseases has been described wherein a secondary loss of immunoglobulins may occur at ages ranging from 2 to 80 years. Generally, such patients have more IgG than is seen in Bruton's syndrome, and, usually, such patients also demonstrate variable deficits in cellular immunity as well as amongst the different immunoglobulin classes. The patterns of immunoglobulin deficiency are not constant; thus Janeway et al. have classified the dysgammaglobulinaemias into a number of sub-types, according to the pattern of immunoglobulin deficits present in a given patient. The usefulness of this sub-classification may thus reasonably be queried.

All of these patients have sufficient IgG to permit isolation and characterisation. Interestingly enough, the electrophoretic mobility of the IgG from patients with acquired dysgammaglobulinaemias is restricted, appearing similar to a monoclonal immunoglobulin in its narrow electrophoretic banding. Furthermore, aggregate IgG from these patients may exhibit impaired complement fixation.

These patients usually exhibit impaired allograft rejection, impaired development of delayed hypersensitivity, and impaired resistance to viral infections. They also exhibit a high coincidence of lymphomas and mesenchymal diseases, especially rheumatoid arthritis. Many patients with acquired dysgammaglobulinaemia exhibit lymphadenopathy, tonsillar hyperplasia, splenomegaly, and, at necropsy, enlarged Peyer's patches. Lymphoid tissue may exhibit either aplastic or extremely hyperplastic germinal follicles, in the latter case often accompanied by a paucity of plasma-cells.

Dysgammaglobulinaemic patients are at high risk to both Coombs' positive and Coombs' negative haemolytic anaemias, and to pernicious anaemia. They are also at high risk to develop amyloidosis. In spite of regular gamma globulin replacement therapy, these patients often succumb eventually to sino-pulmonary infections or to lymphomas.

Transient Hypogammaglobulinaemia of Infancy

A self-limited deficit in circulating immunoglobulins may appear between the 6th and 18th month of age in infants. This condition is often nearly indistinguishable from Bruton's Agammaglobulinaemia, except in that it occurs in infants of both sexes and in that it is self-limited and resolves spontaneously. It appears to result from delayed maturation of the lymphoid system, and, although the immunoglobulin levels usually return to near-normal or normal in these patients, their response to infections following the return of circulating immunoglobulins is not always completely normal. Nonetheless, the degree of spontaneous improvement is always remarkable in these infants.

Lymphopenic Agammaglobulinaemia (Swiss-Type Immune Deficiency Syndrome, Glanzman-Riniker Syndrome)

This is a familiar disease, first described in Switzerland, and transmitted by an autosomal recessive gene. It usually becomes manifest during the first weeks of life in affected (homozygous) infants; however, the mothers and fathers carrying the heterozygous trait are phenotypically normal.

Homozygous infants are unable to express either cellular or humoral immunity; both the T-cell division and the B-cell division of the lymphoid system fail to develop normally. Since development of both systems is impaired, the defect lies either in an absent or defective common lymphoid precursor cell ("stem-cell") or in an absent or defective common maturational factor (*e.g.*, an endocrine factor) upon which the development of both B-cells and T-cells depend.

Severe lymphocytopenia occurs in this disease, accompanied by a gross deficiency of lymphocytes and plasmacytes in bone marrow, lymph-nodes, spleen, connective tissue, and the lamina propria of the G-I tract, an absence of germinal follicles in all lymphoid tissues, and an abnormally-developed, hypoplastic thymus, lacking Hassall's corpuscles, and composed predominantly of reticular epithelial spindle cells.

Lymphopenic agammaglobulinaemia is incompatible with survival; homozygous infants usually die during the first year of life, often from infections with organisms of relatively low virulence.

Since these infants are immunologically incompetent, they are unable to reject allografts (*vide infra*, Chapter 17). Indeed, even blood transfusions may be lethal to these infants, because immunologically-competent donor lymphocytes transfused into these recipients may initiate a fatal systemic graft-vs.-host reaction (*vide infra*, Chapter 17).

Thymic Alymphoplasia

Thymic alymphoplasia is a sex-linked condition, characterised by gross deficits in cellular and humoral immunity. It is similar to, though less severe than (Swiss-type) lymphopenic agammaglobulinaemia (*vide supra*). The thymus is usually hypoplastic, but not atrophic. These children usually present in infancy with severe recurrent infections. Persistent oral *Candidiasis* ("thrush"), *Hecht's giant-cell pneumonia* (on contact with measles virus), *progressive vaccinia* and *vaccinia gangrenosa* (if these patients are vaccinated), *Pneumocystis carinii* infections, or miliary tuberculosis following BCG-vaccination (*"BCG-osis"*) are examples of the various types of grief to which these patients may come as a result of their immunologic incompetence.

These patients exhibit severe lymphopenia, variable deficits (usually severe) in the immunoglobulins, absence of α and β isohaemagglutinins (*vide infra*, Chapter 16), failure to respond to antigens with synthesis of specific antibodies, inability or severely impaired ability to reject skin allografts, and absence of a prominent thymic shadow in A/P radiographs of the chest. As with infants suffering from (Swiss-type) lymphopenic agammaglobulinaemia, blood transfusions may be lethal to patients with thymic alymphoplasia, by virtue of the tendency to result in systemic graft - vs. - host reactions.

Thymic alymphoplasia may result either from a quantitative defect in lymphoid stem-cell maturation, or an abnormal maturation factor, which affects both B-cell division and T-cell division development. Similar to lymphopenic agammaglobulinaemia, this disease is incompatible with survival. Patients usually die within the first two years of life - occasionally surviving to the sixth year before they succumb to viral or fungal infections.

Treatment with gamma globulin and antibiotics, whilst alleviating, somewhat, certain bacterial infections, have not proven adequate to maintain these patients for any length of time.

However, the recent concept of immunologic reconstitution (*i.e.*, grafting immunologically-competent cells antigenically similar to the recipient's cells) appears to enable correction of immunologic deficits in patients with thymic alymphoplasia, with resultant conversion of these patients to a state of immunologic competence, and without inducing fatal graft - vs. - host reactions. Dr. Robert A. Good and his colleagues in

Minneapolis recently transplanted bone marrow and peripheral blood leucocytes successfully from a female sibling donor matched with the patient at the HL-A locus (*vide infra*, Chapter 17). Dramatic conversion of the patient to a state of immunologic competence, with only a transient graft - vs. - host reaction resulted. The child with thymic alymphoplasia who received the graft was thereby rendered "chimaeric" - *i.e.*, bone marrow cells from the donor sister completely replaced the recipient's own bone marrow cells, and the boy assumed his sister's ABO blood type and XX karyo-type in all bone marrow cells*. Although it is still too early to say what the eventual outcome will be, the recipient was thriving, and appeared to be totally normal immunologically nearly twelve months after his blood picture had stabilised following the series of bone marrow and leucocyte grafts.

Di George's Syndrome: Agenesis of the IIIrd and IVth Pharyngeal Pouches

As noted in Chapter 2 (*vide supra*), Di George's syndrome represents an isolated total deficiency of the T-cell division of the lymphoid system, with nearly normal development of the B-cell division. In this condition, the IIIrd and IVth pharyngeal pouches fail to develop in the embryo. These pouches represent the epithelial anlagen from which the thymus, parathyroid glands, and "C"-cells of the thyroid gland develop; consequently, all three tissues are congenitally absent from affected infants. These infants present at birth with neonatal tetany, consequent to hypocalcaemia. Even when the calcium balance is corrected, however, these infants do not survive because of their inability to express cell-mediated immune reactions, which require the presence of the thymus for development. Since these patients lack T-cells, they defend themselves poorly against mycotic, viral, and chronic bacterial infections, in spite of near normally-functioning B-cells and normal levels of circulating immunoglobulins. Normal complements of plasma-cells are present in connective tissue, bone marrow, spleen, and lymph-nodes of these patients, and germinal follicles are present in lymph-nodes and spleen. However, these patients exhibit a profound lymphopenia, and gross depletion of the thymus-dependent regions of the lymph-nodes and spleen.

Immunologic reconstitution of a patient with Di George's syndrome has recently been accomplished by Dr. William W. Cleveland *et al.* in Miami, Florida. This

* *The term "chimaera", derived from Greek mythology, originally connoted a monster with the head of a lion, the body of a goat, and the tail of a serpent. Immunologic chimaerism is a term used to express the concept of a composite individual, the parts of whose body are derived from genetically-different individuals.*

patient received a graft of foetal thymus, derived from an abortus of 13 weeks gestational age. The immaturity of the grafted thymus favoured the development of immunologic tolerance to the tissue antigens of the recipient, thereby preventing a graft - vs. - host reaction from occurring. Since the host could not express cell-mediated immune reactions prior to the thymus graft, he was unable to respond to the graft tissue antigens with an allograft rejection reaction (*vide infra*, Chapter 17).

The Wiskott-Aldrich Syndrome

The Wiskott-Aldrich Syndrome is a sex-linked recessive condition in which a defect in the processing of antigens by macrophages is present, affecting the expression of both cellular and humoral immune reactions by blockading both the T-cell and B-cell divisions of the lymphoid system at their afferent limbs (*vide supra*, Chapter 2). In this disease the deficits in both divisions are not absolute; patients suffering from the Wiskott-Aldrich syndrome respond almost normally to certain antigens (*e.g.*, tetanus toxoid) whilst failing to respond entirely to certain others (*e.g.*, polysaccharide antigens). Cellular immunity is usually present initially (though severely impaired), but the deficiency in this system tends to increase progressively.

The Wiskott-Aldrich syndrome usually presents in early infancy as *thrombocytopenic purpura, severe eczema,* and severe, recurrent episodes of infection caused by many different agents.

Patients with Wiskott-Aldrich disease have a normal thymus throughout the course of their illness. Their peripheral lymphoid tissues, initially normal in appearance, undergo a secondary depletion of lymphocytes within thymus-dependent regions, and a progressive lymphopenia in the peripheral blood. These changes accompany the progressively-increasing deficit in cellular immunity exhibited by these patients.

Although germinal follicles are present in the lymph-nodes and spleen of Wiskott-Aldrich patients throughout the course of their disease, these patients appear invariably to lack the normal ABO blood group isohaemagglutinins and haemolysins (*vide infra*, Chapter 16). As noted above, these patients are unable to respond to any polysaccharide antigens, whilst responses to protein antigens are varied, and, in the case of some antigens, virtually normal.

In the course of their disease, these patients develop *reticulum-cell sarcomas* and *lymphosarcomas* with high frequency; those patients who do not succumb to infective or haemorrhagic processes usually die from neoplastic disease in infancy, childhood, or early adolescence. No survivals to adulthood have been reported in Wiskott-Aldrich patients.

However, immunologic reconstitution of a boy with Wiskott-Aldrich disease has recently been accomplished by Dr. Fritz Bach at the University of Wisconsin. This child was given myelo-obliterative* doses of cyclophosphamide, following which, he received a bone marrow graft from a healthy female sibling, whose tissue antigens were closely matched to those of the patient at the major (HL-A) histocompatibility locus (*vide infra*, Chapter 17). This child, like the *thymic alymphoplasia* patient treated by Dr. Good (*vide supra*), became chimaeric in his marrow and blood cells. Coincident with the establishment of chimaerism, the patient developed normal serum titres of isohaemagglutinins and vastly improved his platelet count. This child has thrived following his bone marrow graft, and has reasonable prospects of being able to lead a normal life in the future.

Good's Syndrome: Benign Thymoma and Agammaglobulinaemia

In 1954, Dr. Robert A. Good described a syndrome in which a broad immunological deficiency accompanied a benign spindle-cell neoplasm of the thymus. These patients demonstrate hypogammaglobulinaemia, impaired cellular immunity, poor humoral responses to antigens, and a frequent absence of eosinophiles. They have a high coincidence of arthritis and other connective tissue diseases.

Although all classes of serum immunoglobulins are deficient in patients with Good's syndrome, they are usually higher than those of patients with *Bruton's Agammaglobulinaemia* or *lymphopenic agammaglobulinaemia*.

As the disease progresses, circulating blood lymphocytes fall to extremely low levels and the immunologic deficits encountered in this condition are uncorrected by excision of the thymoma.

Although the inter-relationships between the various features of this disease remain entirely enigmatic at present, this syndrome is of great historical interest; it initially served to focus attention on a possible role for the thymus in the development of immunological competence.

* *Massive doses, sufficient to destroy all of the patient's bone marrow cells.*

Ataxia-Telangiectasia

Ataxia-Telangiectasia is an hereditary disease, transmitted as an autosomal recessive trait, which consists of a triad of *progressive cerebellar ataxia, prominent arterial telangiectases* on the sclerae, eyelids, earlobes, neck and skin overlying the popliteal and antecubital fossae, and a broad immunological deficit. *Gonadal dysgenesis* and failure of sexual maturation may occur in those patients surviving beyond the first decade. These patients are also at high risk to malignant lymphoreticular neoplasms, including *lymphosarcoma, reticulum-cell sarcoma,* and *reticuloendotheliosis**.

The immunological deficits encountered in patients with ataxia-telangiectasia affect both the T-cell and B-cell divisions of the immune system.

Cellular immunity is profoundly impaired, and peripheral lymphopenia is common. The thymus of a patient with ataxia-telangiectasia is usually hypoplastic, and lacks Hassall's corpuscles. It appears to be poorly differentiated, resembling an embryonic thymus at the start of lymphoid differentiation. Lymph-nodes and spleen demonstrate a decreased complement of lymphocytes. Plasma-cells are present in these lymphoid organs, and the reticular stromal elements are usually prominent.

Humoral immunity is usually less profoundly affected than cellular immunity in ataxia-telangiectasia. Many of these patients respond almost normally to most strong antigens, but produce antibody poorly to many weaker antigens. Serum IgA is usually extremely low or absent in ataxia-telangiectasia, as is serum IgE. Coincident deficiency of both IgA and IgE is the most common pattern of humoral deficit encountered in this disease, and patients exhibiting this pattern usually suffer from repeated sino-pulmonary infections.

The underlying defect in ataxia-telangiectasia is as yet not understood. The peculiar constellation of signs and symptoms may be a reflexion of faulty mesenchymal development or a neuroendocrine disorder which affects lymphoid system differentiation, vascular proliferation, and neurological development.

* *"Reticuloendotheliosis" (or "Histiocytosis X") is a generic term including several clinical diseases, viz.: Hand-Schüller-Christian disease, eosinophilic granuloma, and Letterer-Siwe disease.*

Hereditary Angioneurotic Oedema

Hereditary Angioneurotic Oedema is a genetic disease, inherited as a Mendelian dominant trait, which appears to result from the absence of an inhibitor of the complement system. These patients lack C1 esterase inhibitor, and, in consequence of this, undergo spontaneous activation of the complement system, with resultant attacks of acute, circumscribed, non-inflammatory oedema, unassociated with specific allergic stimulation. Attacks are thus unpredictable, and may occur in the apparent absence of any precipitating factors, or accompanying minor trauma, infections, or menstruation. The condition may be life threatening if the oedema occurs in the glottis or larynx, because acute respiratory obstruction, with rapid death from asphyxia, may result. Treatment, though non-specific, must be decisive and rapid; subcutaneous injection of 0.8-1.0 ml. with adrenaline chloride (1:1000) and concomitant administration of an antihistamine and/or a corticosteroid will usually terminate an attack within minutes. In rare instances, emergency tracheostomy may be required to relieve total airway obstruction. Transfusion of fresh plasma, presumably as a source of C1 esterase inhibitor, will frequently terminate clinical crises.

Miscellaneous Diseases Accompanied by Secondary Immunological Deficits

(a) Hodgkin's Disease: Patients with Hodgkin's Disease frequently develop profound impairment of cellular immunity, whilst often maintaining normal antibody responses to most antigens. These patients may develop severe infections of the type associated with defective cellular immunity, such as *Cryptococcal meningitis*, other disseminated mycoses, severe *herpes zoster*, disseminated *herpes simplex*, *cytomegalic inclusion disease*, *Pneumocystis carinii* pneumonitis, and tuberculosis. Impaired cellular immunity develops early in the course of Hodgkin's Disease, and is usually more profound in patients with disseminated disease than in patients with local disease. Complete clinical remissions, induced by radiotherapy, are often associated with return of specific cellular responsiveness to normal.

(b) Chronic Lymphatic Leukaemia: Immunologic deficiencies in both T-cell and B-cell divisions of the lymphoid system are associated with chronic lymphatic leukaemia. Hypogammaglobulinaemia is a common feature of this disease, especially in the later stages, and the antibody response to many antigens is likely to be poor Rejections of skin allografts is usually slow in these patients, reflecting the impairment of the T-cell division of the immune system. Chronic lymphocytic leukaemia is generally considered a contraindication to smallpox vaccination because of the propensity of these patients to develop *progressive vaccinia* and *vaccinia gangrenosum*, stemming from their immunological deficiencies.

(c) Multiple Myeloma: Accompanying the monoclonal increase in immunoglobulin which is highly characteristic of this disease, is a severe quantitative deficiency in all classes of physiological immunoglobulins. These patients consequently have poor B-cell responses to most antigens, whilst maintaining normal T-cell function throughout most of the course of their disease. The immunological deficiencies encountered in multiple myeloma thus contrast clearly to those encountered in Hodgkin's Disease; the former impairs selectively the expression of humoral immunity, whilst the latter impairs selectively the expression of cellular immunity.

(d) Sarcoidosis: Sarcoidosis is a chronic, granulomatous, systemic, inflammatory disease of unknown aetiology. It is characterised by proliferative, non-caseating tubercles, most commonly encountered in liver, lungs, skin, the uveal tract of the eye, and the reticuloendothelial system, but occurring sporadically in any organ of the body. It occurs most commonly in young adults, but cases have been reported in every age group. Although the clinical features of this disease are highly variable, most individuals present with mild constitutional symptoms, and the disease follows a rather benign course.

Polyclonal hypergammaglobulinaemia is present in most patients with sarcoidosis, and rheumatoid factor tests (*vide supra et infra*, Chapters 6 and 19) are commonly positive as well. Serologic tests for syphilis also may be falsely positive in this disease.

Generally, the B-cells function normally in response to specific antigenic stimulation in patients with sarcoidosis, but a large number of patients with this disease have impaired T-cell function, as evidenced by tuberculin anergy*, and failure to respond to skin sensitisation with contact allergens such as DNCB or picroyl chloride.

* *A state of immunologic non-reactivity.*

The T-cell deficit tends to be relative (rather than absolute) in sarcoidosis. Moreover, patients with this disease tend to develop a peculiar delayed hypersensitivity reaction to a standardised extract of sarcoid tissue known as *Kveim antigen*. This reaction is the basis of a diagnostic test for sarcoidosis known as the Kveim test, but the correlation between a positive Kveim test and a positive diagnosis of sarcoidosis is not absolute.

Chapter 14

NATURE'S EXPERIMENTS IN IMMUNITY: THE MONOCLONAL GAMMOPATHIES

As has been noted elsewhere (*vide supra et infra*, Chapters 2, 5, 20, 21 and 22) the study of monoclonal immunoglobulins produced by functional malignant neoplasms of B-cells as "Nature's Experiments" in immunity has influenced profoundly our current concepts of immunoglobulin structure, function, biosynthesis, and genetics.

Several clinical forms of monoclonal gammopathies (or monoclonal immunoproliferative dyscrasias) have been described; the two most important types are multiple myeloma and Waldenström's Essential Macroglobulinaemia. These will consequently be considered in more detail than the rarer forms of immunoproliferative disease.

Multiple Myeloma

Multiple myeloma is a multifocal osteolytic neoplasm of bone marrow, characteristically occurring in later life, and extremely rare in individuals under the age of forty. It occurs in twice as many male patients as females. The neoplastic cells are generally identifiable morphologically as members of the plasma-cell series.

Protein Dyscrasias Occurring in Multiple Myeloma

The neoplastic plasma-cells in multiple myeloma characteristically remain functional, synthesising and secreting a monoclonal immunoglobulin and/or the excess free light chains of this immunoglobulin into the circulation. The latter products, being small enough to pass the glomerular filtration barrier, concentrate in the urine of myelomatous patients, where they are designated as Bence Jones proteins.

Bence Jones proteinuria results in characteristic renal pathology; tubular casts, syncytial giant cells within the tubules, and glomerular degeneration being amongst the more constant features of this renal disease. Moreover, the renal disease resulting from Bence Jones proteinuria is progressive, and ultimately results in chronic renal failure. Understanding of the nature of the Bence Jones defect may be gained by reviewing the kinetics of immunoglobulin synthesis summarised in Chapter 21 (*vide infra*).

Clinical Features

The clinical presentation of multiple myeloma is variable. Symptoms of anaemia may be the only complaints (*e.g.*, lassitude, dyspnoea on exertion, palpitations, angina pectoris, tachycardia, etc.) - or the patient may present with severe bone pain - usually multi-focal - and characteristically aggrevated by motion. Tenderness, especially over focal regions of the calvaria and back, is a common finding, and pathologic fractures are not infrequent. Hepatosplenomegaly is rare. Marked weight loss is a common feature, and recurrent bouts of pneumonia are likewise frequent. Occasionally, extramedullary plasmacytomata may be evident clinically in patients with multiple myeloma. These may occur in the oropharynx, on the skin, or these tumours may produce neurological signs and symptoms with radicular distribution when a solitary plasmacytoma impinges on and compresses a peripheral nerve root. Symptoms of renal insufficiency are common manifestations of multiple myeloma, and often become increasingly prominent as the disease progresses. Such symptoms - virtually invariant in patients with Bence Jones proteinuria - may also occur in patients who do not produce Bence Jones protein. In latter cases, they may be due to increased viscosity of serum leading to impaired renal perfusion or due to deposition of paramyloid* in the kidney.

Laboratory Investigations of the Suspected Myeloma Patients

Though the diagnosis of multiple myeloma may be tentatively made on clinical evidence, it must be confirmed by laboratory studies.

A normochromic anaemia is usually present and the reticulocyte count is usually low. There are no distinguishing features in the white count or platelets as a rule. Rarely, plasma-cells are present in the peripheral blood, and very rarely, the picture is one of a plasma-cell leukaemia. A greatly elevated erythrocyte sedimentation rate (ESR) is common.

Urinalysis often reveals proteinuria and the presence of granular and hyaline casts. Bence Jones protein, recognisable by its precipitation at 60°C and solubility at 100°C, may be found in 40-50% of cases. When renal failure is present, there is the expected elevation of blood urea nitrogen, creatinine and uric

* *"paramyloid" is a term used to denote the proteinaceous deposits that occur in many tissues of some patients with multiple myeloma. It is thought to represent deposition of a degradative product of myeloma globulin or a precursor-derivative within tissues.*

FIG.1 DIFFERENTIAL DIAGNOSIS OF HYPERGAMMAGLOBULINAEMIAS FROM SERUM ELECTROPHEROGRAMS

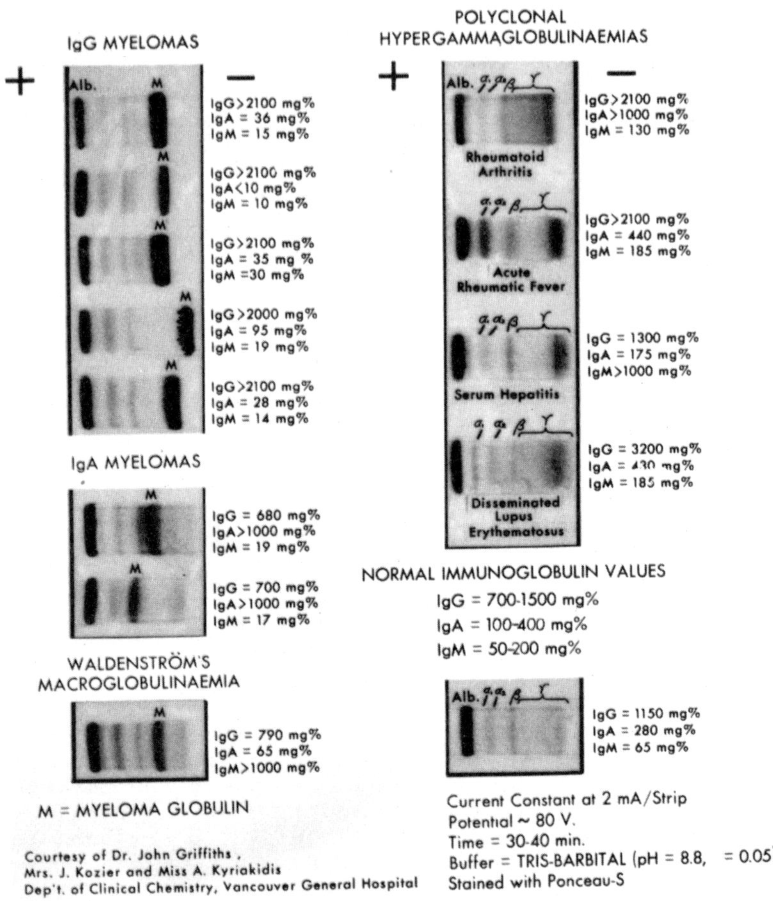

acid.

Increased immunoglobulin in the serum is, of course, usual and characteristically of the monoclonal type. Immunoelectrophoresis will demonstrate this to be confined to only one of the immunoglobulin classes: IgG, IgA, IgD or IgE. This monoclonally-increased immunoglobulin is known as "M-protein", "myeloma globulin", "myeloma protein" or "paraprotein".

Radiographs of the bones in painful or tender areas may reveal localised areas of rarefaction, generalised rarefaction, and either pathological or compression fractures. Multiple "punched-out" areas in the skull are characteristic, and compression fractures of vertebral bodies are common.

The definitive diagnosis is made from the demonstration of "myeloma" plasma-cells in smears of the bone marrow. When immature or bizarre plasma-cells (or sheets of plasma-cells) are seen, the disease is easily differentiated from benign plasmacytosis of the marrow occurring in diseases where marked immunologic stimulation occurs.

Therapy and Prognosis

Multiple myeloma is almost always generalised or multifocal; therefore, systemic chemotherapy is required. Rarely, local excision or localised radio-therapy of individual lesions is performed. Melphalan (Alkeran), an alkylating agent, is the drug of choice; about 50% of patients with this disease may be expected to respond to chemotherapy, usually with both subjective and objective signs of improvement. The latter are, unfortunately, generally of short duration; the average survival time after diagnosis is 1½ to 2 years. Occasional patients may survive many years after diagnosis, but long survival is not to be expected. Patients producing Bence Jones proteins in their urine generally have the worst prognosis - largely on account of their tendency to develop severe nephropathy.

Waldenström's Essential Macroglobulinaemia

The Waldenström syndrome is a chronic neoplastic disease of bone marrow, clinically similar to chronic lymphatic leukaemia, but in which the neoplastic cells produce a monoclonal immunoglobulin of the IgM class. This disease generally develops in patients over fifty years of age, more frequently in males than in females. It may present clinically with symptoms of an anaemia (*e.g.*, lassitude, exertional dyspnoea, angina pectoris,

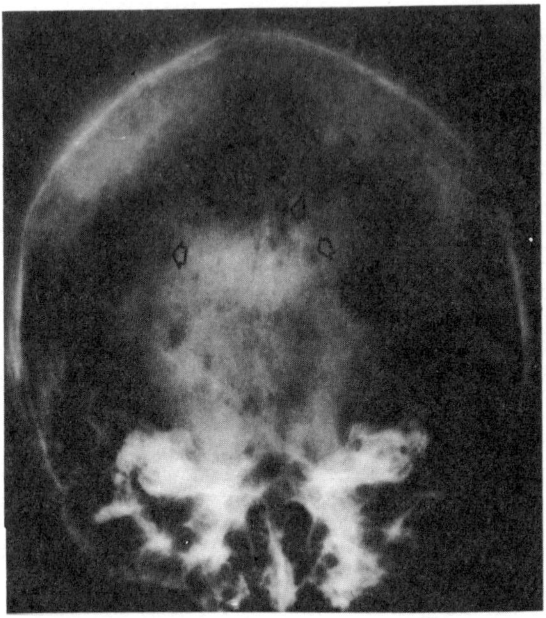

Fig. 2 Radiograph of Skull showing 'punched-out' radiolucencies characteristic of Multiple Myeloma

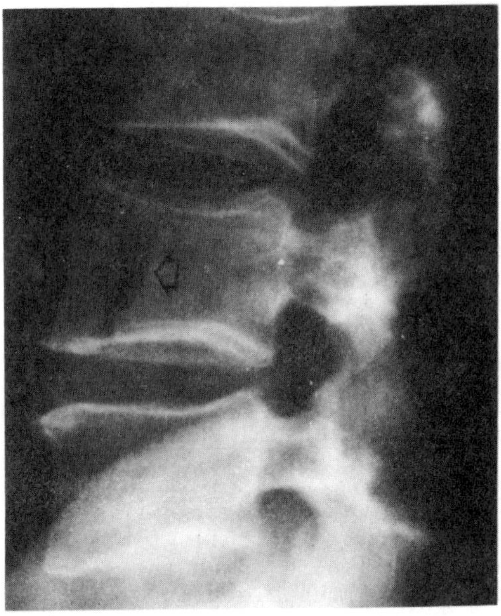

Fig. 3 Radiograph of Lumbar Spine showing 'punched-out' radiolucency characteristic of Multiple Myeloma

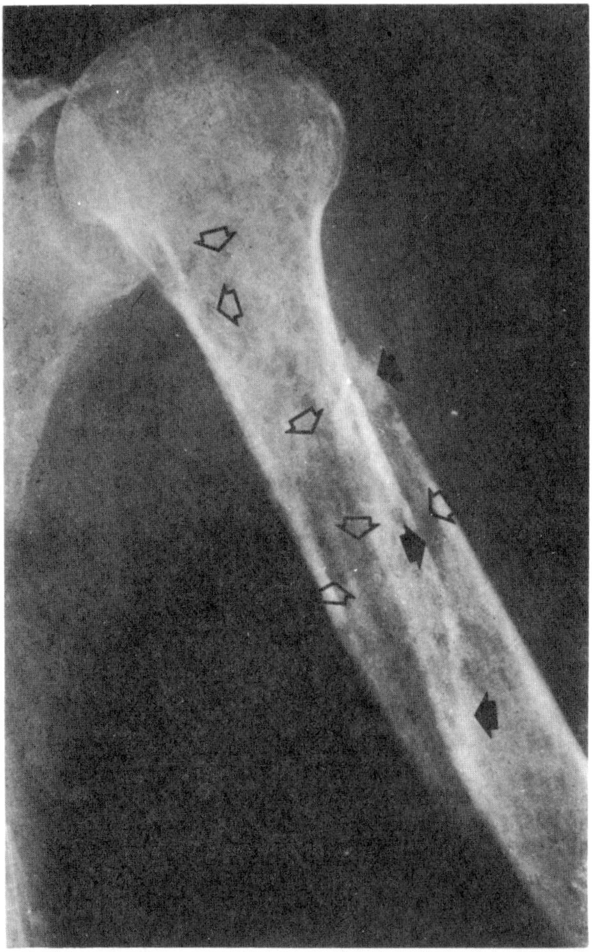

Fig. 4 Pathological Fracture of the Humerus in Multiple Myeloma. Note 'moth-eaten' appearance of bone around fracture site

Figures 2, 3, and 4
Courtesy of:
Dr. W.R. Boyd
Dep't Radiology
The Vancouver General Hospital

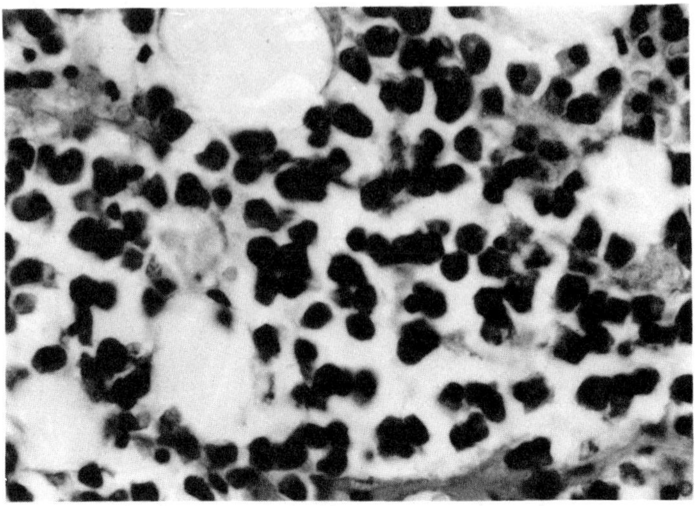

Fig. 5 Multiple Myeloma Marrow Section (H and E)

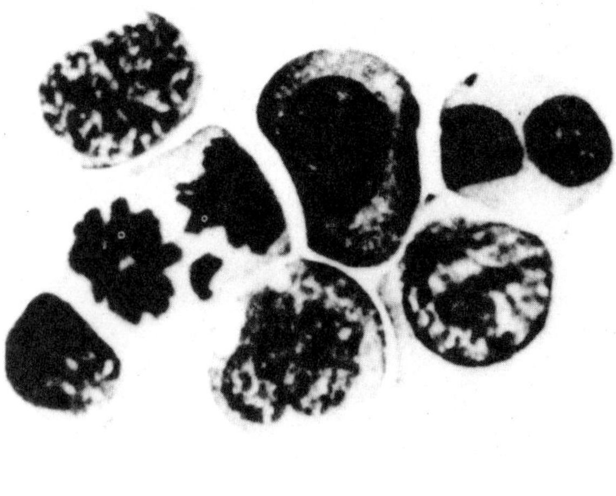

Fig. 6 Multiple Myeloma Bone Marrow Squash
(May-Grünwald-Giemsa)

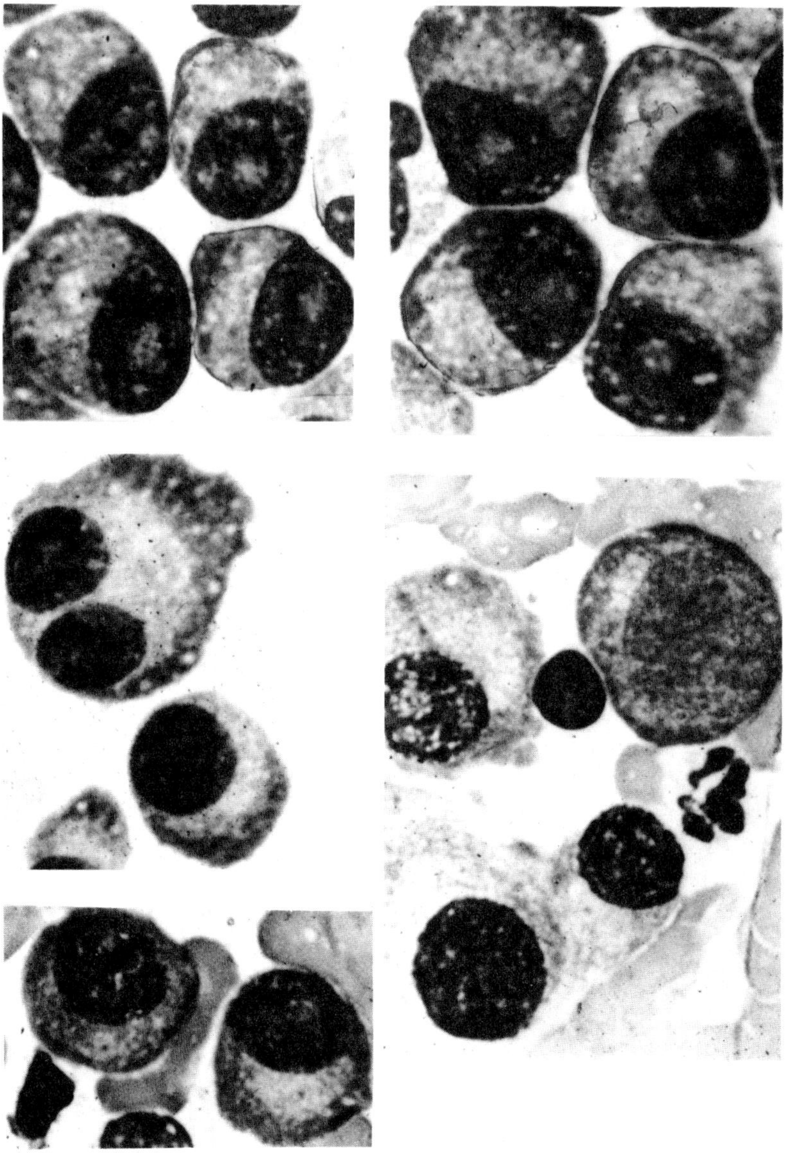

Fig. 7 Bone Marrow Squashes Multiple Myeloma
(Wright's)
(Showing detail of Neoplastic Plasma Cells)

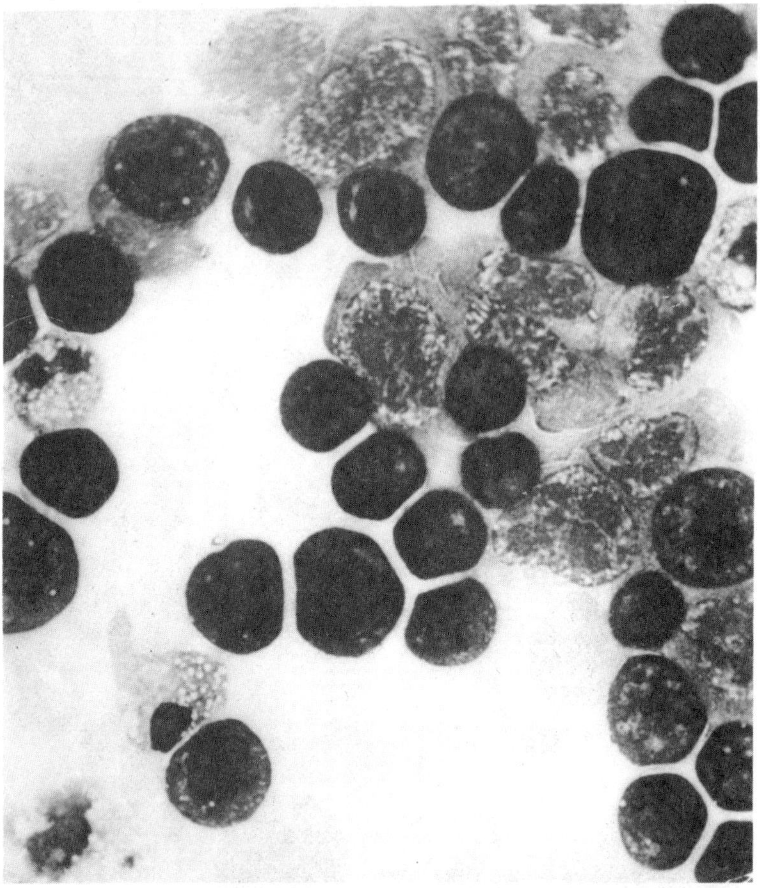

Fig. 8 Waldenstrom's Macroglobulinaemia
Bone Marrow Squash
(May-Grunwald-Giemsa)

palpitations, vertigo, tachycardia, etc.) with or without pyrexia and loss of weight. Hepatosplenomegaly and generalised lymphadenopathy are common stigmata of this disease, in contrast to multiple myeloma. Bence Jones proteinuria occurs in ~10% of patients with Waldenström's macroglobulinaemia, but osteolytic lesions like those encountered in multiple myeloma are rarely seen in this disease. Pancytopenia, granulocytopenia with relative lymphocytosis and haemorrhagic purpura, especially involving mucous membranes, are common stigmata of this disease. As the disease progresses, the increasing serum viscosity frequently leads to circulatory problems and heart failure.

The neoplastic cells in Waldenström's disease may resemble either lymphocytes or plasma-cells in their morphology; frequently they demonstrate morphological features characteristic of both, and are sometimes referred to as "plasmacytoid lymphocytes".

The occurrence of large numbers of circulating morphologically-abnormal neoplastic cells in peripheral blood is rare in macroglobulinaemia; this disease is usually aleukaemic throughout its course.

Marked rouleaux formation and a highly significant elevation of the ESR are common in Waldenström's disease.

Since IgM globulins are classifiable as euglobulins, the Sia water test for euglobulins is usually positive in patients with macroglobulinaemia.

Laboratory tests useful in confirming the diagnosis of macroglobulinaemia include serum electrophoresis (in which a monoclonal globulin elevation is demonstrated), serum immunoelectrophoresis (which demonstrates the monoclonal protein to be of the IgM class), and quantitative immunoglobulin determination (showing an elevation in IgM and normal or low values for IgA and IgG). The electrophoretic pattern in macroglobulinaemia will be altered by treatment of the serum with penicillamine, an agent which splits IgM molecules into smaller fragments of differing electrophoretic mobility.

Therapy and Prognosis

The Waldenström syndrome is usually treated by chemotherapy with alkylating agents. Chlorambucil (Leukeran®) is the drug of first choice, with Melphan (Alkeran®) and cyclophosphamide (Cytoxan®, Procytox®) as alternative agents. Treatment with these agents is directed toward relief of symptoms - asymptomatic or mild cases should not be treated with alkylating agents.

The prognosis in this condition is better than in multiple myeloma; four years from diagnosis being the average time for survival of treated cases. Plasmapheresis (removal of blood from patients followed by replacement of cellular elements) is often helpful in lowering the viscosity of the blood and improving circulatory status; in fact, this may be the only therapy necessary for most of the course of this disease.

Solitary Extramedullary Plasmacytoma

Solitary plasma-cell neoplasms arising in soft-tissue sites occur most commonly in the respiratory tract. These tumours are frequently more benign than multiple myeloma, remaining localised *in situ* for many years, during which they grow slowly. However, these tumours may eventually metastasise to bone marrow, and produce a syndrome of secondary multiple myeloma. It has been suggested that this disease represents a partially-autonomous clone of plasma-cells, which may become eventually totally autonomous, and the tumour thus assumes a malignant course;alternatively, the clone may remain partially-subject to the body's homeostatic mechanism, and the tumour consequently follows a benign course.

Other Lymphoproliferative Diseases Occasionally Associated With Production of a Monoclonal Immunoglobulin

A monoclonal immunoglobulin of the IgG type in the serum may occur occasionally in patients who demonstrate the clinical features of the following neoplastic diseases, *viz:* chronic lymphatic leukaemia, malignant lymphoma, lymphosarcoma, and reticulum cell sarcoma. (Malignant lymphomas and lymphosarcomas which produce monoclonal IgM proteins would be classified as variants of Waldenström's Disease). All of these conditions, however, are distinct rarities when compared with multiple myeloma and Waldenström's Macroglobulinaemia.

Heavy-Chain Diseases

Heavy-chain diseases are a series of diverse clinical entities, in which neoplastic cells produce and secrete portions (constant regions) of heavy chains into the blood stream. Variants of this type of disease have been described which produce fragments of γ-chains, α-chains, and μ-chains. (*Vide infra,* Chapters 21, 22 and 23).

Franklin's Disease (γ-Chain Disease)

At least 13 cases of this peculiar immunoproliferative dyscrasia have been reported. These patients all presented as recurrent pyrexia, lymphadenopathy, and hepatosplenomegaly. Twelve of these cases occurred in men above the age of forty. In some patients, this disease develops insidiously, whilst in others it is rapid in onset and progressive. The clinical features are those of malignant lymphoma, oedema of the soft palate, recurrent infections, normochromic anaemia, eosinophilia, neutropenia, and marked proteinuria. The urinary protein is the γ-chain fragment itself - and not Bence Jones protein. This feature is the diagnostic finding in γ-chain disease.

Normal serum immunoglobulins are decreased, and a monoclonal globulin peak, representing the γ-chain fragment, can be observed on serum electropherograms and immunoelectropherograms at some point during the course of the disease.

α-Chain Disease

Six patients with rapidly-progressive malignant lymphomas of the intestine, associated with malabsorption, and producing a fragment of α-chain (the class-specific chain of IgA immunoglobulins) have now been described. All of these patients have been young persons from the Mediterranean region.

μ-Chain Disease

A patient was described recently in whom the diagnosis of μ-chain disease was made. This patient presented with chronic lymphocytic leukaemia, bone pain (related to neoplastic infiltration of the femur), amyloidosis, Bence Jones proteinuria, marked plasmacytic and lymphocytic infiltration of the bone marrow, and bilateral carpal tunnel syndrome. The plasma-cells in the bone marrow demonstrated bizarre morphological features. An anomalous serum protein was identified, which possessed antigenic determinants of μ-chains; this μ-chain fragment, however, did not appear in the urine. The urinary protein in this patient consisted entirely of the κ-type of light chain - *i.e.,* a typical Bence Jones protein.

Multiple Myeloma Secreting Two M-Proteins

H. H. Fudenberg and his colleagues in San Francisco have reported a patient with multiple myeloma (designated as "*Til*") whose serum contained two distinct M-proteins. One of these was of the $IgG_{2\kappa}$-type and the other of the IgM_{κ}-type. These two M-proteins were entirely distinct electrophoretically, immunologically, ultracentrifugally, and biochemically. However, the amino-acid sequences of these two *paraproteins* were identical in the regions of the molecules containing the antigen-binding sites.

This fascinating experiment of nature sheds important light on the mechanisms and genetics of immunoglobulin synthesis, and, consequently, will be discussed further in Chapter 20 (*vide infra*).

Chapter 15

CYTOTOXIC ANTIBODIES IN HUMAN DISEASE

The effect of an antibody on a target-cell depends upon a number of interdependent factors, some of which are considered below:

Nature of the Target-Cell

It was noted in Chapter 7 (*vide supra*) that the nature of the target-cell is an important factor in determining the effects of antibodies to membrane antigens on these cells. For example, antibodies to erythrocyte membrane antigens are more prone to induce a lytic reaction than are antibodies to similar antigen on leucocytes. Thus, if erythrocytes are mixed with appropriate antibodies in the presence of complement *in vitro*, haemolysis is the expected result, whilst *in vitro* mixture of leucocytes with appropriate antibodies and complement is expected to demonstrate cytotoxicity without leucocytolysis. The latter may occur, however, when the titres of cytotoxic antibodies and complement are high.

In vivo, several clinical entities may develop which are due to interactions of different types of target cells with complement-dependent cytotoxic antibodies. For example:

(1) Intravascular haemolysis may occur during a blood transfusion mismatched for a major blood group antigen (*vide infra*, this Chapter and Chapter 16).

(2) Granulocytopenia may occur in patients who have developed complement-dependent cytotoxic antibodies to leucocyte antigens resulting from multiple blood transfusions. A similar reaction may occur following sensitisation of a mother by multiple pregnancies with maternal-foetal disparity between leucocyte antigens.

The difference in the clinical reactions observed depends somewhat on the differences in structure between erythrocytes and leucocytes.

Location of Antigens on Target-Cells

The location of the antigens on the target-cell is likewise important in determining the effects which antibodies and complement will exert on the target-cell. For example, antinuclear antibodies (*vide supra et infra*, Chapters 6, 10 and 19) are not cytotoxic to living cells, even when they are able to bind complement, because they cannot gain access to the nuclei of living cells.

Ability of Antibodies to Activate Complement

The ability of an antibody to activate the complement system is an extremely important factor in determining its effect upon a target-cell. Ability to activate complement is restricted to IgM antibodies and IgG antibodies (except for the γ_4 subclass). By no means, however, is that the only function mediated by these types of antibodies (*vide supra*, Chapters 5 and 6). Thus, antibodies of the IgM class to the A or B blood group substances of human erythrocytes will mediate an agglutination reaction when mixed with erythrocytes containing the appropriate antigen *in vitro* in the absence of complement, whilst the same mixture will undergo a haemolytic reaction when complement is present (*vide infra*, Chapter 16).

Acute (second-set) rejection of surgically-transplanted organs is mediated by cytotoxic antibodies which are complement-dependent. Where such antibodies are present (having developed as a result of prior rejection of an earlier organ transplant with similar antigenicity) the transplanted organ may be rejected totally within a few minutes (*vide infra*, Chapter 18).

Nonetheless, antibodies not capable of activating the complement system are sometimes able to cause injury to target-cells. Under these circumstances, the injury is usually less profound than when the antibodies activate complement, and the injured cells are usually eliminated from the body by the reticulo-endothelial system and its circulating scavenger cells, when this type of reaction occurs *in vivo*.

Frequently, when antibodies of this type are mixed with a suspension of target-cells *in vitro*, the reaction will be evidenced by agglutination and slow loss of viability of the target-cells. However, this is by no means invariant, and sometimes no visible reaction occurs after mixture of target-cells and antibody. For example, an individual who is Rh negative may develop antibodies to the D antigen of the Rh system after a transfusion of Rh positive blood. When the serum from such an individual is mixed with a suspension of Rh positive erythrocytes, there is often no visible reaction. The anti-D antibodies are bound to the D-antigen on the erythrocytes, but both antigen-binding sites on each antibody molecule are thought to be bound to antigens on the same red cell. For this reason, no agglutination results unless an antibody to human immunoglobulins (prepared in the rabbit) is added to the mixture. This antiglobulin antibody is denoted as Coombs' serum, and the test described is the indirect Coombs' test (*vide supra et infra,* Chapters 6 and 16).

It must be clearly understood that all antibodies to accessible membrane antigens are injurious to their target-cells. In fact, such antibodies may even be protective to target-cells under certain conditions, as exemplified by the phenomena of tumour enhancement and allograft enhancement (*vide infra,* Chapter 17). When these phenomena occur, antibodies to membrane antigens which are present on the surfaces of neoplastic cells or the cells of a transplanted organ will actually promote the survival of these target-cells, so that the tumour grows more quickly or the transplanted organ survives better within an immunologically-competent recipient. The mechanisms by which this paradoxical effect of antibodies may occur will be deferred to Chapters 17 and 18 for more complete discussion.

Cytotoxic Antibodies and Target-Cells *In vivo* and *In vitro*

Finally, the circumstances under which an antibody and a target-cell react greatly affect the nature of the reaction observed. Frequently, there is good correlation between *in vitro* and *in vivo* reactions, but it is not always possible to predict accurately the former from the latter, since conditions within the body cannot be duplicated in the test tube.

The nature of a target-cell-cytotoxic antibody reaction *in vivo* will further depend upon where in the body the reaction has occurred. For example, haemolysis occurring within phagocytes of the reticulo-endothelial system induces a very different clinical response than that induced by intravascular haemolysis (*vide infra,* Chapter 16).

Chapter 16

BLOOD TRANSFUSION

The tissues of each individual in an outbred population (such as exists in man) possess an unique composite of antigens, which makes it impossible to transplant tissues from one individual to another, if the recipient is immunologically-competent. Fortunately, however, the antigenic complexity of human erythrocytes is less than that of other tissues, which makes the transfusion of erythrocytes a practical possibility without the use of immunosuppressive therapy. For example, when the erythrocyte antigens of prospective donor and prospective recipient are properly "matched" to each other, ~97% of transfusions will proceed without difficulty.

Blood Group Antigens

The antigens on human erythrocytes are denoted as "blood groups", and are regulated by a number of genetic loci. Only two of these genetic loci, the *ABO* and *Rh* blood group systems are of major importance as causes of transfusion reactions or in the aetiology of maternal-foetal reactions leading to haemolytic disease of the newborn (*erythroblastosis foetalis*).

It is unfortunate that blood group antigens were discovered in a "piecemeal" fashion; their notation and nomenclature is riddled with inconsistencies. For example, alternative (allelic) antigens may be designated by different letters (*e.g.*, *A* and *B*, *M* and *N*), by large and small letters (*e.g.*, *S* and *s*, *K* and *k*, *D* and *d*) or by symbols with superscripts (*e.g.*, Lu^a and Lu^b, Fy^a and Fy^b, Jk^a and Jk^b, etc.). Fourteen blood group systems are illustrated in Figure 1. Only the *ABO* system and the *Rh* system are of major importance as causes of transfusion reactions or of haemolytic disease of the newborn.

The ABO Blood Group System

Antibodies to ABO antigens are *isohaemagglutinins*, since the antigens are of human origin (*iso* = same species), and because they are ordinarily detected by means of an agglutination reaction against cells of known ABO type. In other words, serum containing antibodies to the A_1, A_2 or *B* antigens will clump erythrocytes containing these antigens on their surfaces.

There are four major *ABO* phenotypes, designated as *O* (red cells with neither *A* nor *B* antigens), *A* (red cells with only *A* antigens), *B* (red cells with only *B* antigen) or *AB* (red cells with both *A* and *B* antigens). The *A* and *AB* groups are further separated into subgroups, denoted as A_1, A_2, A_1B, and A_2B. A_1 is a stronger agglutinogen than A_2 with the usual α agglutinins (*i.e.*, anti-*A* serum), and occasionally subgroup specific antisera occur. For example, α_1 antiserum (*i.e.*, specific anti-A_1 serum) may occur in a few patients with erythrocytes of the A_2 or A_2B subgroups and A_1 or A_1B individuals may produce anti-*H** antibodies, which agglutinate group *O* red cells strongly and subgroups A_2 and A_2B red cells less strongly.

Fig. 1 THE KNOWN BLOOD GROUP SYSTEMS OF MAN

SYSTEM	ANTIGENS (Not Complete List)
1. ABO	A_1, A_2, B, H,
2. MNSs	M, N, S, rs
3. P	P_1, P_2, Pk
4. Rh (Rhesus)	C, C^w, c, D, D^u, d*, E, e
5. Lutheran	Lu^a, Lu^b
6. Kell-Sutter	K, k, Kp^a, Kp^b, Js^a, Js^b
7. Lewis	Le^a, Le^b
8. Duffy	Fy^a, Fy^b
9. Kidd	Jk^a, Jk^b
10. Diego	Di^a
11. I	I, i
12. Auberger	Au^a
13. Xg	Xg^a (sex-linked)
14. Dombrock	Do^a

* N.B.: Anti-d antibodies have never been detected

* *H-substance is a glycoprotein precursor in the synthesis of A_1, A_2, and B antigens (vide infra).*

Only the *O* gene is recessive; it is thought to represent a totally inactive gene, allelic to the *A* and *B* genes which regulate enzymes that convert a glycoprotein precursor (*H*-substance) into the (glycoprotein) *A*-substances and *B*-substance. Since *H*-substance is common to erythrocytes of groups *O*, *A* and *B*, antibodies to it are not usually found in individuals of any of the major *ABO* phenotypes. For this reason, type *O* individuals respond immunologically to both *A*-substances and to *B* substance, whilst individuals of phenotype *AB* do not respond to either *A*-substance or *B*-substance. Since *A*-substance and *B*-substance are widespread in nature, constant low-level immunologic stimulation occurs through life, and natural antibodies are usually present (even in individuals who have not received incompatible blood transfusions) to those *ABO* blood group substances which the individual does not possess.

Antibodies to *H*-substance (the substrate common to types A_1, A_2, B, A_1B, A_2B and *O*) do occur in rare individuals with the so-called "Bombay phenotype", lacking a gene regulating an enzyme which converts a glycolipid precursor to *H*-substance. Such individuals therefore will produce serum antibodies to *H*-substance, *A*-substance, and *B*-substance, *i.e.*, their sera will contain isohaemagglutinins to red cells of types *O*, *A*, *B*, and *AB*; and their red cells will contain no *H*, *A* or *B* antigens.

Fig. 2 THE ABO BLOOD GROUP SYSTEM

ABO BLOOD GROUP	DISTRIBUTION IN POPULATION †	ANTIGENS ON RED CELL	ANTIBODIES IN SERUM
O	46%	H*	ANTI-A (α) & ANTI-B (β)
A	42%	A { A_1, A_2	ANTI-B (β)
B	9%	B	ANTI-A (α)
AB	3%	A_1, A_2 } A & B	—

*ANTIBODIES TO H-SUBSTANCE FOUND ONLY IN INDIVIDUALS WITH 'BOMBAY' PHENOTYPE AND (RARELY) IN A_1 OR A_1B PHENOTYPES

† (WHITE NORTH AMERICAN POPULATION)

The Rh (Rhesus) Blood Group System

The *Rh* blood group antigens were so named because they were initially identified on the red cells of the rhesus monkey (*Macaca mulatta*). The genetics of *Rh* antigens is controversial, and two hypotheses have been advanced to account for their inheritance.

Fisher and Race have explained the data in terms of three closely-linked sets of allelic genes denoted *C*, *D*, and *E*, with allelic forms *c*, C^{w}, *d*, D^{u} and *e*. Each set of allelic genes determines one antigen of the *Rh* system. The linkage groups are expressed as combinations of allelic forms; *e.g.*, *CDE*, *cde*, *CDe*, etc.

On the other hand, Wiener (who is co-discoverer of the *Rh* system) explains the inheritance of *Rh*-antigens as governed by a single genetic locus with multiple (allelomorphic) forms. An enormous number of genotypes are possible, which depend upon the segregation of *Rh* genes in the parental gametes. The Fisher-Race and Wiener nomenclatures of the *Rh* phenotypes are compared in Figure 3.

Fig. 3 PARTIAL LIST OF Rh PHENOTYPES

FISHER-RACE NOTATION	WIENER NOTATION	SHORT NOTATION	FREQUENCY IN ENGLISH POPULATION
CDe	R^1	R_1	41%
cDe	R^0	R_0	3%
cDE	R^2	R_2	14%
CDE	R^Z	R_Z	(v. low)
Cde	r'	R'	1%
cde	r	r	39%
cdE	r''	R''	1%
CdE	ry	Ry	(v. low)

The most frequent *Rh* genotypes in North American Caucasians are expressed in Figure 4.

It is the *D*-antigen that determines whether an individual is *Rh*-positive or negative; individuals of genotype *DD* or *Dd* are *Rh*-positive, whilst individuals of type *dd* are *Rh*-negative. Anti-*D* antiserum is synonymous with anti-*Rh* serum.

Fig. 4 MOST FREQUENT Rh GENOTYPES AMONGST CAUCASIANS

FISHER-RACE NOTATION	SHORT NOTATION	FREQUENCY
CDe/cde	$(R_1 r)$	33%
CDe/CDe	$(R_1 R_1)$	17%
cde/cde	(rr)	15%

Anti-*D* antiserum reacts with the red cells of ~84% of white North Americans (who are therefore *Rh*-positive), whilst the remaining 16% of individuals are *Rh*-negative, since their red cells do not possess the *D*-antigen. The *C*-and the *E*-antigens, whilst closely associated with the medically-important *D*-antigen, are not important causes of transfusion reactions or of haemolytic disease of the newborn. Naturally-occurring anti-*D* antibodies are extremely rarely encountered; when anti-*D* antibodies occur in the sera of patients, they are nearly always the result of previous incompatible blood transfusions or following delivery of several *D*-positive babies from a *D*-negative mother.

Potential Risks Associated with Blood Transfusion

The indications and contraindications for blood transfusion, whilst not a part of the present discussion, should be clearly considered for each patient individually before a transfusion is administered. Although blood transfusions are no longer the formidable procedures that they were a few decades ago, they are still attended by a significant morbidity and mortality. It has been estimated that two transfusion reactions occur in every hundred transfusions administered, and one death in every three thousand. The significance of the risk of transfusion may be appreciated better after noting that more than 4.5 million transfusions per year are administered in the United States, and about one-half million per year in Canada; thus, transfusions should never be given except in the presence of clear indications.

Selection of Blood Donors

Each donor is initially screened by careful history and physical examination, with special attention paid to the following:

(a) Does the prospective donor carry any disease that might be transmitted via transfusion? (Examples: *malaria, syphilis, hepatitis,* etc.).

(b) Might the blood of the prospective donor be likely to cause transfusion reaction in recipients? (For eample, has the prospective donor received a large number of transfusions in the past?)

(c) Might the withdrawal of 450 ml. of blood for transfusion be likely to have an adverse effect upon the prospective donor? (For example, is the donor anaemic?)

Prior to withdrawal of a unit of blood for transfusion, a small sample is drawn from each prospective donor, and this sample is subjected to haemoglobin determination and *V.D.R.L.* serology. If the haemoglobin is 12.5 grammes % or less, or if the *V.D.R.L.* serology is positive, the prospective donor is immediately rejected. Routine screening of prospective donors for the Australia antigen (a recently-discovered serum antigenic determinant associated with the virus of serum hepatitis) has now been adopted in both Canada and the U.S.A., and all prospective donors positive for this antigen are likewise rejected immediately. Presently, prospective donors are also rejected if they have any evidence (historical, clinical or laboratory) of present or recent infective processes of any type (including colds), or if they have any past history of *malaria, lues*, or *hepatitis*.

Determination of Blood Types of Prospective Donors and Recipients of Blood Transfusions

In the routine blood typing of prospective donors and recipients, only the *ABO* and *Rh* (*C*, *D*, and *E*) antigens and the α- and β-isohaemagglutinins are tested for. However, in individuals belonging to types *A* and *AB*, it is desirable to determine the correct subgroup, since occasional A_2 and A_2B patients produce significant titres of α_1-isohaemagglutinins, which react with erythrocytes of A_1 or A_1B individuals, and may thus induce severe transfusion reactions when incorrectly matched. Usually, these reactions are mild on first transfusion, but the antigenic stimulus provided by the transfusion results in an increased isohaemagglutinin titre in the recipient, so that subsequent transfusions may induce severe or fatal reactions.

Direct Compatibility Testing of Donor and Recipient: The Cross-Match

In spite of the fact that extreme caution has been observed in the typing of both donor and recipient, the possibility of a severe transfusion reaction is still present for several reasons:

(a) Either the blood typing or recording of the blood type may be in error.

(b) Either donor or recipient may contain high titres of antibody against minor blood group antigens, which have not been typed.

(c) Antibodies may be present in the serum of some patients that do not agglutinate erythrocytes *in vitro* directly, but which may be demonstrated by techniques like the indirect Coombs' test (*vide supra*, Chapter 6) wherein serum from the prospective recipient is mixed with erythrocytes from the prospective donor, and rabbit antiserum to human globulins (*i.e.*, Coombs' serum) is added to the system to promote the agglutination of antibody-coated erythrocytes.

The cross-match of donor and recipient may consist of two parts, denoted as major and minor sides. The major side consists of mixing the donor's cells with the recipient's serum, both in the presence and absence of Coombs' serum, whilst the minor side (not routinely done in most centres in the U.S.A. and Canada) consists of mixing the recipient's erythrocytes with the donor's serum, with and without Coombs' serum. The major side is referred to in that way because it tests for antibodies present in the recipient's serum, which represent the most common causes of severe or fatal haemolytic transfusion reactions. When transfusion reactions are due to incompatibility in the minor side of the cross-match, they tend to be mild.

Use of Unmatched "Universal Donor" Blood

In extreme emergencies, where *stat* blood transfusions are required to maintain the life of a patient, it is not possible to await the results of a cross-match, and unmatched "universal donor" blood may be used. This is type *O*, *Rh*-negative for females of reproductive age or lower and for men, and type *O*, *Rh*-positive for post-menopausal women (the latter being employed because of the scarcity of type *O*, *Rh*-negative blood). Universal donor bloods are chosen by the Red Cross (or the Blood Bank) for unusually low titres of α- and β-haemolysins (to minimise the risk of minor-side incompatibility reactions). However, although "universal donor" blood may be life-saving in emergent situations, it must never be employed where there is time for a cross-match to be performed. The time required for an accurate cross-match to be performed is two hours, but an emergency cross-match, requiring only twenty minutes, can be performed as well. Although this is less accurate than a routine cross-match, it is preferred to using unmatched "universal donor" blood wherever possible.

Transfusion Reactions

Five types of transfusion reactions occur, of which three are of direct immunological interest. These general types of reactions include:

(a) Haemolytic Reactions
(b) Febrile Reactions
(c) Allergic Reactions
} (of immunological interest)

(d) Circulatory overloading Reactions

(e) Transmission of Disease

(a) Haemolytic reactions: These reactions are the most serious complications of blood transfusions, resulting from:

(1) *ABO* blood group incompatibility (usually from clerical or laboratory error)

(2) Minor blood group antigen incompatibilities (usually *Kell* or *Duffy*)

(3) *A*- or *AB*-subgroup incompatibility or *Rh*-incompatibility

(4) Minor side incompatibility in anti-*ABO* or anti-*Rh* antibodies

(5) Transfusion of outdated or haemolysed blood

Severe haemolytic reactions occur immediately, *e.g.*, after one or two hundred ml. of blood have been administered. The severity of this type of reaction makes its early recognition mandatory, for the infusion must be stopped immediately if the patient is to survive. The patient usually complains of pain in the lower back, diffuse pain in the muscles, headaches, substernal oppression and nausea, often proceeding to vomiting. A severe racking chill with frank rigors and followed by a sharp rise in temperature is common. The patient may then go into a state of shock. If the immediate reaction is not fatal, the patient will develop signs of acute renal failure and severe haemorrhagic tendency, either or both of which can be fatal themselves. The renal failure results from *acute tubular necrosis*, secondary to *disseminated intravascular thrombosis (consumptive coagulopathy)* whilst the haemorrhage is of similar aetiology.

Damage to erythrocyte membranes (*e.g.*, by isohaemolysins and complement) results in the acquisition of thromboplastic activity by the damaged membranes. Thus, these membranes are able to activate blood clotting factors continuously, which are consumed within the vascular bed at a rate greater than new factors can be synthesised. Increasing consumption of clotting factors thus leads to their eventual depletion, and results in a generalised bleeding tendency.

When a haemolytic transfusion reaction is suspected, the transfusion must be stopped immediately and the following investigations undertaken at once:

(1) A blood sample is taken as soon as possible after the onset of reaction and the serum is compared with a pre-transfusion specimen. Spectrophotometric analysis is performed for free haemoglobin and for bilirubin. The presence of free haemoglobin or an increase (over the pretransfusion specimen) in serum bilirubin confirms a haemolytic reaction.

(2) A urine sample is collected as soon as possible after the onset of the reaction. This specimen may contain haemoglobin and albumin, and often contains red cells as well. Pigmented casts may not appear until later. When renal damage is severe, persistent oliguria or complete anuria are expected, and continuously-increasing azotaemia and uraemia will be noted. Unless definitively treated, the uraemia will progress to death.

(3) All of the typing and cross-matching procedures must be rechecked and repeated immediately to determine the cause of reaction.

(4) Where an unmatched "universal donor" blood was used, an immediate cross-match must be performed.

If minor side incompatibility is detected, the haemolysin titre of the donor serum must be determined.

(5) The remaining blood used for the transfusion is examined for its date of collection, the presence of free haemoglobin, and the presence of bacterial contamination. Complete review of blood bank records for irregularities in collection or storage must be made.

(b) Febrile reactions: Many febrile reactions are due to leucocyte and platelet antigens being mismatched. Smaller numbers are due to minor blood group mismatches or to miscellaneous plasma factors. When febrile reactions occur, the same types of investigations and rechecks as outlined above in the preceding section should be performed, so that the ultimate cause of the reaction can be determined, if possible. This is desirable because a febrile reaction on one transfusion may presage the development of a haemolytic reaction on a subsequent transfusion, since the transfused blood will be likely to stimulate the development of a secondary response to the mismatched antigens, (*vide supra,* Chapter 8) with a consequent rapid rise in antibody titre.

Repeated transfusions are likely to stimulate an individual to develop antibodies to the minor blood group antigens and to leucocyte and platelet antigens. Leucocyte and platelet antigens are representative of the nucleated-cell antigens of the body, and fall into a group known as the HL-A (human leucocyte antigen) system, which will be discussed at length in Chapter 17 (*vide infra*). Development of specific circulating antibodies against HL-A antigens in certain patients who have received multiple transfusions has provided the laboratory with a means of typing these nucleated-cell antigens. This method, described in the following chapter (*vide infra,* Chapter 17), is employed to "type" tissue antigens prior to surgical transplantation of solid tissues.

A febrile reaction can also be initiated by the introduction of bacteria or other pyrogens via a contaminated bottle of blood.

(c) Allergic reactions: Atopic reactions to transfused blood usually take the form of mild urticaria, but may occur as frank anaphylactic shock. The signs and symptoms are typical of either of these conditions; *i.e.,* the patient may break out in hives, or may exhibit itching of the palms followed by rapidly-developing bronchoconstriction with dyspnoea, wheeze, and complete or partial cardiovascular collapse, with rapid and profound fall in blood pressure. The incidence of allergic reactions is lowered by concomitant or prior administration of antihistamines. If anaphylactic shock occurs, however, this must be treated by *stat* injection of adrenaline chloride (1:1000).

Haemolytic Disease of the Newborn (Erythroblastosis Foetalis)

Naturally-occurring "mismatch" between mother and foetus related to the *ABO* blood group antigens and leading to clinical disease in the foetus is extremely rare, since most isohaemagglutinins of the *ABO* system are IgM antibodies, which do not cross the placental barrier.

This is not the case, however, where the mother is *Rh*-negative (*D*-negative) and the child is *Rh*-positive (*D*-positive). In this situation, upon stimulation resulting usually from several pregnancies, the mother develops anti-*D* antibodies. Although these, too, are initially of the IgM type, and therefore incapable of crossing the placental barrier, continued antigenic stimulation favours the development of IgG antibodies, which cross the placental barrier readily.

Maternal anti-*D* antibodies of the IgG type, thus, may haemolyse the erythrocytes of the developing foetus, leading to *haemolytic disease of the newborn*, or *erythroblastosis foetalis*. Such infants develop severe *anaemia*, *cardiomegaly*, and *hepatosplenomegaly*, from the massive destruction of blood *in utero* and immediately *post partum*. Unless adequately-treated (by total exchange transfusion), *congestive heart failure* and/or *kernicterus* develop. When anti-*D* antibodies of the IgG type are demonstrated in a mother during pregnancy, the severity of the haemolytic process occurring in the foetus may be monitored by repeated amniocentesis. Whenever the amniotic fluid is heavily stained with bilirubin (which indicates a severe degree of haemolysis) a catheter may be inserted into the foetal peritoneum through the mother's abdomenal wall and uterus, under radiological guidance. Packed *D*-negative erythrocytes are injected into the peritoneum of the foetus, and from there are absorbed into the foetal circulation. When intra-uterine transfusions of this type have been performed, the baby may be born with only *Rh*-negative cells in its circulation.

Recently, it has become possible to prevent this disease. Since the sensitisation of the mother mainly occurs just at the time of birth, injection of anti-*D* antibodies (*RhoGam*®) into the *Rh*-negative mother just after delivery of an *Rh*-positive infant will coat any foetal (*D*-positive) cells circulating in the mother. Antibody-coated cells are rapidly removed from the maternal circulation. Under these circumstances, the mother is prevented from developing her own antibodies to foetal cells; this failure probably results from antibody-coated *D*-antigens being unavailable to stimulate the lymphoid system of the mother (*i.e.*, afferent inhibition of the lymphoid system), rather than from rapid removal of foetal red cells from the maternal circulation *per se*.

Chapter 17

TISSUE TRANSPLANTATION

Transplantation refers to the grafting of organs or tissues from one individual to another. When this is done between immunocompetent individuals who are genetically different, the grafted tissue will be rejected in about two weeks by immunological mechanisms which depend on the antigenic differences between donor and host.

Definitions

Allograft or Homograft	Transplants between genetically non-identical individuals of the same species.
Isograft	Transplants between donor and recipient of an inbred strain, or between identical twins (*i.e.*, genetically-identical individuals); sometimes called a syngeneic allograft.
Xenograft	Tissue grafts between a donor and a recipient of different species.
Autograft	Tissue transplants within a single individual.
Orthotopic Graft	Tissue transplanted into its normal anatomical position.
Heterotopic Graft	Tissue transplanted into an unnatural anatomic position.
Histocompatible	A state whereby donor and recipient individuals have an identical complement of tissue antigens, and are mutually able to accept tissue grafts from each other without resultant stimulation of the immune system.
Histoincompatible	Antonym of "histocompatible".

Heterogenetic or Heterophile Antigens

Identical or cross-reacting antigens common to organisms of different species. Some of these are clinically important:

(1) Forssman's antigen: A peculiar hapten, widely and somewhat erratically distributed in nature amongst animals, plants, and bacteria. Amongst vertebrates in which it is present, it may occur in tissues or in erythrocytes; in some cases it is present in one but not the other. For example, in the guinea pig, this antigen occurs in the tissue but not in the red cells, whilst in the sheep it is found only in the erythrocytes, and in the dog, cat, tortoise, and fowl it occurs in both locations. It is found in human erythrocytes of types *A* and *AB* but not in human erythrocytes of other types. This substance is of academic interest only in the context of this chapter.

(2) Paul-Bunnell test for *infectious mononucleosis*: A person with *infectious mononucleosis* develops antibodies which agglutinate sheep red blood cells, but are not directed against the Forssman antigen. Presumably, the virus of *infectious mononucleosis* shares a heterophile antigen other than the Forssman antigen with sheep red blood cells. (*Vide supra*, Chapter 6).

(3) Weil-Felix test: *Rickettsi prowazeki* and *R. mooseri*, the aetiologic agents of epidemic and endemic *typhus*, share antigens with the OX19 strain of *Proteus vulgaris*, and thus, patients recovering from *typhus* develop circulating antibodies which will agglutinate *Proteus*.

Species-Specific Antigens

Each species of organism has an unique complement of tissue antigens shared by all individuals of these same species. Cross-reactivity between tissue antigens is maximal in closely-related species, and diminishes as evolutionary separation increases. However, certain primitive tissue components (such as collagen) have similar antigenic structure even in widely-separated species.

Organ-Specific Antigens

Most organs contain a large number of antigens. Many of these are shared by other tissues, but some are specific for particular organs. For example, one can make an organ-specific anti-kidney serum, or an antiserum specific for thyroglobulin.

Isoantigens

Antigenic differences between individuals of a species are known as isoantigens. Isoantigens are of greatest importance in the rejection of allografts. In the human, in addition to the red cell isoantigens discussed in Chapter 16 (*vide supra*), the most important tissue isoantigens are determined by a genetic locus containing two closely-linked groups of several alleles (*i.e.*, two subloci). The antigens determined by these alleles are known as *HL-A* antigens, and are listed in Figure 1.

The term *HL-A* is derived from *Human Leucocyte Antigens;* these antigens were first studied in human peripheral blood leucocytes. However, *HL-A* antigens are now known to be shared by most nucleated cells of the body. Antigens of both subloci are inherited in a straightforward Mendelian manner; most individuals have 4 *HL-A* antigens (2 in each sublocus), and there is approximately a 1:4 chance that two (dizygotic) siblings will have histocompatible phenotypes at both of these subloci, as may be seen in Figure 2.

The complexity of human tissue isoantigens is not surprising in view of the multi-allelic polygenic systems that determine the total complement of isoantigens in man. The chances, therefore, are virtually infinitesimal that two unrelated individuals would inherit identical sets of alleles at all of these loci, and consequently demonstrate identical antigenic phenotypes. For this reason, tissue allografts between an unrelated donor and recipient are usually accompanied by the development of rejection phenomena. Monozygotic (identical) twins have identical patterns (genotypes), since they began life as a single individual (zygote). The likelihood of histocompatibility occurring at both *HL-A* subloci amongst dizygotic siblings, is about 1:4 as has already been noted.

The Mechanism of Transplantation Rejection

Skin Allografts

A. First-Set Rejection: In an initial rejection (*i.e.*, a "first set" rejection), sensitised lymphocytes are found in the lymph-nodes which drain the site of the graft. These sensitised cells appear within 6-10 days after the graft has been put in place. The appearance of these cells is dependent on antigens from the grafted skin entering the lymphatics and stimulating an immune response in the regional lymph-nodes. These lymph-nodes enlarge and undergo certain characteristic changes (*e.g.*,

Figure I. THE HL-A ANTIGENS

1st sublocus (LA)	2nd sublocus (Four)
HL-A1	HL-A5
HL-A2	HL-A7
HL-A3	HL-A8
HL-A9	HL-A12
HL-A10	HL-A13
HL-A11	
W19.1	W 5
W 19.3	W 10
W 19.4	W 14
W 19.5	W 15
W 19.6	W 16
W23	W 17
W24	W 18
W25	W20
W26	W21
W28	W22
	W27

The nomenclature used here is that which was agreed upon at the 19th meeting of the World Health Organisation. The HL-A designation is for established specificities. The "W" designation is for new specificities, which, when better defined, will be given an HL-A designation.

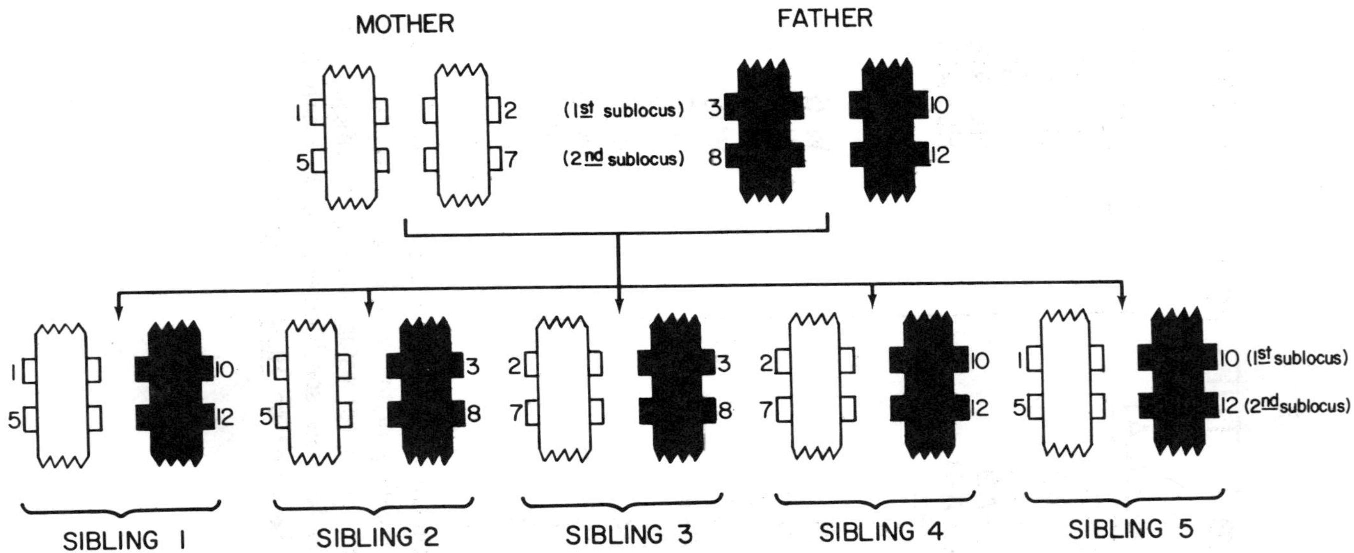

Figure 2. THE GENETICS OF HL-A INHERITANCE

proliferation of lymphoblasts and pyroninophilic cells). In skin grafts, vascularisation of skin graft coincides with these changes. The first clinical signs of rejection appear somewhat later, usually at 10-14 days. At this time, increasing numbers of sensitised lymphocytes are released into the circulation by the stimulated regional lymph-nodes. These sensitised lymphocytes are the primary mediators of first-set allograft rejections. They infiltrate the graft bed, where they are found in large numbers. Destruction of the graft is due to vascular damage, leading to thrombosis. The precise manner in which the vascular injury is produced is not entirely known.

B. Second-Set Rejection: If a second skin graft from the same donor is applied to the recipient after a first such graft has been rejected, accelerated destruction of the graft will occur, because the recipient has been sensitised to graft antigens during the first exposure. "Second-set" rejections are therefore much more rapid than "first-set" rejections. Individuals who have rejected one graft often have high titres of circulating cytotoxic antibodies to graft antigens, which usually appear after the first graft has been completely rejected. These antibodies appear to play no role in first-set rejections, but they are capable of initiating immediate cytotoxic effects upon second grafts in the presence of complement (*vide supra*, Chapter 15). Second-set rejection may occur so rapidly that the graft never becomes vascularised. For this reason these are often referred to as "white grafts".

Organ Grafts

In organ transplantation (such as heart or kidney), vascular anastomosis is accomplished by the surgeon; contact between cells of the donor and recipient occurs immediately. This represents the principal difference between organ and skin allografts; in skin grafts, vascularisation requires several days to establish itself. In other respects, the processes and mechanisms of rejection of both skin and organs are similar. Transplanted organs undergoing first-set rejections become infiltrated with mononuclear cells, which are believed to represent (at least in part) sensitised cells, produced by the recipient as a result of stimulation of the recipient's lymphoid system by antigens released from the transplanted tissue. It is not yet established whether these sensitised lymphocytes are primarily generated within the lymphoid organs of the recipient or within the perivascular spaces of the grafted organ itself. Regardless of the site of lymphocyte generation and transformation, the perivascular spaces around the post-capillary venules become heavily infiltrated with large mononuclear cells. Many of these cells show mitosis and evidence of active protein synthesis. Plasma-cells also appear. The organ becomes boggy, oedematous, and shows damage to its venule endothelium. Endothelial damage activates clotting factors, leading to intravascular thrombosis and ischaemic necrosis of the graft. Thus, first-set rejection of transplanted kidneys (like first-set skin rejections) depends on cellular (rather than humoral) immune mechanisms. However, where the recipient has become sensitised to graft isoantigens by previous grafts or multiple blood transfusions, circulating complement-activating cytotoxic antibodies may be present which can result in immediate injury to the graft. Clinical evidence of rejection may occur within hours or minutes. This is known as hyperacute rejection (*vide supra*, Chapter 15). The presence of such cytotoxic antibodies must be excluded in potential recipients before organ grafts are attempted, by careful cross-matching of prospective donors with potential recipients.

Chronic Rejection

The judicious use of immunosuppressive agents (*vide infra*, this chapter) can delay or prevent many features of acute graft rejection. However, in spite of their continued use, evidence of disease in the graft may appear after months (or even years) of successful graft function. In kidneys, chronic rejection usually manifests itself as gradual loss of renal function. Renal biopsy will often show sclerotic glomeruli, mild perivascular lymphoid infiltrates, (lymphocytes and plasma-cells) and prominent fibrous thickening of the intima of small arteries. Coronary intimal fibrosis has been noted similarly in long-standing heart transplants. These changes are evidence of chronic, smouldering graft rejection, modified by the use of immunosuppressive agents. The precise mechanisms of development of such modified rejection reactions, however, are not yet completely understood.

Graft-Versus-Host (GVH) Reactions

In the transplantation of immunocompetent tissues between individuals, the immunocompetence of the donor tissue as well as that of the recipient must be considered carefully. The importance of this has already been alluded to in Chapter 13 in connection with the concept of immunologic reconstitution of individuals with certain immune deficiency diseases (*vide supra*), and in the introduction to cellular responses in Chapter 2 (*vide supra*). Not only can recipient T-cells recognise donor antigens in transplanted tissue, but donor immunocytes present in the tissue graft can also respond to recipient isoantigens. In other words, not only can the host reject the graft, but the graft can also reject the host. The latter type of response has been termed a "graft-versus-host" (*GVH*) reaction.

Stigmata characteristic of *GVH*-reactions include: anaemia, leucopenia, thrombocytopenia, anorexia, cachexia, diarrhoea, alopecia and dermatitis. Unless vigorously treated with adequate doses of immunosuppressive therapy, a *GVH* reaction may terminate fatally.

Tissue Typing

In order to minimise the immune response to transplanted tissues, various tests have been developed to match, as closely as possible, the tissue antigens of the donor and the recipient. The matching begins with the *ABO*- and the *Rh*-antigens (for techniques employed, *vide supra*, Chapter 16). Next, the *ABO*- and *Rh*-matched prospective donor and recipient are matched for *HL-A* antigens. As each individual has from two to four *HL-A* antigens, and there are a multitude of antigens found in the human population (*vide supra*), it is difficult to find a donor and recipient pair with all four antigens matched. Statistical studies have indicated that, of the two subloci, matching of the 2nd sublocus antigens is more important in minimising the host-vs.-graft response. When the best possibly matched donor-recipient pair has been determined, a direct crossmatch test, using the potential recipient's serum and the prospective donor's lymphocytes, is performed to detect any circulating cytotoxic antibodies to the donor cell type in the recipient.

The determination of *HL-A* antigens is referred to as tissue typing. In tissue typing, a panel of sera from patients who have received multiple blood transfusions, or from grand multiparas, with known titres of anti-*HL-A* cytotoxic antibodies, are allowed to react with a sample of the patient's peripheral blood lymphocytes in the presence of rabbit complement. The antibodies in each serum sample have been previously characterised by the use of a cell panel containing all known specificities. The death of the lymphocytes upon reaction with a particular serum indicate the presence, on the cell surface, of the *HL-A* antigens to which the serum antibodies are directed.

The Mixed Leucocyte Reaction

If peripheral blood lymphocytes from two different individuals are mixed together in tissue culture, a certain number of them will transform into blasts and undergo mitosis. This is an immunological reaction, dependent on isoantigenic differences on the surfaces of each individual's cells. The degree to which the cells react corresponds fairly well with the level of histoincompatibility between the two individuals.

If the lymphocytes have broadly different isoantigen patterns, they respond (when mixed together in tissue culture) with a high level of blast cell transformation and mitotic activity; if, however, they have less profound differences in isoantigens, less blast transformation and mitotic activity occurs. Lymphocyte stimulation observed in mixed leucocyte cultures can therefore be used as a parameter of histocompatibility. However, the situation described above is a two-way reaction; the cells of each individual react against isoantigen differences in the other's cells. When matching potential organ donors with prospective recipients, therefore, it is usual to irradiate (or otherwise inactivate) the potential donor cells so that a one-way mixed leucocyte reaction which represents only the prospective recipient's reaction to the tissue isoantigens of the potential donor is obtained. Stimulation in mixed leucocyte reactions is usually assayed in the laboratory by measuring the uptake of H^3-Thymidine by recipient lymphocytes when mixed with inactivated donor lymphocytes.

The reversed one-way mixed leucocyte reaction (*vide supra*, this chapter) can be utilised as a parameter of *GVH*-reaction potential. To accomplish this, the leucocytes of the prospective recipient are inactivated prior to testing. Under those conditions, the uptake of H^3-Thymidine by transformed donor leucocytes will enable one to estimate the probability of serious *GVH*-reactions occurring following the transplantation of an organ containing immunologically-competent lymphoid cells.

The one-way mixed leucocyte reaction is practical for assessing histoincompatibility in the clinical laboratory, because only peripheral blood leucocytes are required; however, it cannot be used in situations where matching must be accomplished within a few hours. It has been employed profitably to assess the degree of histocompatibility of potential recipients with living prospective donors, where removal and storage of kidneys are not emergent problems.

Grafts in Privileged Sites

Certain areas appear to be peculiarly "privileged" since tissue grafts grow quite readily at these sites. For example, eyes of human cadavers, stored at low temperatures for periods of up to several days (in "eye banks") can be used as sources of corneal tissue for transplant into certain blind patients. The cornea is removed from the donor eye in the operating theatre, and grafted onto a patient blind from corneal opacification. Dramatic restoration of eyesight can result in suitably chosen recipients, usually without initiating rejection of the corneal graft. The principal reason for the lack of rejection is the relative avascularity of the corneal area; consequently, corneal isoantigens are less likely to reach the recipient's lymphoid system than similar tissue isoantigens grafted onto more vascularised regions of the body.

Another example of a "graft at a privileged site" is the human trophoblast and foetus *in utero*. During pregnancy, foetal chorionic villi, antigenically foreign to the mother, remain in intimate contact with the maternal circulation during the entire period of gestation. Moreover, abundant evidence exists that trophoblastic tissue is shed regularly into the maternal circulation during the second and third trimesters of pregnancy, and these trophoblastic emboli are destroyed by the mother, usually within the capillary beds of the lungs. Thus, it is virtually certain that foreign antigens from the foetus continually are released into the circulation of the immunologically-competent mothers, but fail to initiate significant maternal immune responses against the trophoblast and foetus *in utero*, although antibodies are often produced to the paternal antigens present in the foetus. The reasons for this are entirely unclear.

Other Deficiencies in Graft Rejection

Since cellular immunity is so intimately involved in rejecting grafted tissue, one might suspect that impairment of cellular immunity would result in impaired first-set allograft rejections. This is, in fact, the case; individuals with Di George's syndrome are virtually incapable of initiating primary graft rejection. Similarly, patients with Hodgkin's Disease (which impairs severely the function of the cellular [T-cell] division of the lymphoid system), reject allogeneic skin grafts extremely poorly; consequently these patients retain such grafts for prolonged intervals.

The Clinical Suppression of Allograft Rejection

As noted previously, it is important to match prospective donors and recipients of grafts as closely as possible to minimise immune responses against grafted tissue. Unfortunately, really close matches are rarely possible, and one must, therefore, suppress the recipient's immune system to prevent graft rejection. Clinical immunosuppression is presently accomplished in three different ways:

(1) Antimetabolites and Alkylating Agents: These drugs exert maximal effects against cell populations having rapid rates of multiplication. They are not highly selective for cells of the T-cell division of the lymphoid system, but may affect these cells somewhat more profoundly than cells of the B-cell division. Nonetheless, these drugs do exert profound effects on cells of the B-cell division, on haematopoietic tissue generally, and other mitotically-active cells (such as the mucosal cells of the gastrointestinal tract). Azathioprine (Imuran®) has been the antimetabolite of choice in clinical immunosuppression; it is the least toxic antimetabolite which still maintains adequate suppression of the T-cell division of the lymphoid system. Maintenance doses of azathioprine generally vary between 1.0 - 2.0 mgm/kg/day, when employed on a long-term basis. 6-Mercapto-purine (6-MP, Purinethol®) and cyclophosphamide (procytox, Cytoxan®) may be employed also for clinical immunosuppression.

(2) Adrenal Corticosteroids: The glucocorticoids (especially prednisone) are known to be anti-inflammatory and lymphocytotoxic. They have been used extensively in attempts to prevent first-set rejections by sensitised lymphocytes. Although cellular immunity is more profoundly suppressed than humoral immunity by corticosteroids, antibody synthesis is also inhibited, and many other untoward side-effects are associated with the use of these drugs in the high doses (20-300 mgm/day) needed to achieve adequate immunosuppression. These include the development of Cushing's syndrome, psychosis, aseptic necrosis of bone, hypertension, fluid retention, aggrevation of diabetes, peptic ulcers and severe infections. These complications of steroid therapy may be so severe that adequate doses of prednisone or other corticosteroid cannot be continued. It is customary to use both azathioprine and prednisone together to achieve immunosuppression, as they appear to exert a synergistic effect.

(3) Antilymphocytic Serum (ALS): Antiserum directed against human lymphocytes may be prepared by immunising horses with human lymphoid tissues. The globulin fraction of this antiserum (antilymphocyte globulin or *ALG*) is effective in suppressing graft rejection, without significant impairment of the B-cell division of the lymphoid system. Consequently, humoral immunity is not abolished by *ALS* or *ALG* treatment. It is not known precisely how *ALG* works, but its activity does not depend on cytotoxic effects upon lymphocytes. The most

potent preparations of *ALG* are made by immunising horses with human foetal thymocytes, derived from abortuses. Antisera to thymocytes appear to prevent antigen-reactive T-cells from responding to the foreign antigens of the graft, perhaps by blocking antigen recognition sites on the membranes of sensitised lymphocytes.

Since *ALS* is a mixture of foreign proteins, it is antigenic to man. Thus, immune responses will occur after injection of *ALS*, as evidenced by the production of precipitating antibodies against horse serum proteins in patients treated with *ALS*. Since *ALG* contains less foreign protein per equivalently-active dose, it is somewhat less antigenic than *ALS*. Nonetheless, reactions to *ALG* are by no means uncommon. Arthus reactions (*vide supra*, Chapter 10) can occur, and pain at the site of injection is a frequent (and often serious) handicap to the clinical use of *ALG*.

<u>Other Immunosuppressive Drugs</u>: Although many other drugs are available for immunosuppression, none have yet proven generally superior to azathioprine, prednisone and *ALG* in the clinic.

<u>Risks of Immunosuppressive Therapy</u>: Since none of the clinically-available immunosuppressives are specific in their action for only graft tissue isoantigens and immune responses against them, many undesired effects may result in consequence of treatment with these agents. Thus:

Infection is the principal cause of death in patients on long-term immunosuppressive therapy to support allogeneic organ grafts.

Secondly, such patients have a significantly elevated risk of developing lymphoreticular malignancy, perhaps from impairment of immune surveillance mechanisms, which ordinarily serve to control neoplastic growths (*vide infra*, Chapter 18).

To suppress rejection of allogeneic tissue, whilst allowing sufficient immunologic competence to remain for adequate control of infections and neoplasms is an extremely delicate problem in therapeutic management, which unfortunately has remained largely unsolved at present.

Tolerance

Whilst present efforts to avoid graft rejection lie in having a good tissue match and adequate immunosuppression, the frequent complications associated with immunosuppression and the development of chronic rejection syndromes after several years of apparently successful function have led to a search for better ways to prevent rejection. It seems likely that serious attempts will be made to utilise the phenomenon of immunological tolerance for this purpose (*vide supra*, Chapter 9). Specific acquired immunologic tolerance is a state wherein an individual manifests an inability to respond immunologically to a specific antigen, without impairment of immunologic responses to other antigens. Such states can be induced in experimental animals by three methods.

Neonatal Injections of Antigen

Newborn mice exposed to an antigen are rendered specifically tolerant to that antigen. This tolerance may persist for many months, although it tends to be lost gradually unless contact with the antigen persists. It is difficult to envision any direct application of this phenomenon to the human transplantation problem, (*vide supra*, Chapter 9).

High Dose Tolerance

Very large doses of certain antigens (especially polysaccharides) will result in "paralysis" of the immune system. Maintenance of this type of tolerance requires repeated injections of the antigen; immune responses to the antigen tend to occur when the antigen concentration declines. This also has not found practical application.

Low Dose Tolerance

Very small amounts of a purified, soluble antigen, given intravenously will sometimes inhibit the immune response to subsequent (larger) doses of the same antigen. This type of antigen-specific inhibition may occur even if subsequent injections are made strongly immunogenic by the use of adjuvants. The mechanism of this phenomenon is not now known. However, it appears to depend on bypassing macrophages, which ordinarily "process" primary doses of antigen. Initiation of low-dose tolerance has been used successfully to prolong allograft acceptance in animal experiments.

"Naturally-Occurring Non-Responders"

Certain individuals, without any previous desensitisation therapy, do not produce cytotoxic antibodies when exposed to certain HL-A antigens (other than their own). This non-reactivity appears to be selective: a patient may respond to all foreign HL-A antigens except one or two. A patient who fails to produce cytotoxic antibodies to a given antigen is referred to as a "non-responder" to that antigen.

This phenomenon could prove to be useful in organ transplantation. The patient, generally requiring multiple blood transfusions before transplantation, could be given blood of selected, known, HL-A types. Antibody response to the antigens would then be noted, allowing the determination of the antigens to which the patient does not respond. Tissue could then be transplanted to the patient even though there were antigenic differences, as long as the differing antigens on the donor tissue were among those to which the patient is a "non-responder".

Although none of the previously-discussed methods of inducing or observing specific tolerance has yet been employed successfully in human transplants, it is hoped that rapid progress in understanding the mechanisms of immune tolerance and immunity will hasten development of practical methods for inducing specific tolerance to graft antigens in the clinic.

Enhancement

A tumour from one strain of rat implanted into an individual of another (histoincompatible) strain will grow briefly, and subsequently be destroyed by the recipient's lymphoid system. Destruction of the tumour occurs because of its derivation from a histoincompatible strain of animals, differing antigenically from the recipient. A similar tumour transfer, this time accompanied by an injection of rabbit antibody to the tumour, may, in fact, prevent such tumour rejection. In fact, in the latter situation, the tumour may grow progressively and eventually kill the second host. This rather surprising effect, where antibody protects histoincompatible tumour cells from rejection, is known as "enhancement". Enhancing antibodies are usually not complement-fixing and not cytotoxic. The mechanism of enhancement is incompletely understood, but is thought to depend on antibody coating the transplanted tumour cells. These coated cells often may not stimulate the recipient's lymphoid system (inhibition at the afferent limb of the immune response). Moreover, when the lymphoid system is stimulated to produce sensitised lymphocytes, these effector cells may be prevented from contacting the target-cell antigens (efferent limb inhibition of immunity). Direct contact of sensitised lymphocytes with target-cells is necessary for cell-mediated cytolysis to occur.

The application of enhancement to tissue or organ grafts is promising. It has already been applied successfully to renal transplants in rats, wherein injection of non-cytotoxic antibody to kidney graft isoantigens markedly inhibits allograft rejection. It is possible, moreover, for recipients to develop non-cytotoxic antibodies to the antigens of transplanted organs; such non-cytotoxic antibodies may, in fact, help in preventing allograft rejection by sensitised lymphocytes. It yet remains to be seen whether enhancement phenomena will be able to be harnessed as practical methods of controlling allograft rejection in man.

Enhancement is not tolerance; in enhancement, immunologic responsiveness of the recipient is not impaired, but the effectors of graft rejection (*i.e.*, sensitised cells) are prevented from causing tissue injury because they cannot gain access to their target antigens. The preservation of all immune responses is a great advantage to organ-graft recipients, provided that these patients can be prevented from destroying the grafted organs.

Chapter 18

THE IMMUNOLOGY OF CANCER

The possibility that neoplastic growth may be susceptible to immunological control has intrigued investigators for many years. Thus, this field is presently under intensive investigation, in the hope that new, clinically-useful approaches to the problem of cancer therapy may be developed as knowledge of tumour immunity increases.

Most neoplasms can be regarded as antigenically-altered somatic cells. As described in Chapter 1, it seems likely that a major function of the immune system is to seek out and destroy such neoplastic cells arising during the life of the organism. Effective immunologic surveillance depends on tumour-specific antigenic determinants being present on the surfaces of neoplastic cells, which enable these altered cells to be recognised as "non-self" and destroyed by immunological reactions.

Tumour-specific antigens can often be demonstrated on the cell surfaces of neoplastic cells. In fact, tumours may be regarded as "autogenous tissue grafts", capable of stimulating immunological responses by virtue of their *tumour-specific transplantation antigens(TSTA)*.

In some cases, however, no immune responses by the patient to a growing tumour can be detected; thus, it would appear that the patient's immune response to tumour may be suppressed or circumvented. In fact, there is increasing opinion that tumours become established and grow progressively only when natural immune responses against them are inhibited, altered or suppressed in some way - *e.g.*, if the patient develops immunologic deficiencies which impair recognition of tumour-specific transplantation antigens.

Tumour Immunity in Animals

Immune responses to spontaneous, carcinogen-induced, and transplanted neoplasms in animals have been studied extensively as model systems for human cancer. Human experimentation is often not ethically possible; moreover, the marked heterogeneity of tissue isoantigens amongst unrelated individuals would frequently be expected to overshadow and obscure the weak responses to tumour-specific antigens in cases of allogeneic human tumour transplants.

Tumour Antigens of Viral-Induced Neoplasms in Experimental Animals

Viral-induced tumours possess a group of transplantation antigens determined by the viral genome; these antigens are not related to any other transplantation antigens of the species, strain, or organ in which the neoplasm originated. Three types of virus-specific antigens have been distinguished, and are illustrated in Figure 1.

(a) Surface Antigens: Surface antigens determined by the viral genome may be present on the cell membranes of neoplastic cells; furthermore, these antigens may be capable of acting as transplantation antigens. For example, mice inoculated with polyoma virus-induced tumour cells of xenogeneic, allogeneic or isogeneic origin will develop increased resistance to subsequent challenge with any tumour induced by the polyoma virus, whether or not infection of the recipient is established. In other words, all tumours induced by polyoma virus develop a virus-specific group of common surface antigens capable of provoking specific immune responses. These antigens, although not present on the naked polyoma virion itself, nonetheless represent viral gene products, encoded in the *DNA* of the polyoma virus.

(b) Intracellular Antigens: Intracellular antigens (denoted as T-antigens) can be identified in virus-induced animal tumours by immunofluorescent staining or by complement-fixation reactions. Like the surface antigens discussed above, T-antigens are encoded in viral *DNA* and are shared by all cells infected by a given virus, irrespective of the species of animal infected, or whether infection leads to oncogenesis. Thus, T-antigens can be recognised in carcinogenic, abortive or cytolytic infections by potentially-oncogenic viruses. The role of T-antigens in host resistance to virus-induced tumours is presently undetermined, but it is thought by many investigators to be rather inconsequential.

(c) Antigens Present on the Infective Viral Particle (Virion-Specific Antigens): In addition to the two types of antigens discussed above, viral-induced neoplasms may be accompanied by the development of specific antibodies to the antigens of the virion itself. Antigens of the virion are, of course, not transplantation antigens. Although antibodies to virion antigens generally do not affect the growth of the primary tumour, they are able to neutralise viral infectivity, thus preventing reinfection by the same agent. For example, rabbits infected with Shope papilloma virus develop circulating antibodies against the Shope virion during the course of their infection, which are capable

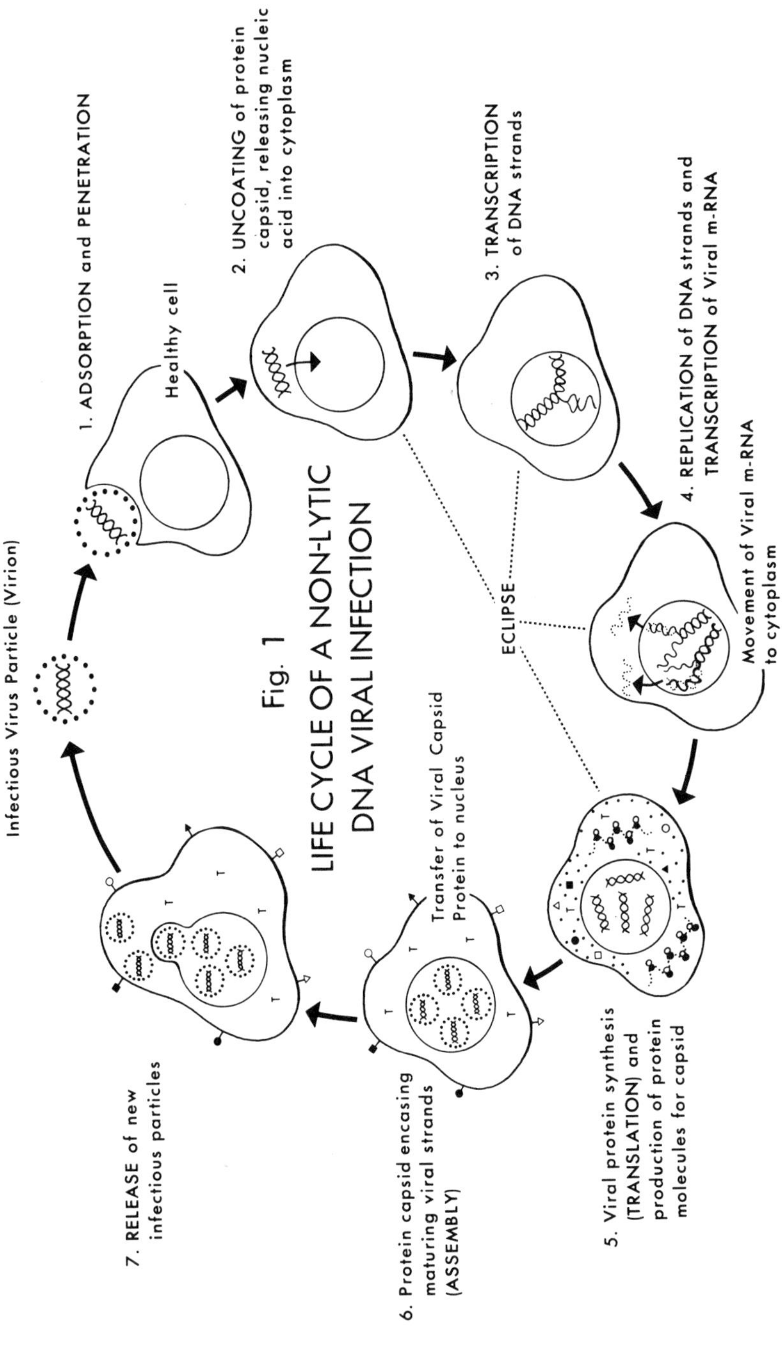

Fig. 1

LIFE CYCLE OF A NON-LYTIC DNA VIRAL INFECTION

of conferring further protection against second infections by the Shope virus, and are able also to effect passive transfer of resistance to Shope virus infection into uninfected recipient rabbits. As noted, however, such antibodies do not affect the growth of the original papilloma, since the virus is entirely in an eclipse phase within the papilloma (*vide supra*, Figure 1).

Immunologic Resistance to Virus-Induced Neoplasms of Experimental Animals

Some viral-induced tumours will grow only when a state of specific immune tolerance to virus-specific antigens is present. For example, the mouse mammary tumour virus (*MTV* or Bittner virus), secreted in maternal milk, infects suckling mice before they develop immunologic competence. These mice become tolerant both to the virus and to transplanted (*MTV*-induced) tumours. Thus, (otherwise susceptible) mice suckled by virus-free mothers are able to resist later transplantation of mammary tumours, whilst similar mammary tumour implants grow readily in other mice of the same strain suckled as neonates by *MTV*-infected mothers. Virus-free mice resist tumour implants because they respond immunologically to *MTV*-specific transplantation antigens, thus inhibiting the growth of tumours induced by this virus. Mice infected during the neonatal period, on the other hand, are unable to respond immunologically to tumour implants because they have developed tolerance to transplantation antigens determined by the *MTV*.

Surface antigens appear to be the transplantation antigens of greatest importance in enabling experimental animals to resist challenges with viral-induced tumours; *i.e.*, resistance to implants of viral-induced tumours in normal animals seems to be dependent largely upon the development of immunologic responses to surface antigens of virus transformed tumour cells.

Tumour Antigens of Neoplasms Induced by Physical or Chemical Carcinogens in Experimental Animals

Tumours induced by physical or chemical carcinogens may have individually-unique antigenic profiles. Thus, a series of similar tumours induced in a single genetically homogenous strain of animals by a single carcinogenic agent may not share common transplantation antigens of the sort characteristic of tumours induced by a single oncogenic virus. Although these tumour-specific transplantation antigens are different from membrane-bound antigens found on the surface of normal cells (*i.e.*, the tissue isoantigens discussed in previous chapters; *vide supra*, Chapters 16 & 17), they constitute relatively weak antigens. For this reason, tumour-cells of this nature can easily be transplanted from one animal to another provided the two individuals

Fig. 2

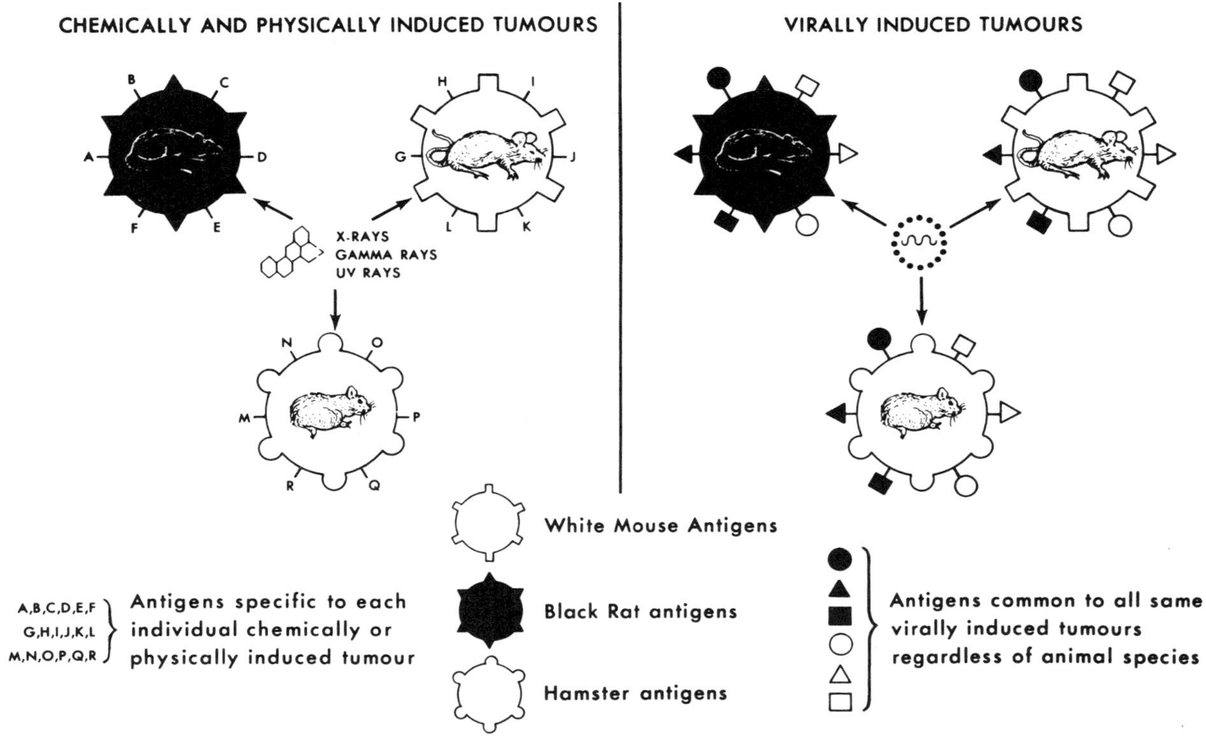
CHEMICALLY AND PHYSICALLY INDUCED TUMOURS
VIRALLY INDUCED TUMOURS
A
B
C
D
E
F
G
H
I
J
K
L
M
N
O
P
Q
R
X-RAYS
GAMMA RAYS
UV RAYS
White Mouse Antigens
Black Rat antigens
Hamster antigens
A,B,C,D,E,F
G,H,I,J,K,L
M,N,O,P,Q,R
Antigens specific to each individual chemically or physically induced tumour
Antigens common to all same virally induced tumours regardless of animal species

share common tissue isoantigens, without problems of rejection becoming apparent. Research on chemically-induced neoplasms in animals has been carried out predominantly in highly-inbred strains of mice or rats, since transfer of tumour-cells, and resultant tumour development is greatly facilitated under these conditions. Antigenic profiles characteristic of viral and carcinogen induced tumours are compared in Fig. 2.

An animal bearing a transplanted tumour often does not demonstrate any measurable immune response to the tumour; *i.e.*, no circulating antibodies against tumour antigens can be detected and no "sensitised" lymphocytes capable of reacting with tumour-cells are found in the blood or lymph-nodes. However, there is evidence for the presence of *TSTA* even under these conditions. If the tumour is excised before it kills the animal, or if only small tumour-cell grafts (cell numbers insufficient to cause tumour development) are given, or if the animal receives immunisation with inactivated tumour-cells prior to tumour-cell graft, the animal may develop increased resistance to challenge with subsequent tumour implants. Tumour specific immunity has thus developed, which provides effective resistance to the growth of the same tumour. However, immunity to other tumours induced by the same agent would not necessarily be expected.

Immunity to such tumour transplants can be transferred passively by injection of lymphocytes from immune donor animals into normal (isogeneic) recipients, but not by injection of immune donor serum. Effective immunity is therefore thought to be cellular rather than humoral. This concept is further supported by the demonstration that lymphocytes from animals with acquired resistance to a tumour will show cytotoxic effects against tissue-culture cells derived from the same tumour. The tumour-cells are destroyed by the "sensitised lymphocytes" in a process requiring cell-to-cell contact. Moreover, delayed hypersensitivity (another cell-mediated immune reaction) can sometimes be demonstrated by intradermal injections of tumour extracts in animals with acquired resistance to a tumour.

Whilst many cell-mediated immune reactions to tumours have been described in experimental animals, and some of these are known to confer resistance to neoplastic growth, the role of serum antibodies to tumour antigens in conferring protection against tumour growth is far less clear. It is known that an animal which has developed a tumour, and subsequently has become immunised to it, may demonstrate circulating antibodies to tumour antigens, detectable by agglutination, cytotoxicity, immunofluorescence or complement-fixation. In fact, antisera possessing high titres of specific anti-tumour antibodies can be produced by repeated immunisations with tumour antigens. However, such antisera unfortunately exert unpredictable effects on tumour growth when tested in animals bearing transplanted tumours. For example, such antisera may inhibit, enhance or exert no effect on tumour growth, the ultimate effects depending partly on the nature of the tumour, including its relative size and structure, and partly on the nature of the antibodies. Generally, *solid tumours* are more resistant to cytotoxic antibody, even in large doses, than are ascites tumours.

It is evident from the foregoing discussion that animal tumours possess specific antigenic determinants capable of eliciting immune responses in (non-tolerant) susceptible animals. However, naturally-occurring immune responses to tumour antigens are usually weak - in fact, often undetectable - unless the tumour is excised and the animal tested after excision. Such ineffectual responses usually exert little or no influence on the development and clinical course of the tumour. When immunological resistance to tumour transplantation is demonstrable, cellular (rather than humoral) immunity appears to be the primary effector of tumour resistance.

Human Tumours

The antigenic structure of human tumours and the nature of immune responses to them in many cases is still poorly understood. To some extent, the lack of understanding is due to the great difficulties inherent in conducting human experimentation. Thus, the status of human *TSTA* are at present somewhat unclarified. In a number of human neoplastic conditions, including *Burkitt's lymphoma, malignant melanoma, osteogenic sarcoma,* certain types of *leukaemia, neuroblastoma* and *transitional cell carcinoma of the bladder,* tumour specific antigens common to each tumour type have been demonstrated. Moreover, accumulating evidence suggests that other human tumours may demonstrate similar group-specific transplantation antigens as well. The presence of common group antigens has been offered as evidence for the viral aetiology of such tumours. However, viral aetiology has never been established incontrovertibly for any human tumour, and common tumour antigens may also reflect derepression of genes in certain types of cancer which encode information for foetal antigens.

Many clinical and laboratory observations suggest that immune mechanisms may play an important part in resistance to some human tumours. For example, certain human tumours, which are heavily-infiltrated with lymphocytes and inflammatory cells, or which are accompanied by reactive hyperplasia in draining lymph-nodes, have slower rates of growth and better prognoses than similar tumours unaccompanied by such phenomena. Medullary carcinoma of the breast represents one example of this type of situation, in which lymphoid infiltrates or lymph-node hyperplasia appear to represent immune reactions against the neoplasm.

The ability to, or the manner in which, cancer patients respond to the *TSTA* on their own tumours or on other similar tumours may be measured in several ways:

a) The patient may be tested directly by intradermal injections of extracts or killed cells from an autologous or heterologous tumour.

b) The patient's lymphocytes may be tested *in vitro* for their ability to inhibit the growth of autologous or related tumour cells.

c) Tumour extracts or preparations of tumour cell membranes may be tested for their ability to stimulate the production of MIF in the lymphocytes from cancer patients (*vide supra*, Chapter 4).

d) The patient's serum may be tested for its ability to kill preparations of autologous or heterologous living tumour cells in the presence of complement *in vitro*.

e) The patient's serum may also be tested for its ability to inhibit the cellular response of that individual to his own tumour cells (the presence of blocking factors).

Numerous studies similar to those enumerated above have been carried out, with widely varying observations. However, a general consensus at present would appear to indicate the following:

a) A significant number of patients exhibit cellular immunity to their own as well as to related tumours. The most comprehensive data of this type comes from Karl-Eric and Ingegerd Hellström, who have utilised colony formation by tumour cells, primarily derived from neuroblastomas, as an *in vitro* assay for cell-mediated immunity to those neoplastic cells. Their data suggest that the "blocking factors" observed may constitute complexes of antibody and soluble tumour-antigens which in some way serve to prevent access of sensitised lymphocytes to the neoplastic target-cells. Serum taken from patients following surgery or other therapeutic measures which decrease effectively the numbers of tumour cells in the body (*i.e.*, induce temporary or complete remission) does not contain such "blocking factors". Such serum should not inhibit (and may augment) the killing of tumour cells by sensitised lymphocytes.

Immunotherapy in Human Cancer

Efforts have been made to stimulate immunological responsiveness in cancer patients, in the hope of suppressing progressive growth of their tumours. Such efforts have included both specific and non-specific immunologic stimulants. Specific immunotherapy involves repeated injection of the patient with preparations derived from autologous tumour, such as irradiated tumour cells, chemically-modified tumour cells (or tumour extracts), or tumour cells inactivated by enzyme treatment. The results of such experiments have generally been equivocal. However, rather interesting data has now begun to appear about the use of immunotherapy with tumour cell preparations treated with the enzyme *neuraminidase*. Neuraminidase, an enzyme derived from *V. Cholerae*,removes sialic acid residues from the surfaces of cell membranes. This is thought to reduce the surface electronegativity of the tumour cells, thus allowing increased surface interactions with sensitised lymphocytes to occur. However, an alternative explanation - *i.e.*, that neuraminidase treatment may expose previously-sequestered *TSTA*, is also feasible.

Non-specific immunotherapy has involved repeated administrations of non-specific immunologic stimulants, the most common of which have been B.C.G. and vaccinia virus. Although studies at present are somewhat limited and often inadequately controlled, they do indeed suggest that beneficial effects can be obtained in patients with malignant melanoma, a variety of haematologic malignancies, bronchogenic carcinoma, carcinoma of the breast, and other types of cancer. Non-specific immunotherapy appears to work best under conditions where partial or complete remissions have been induced by appropriate surgery, intensive chemotherapy, and/or radiotherapy - *i.e.*, where a relatively small number of neoplastic cells remain in the body. Under these conditions, the response to non-specific immunotherapy appears to augment the body's specific immune responses to tumour cells.

The use of dinitrochlorobenzene (*DCNB*) in treating certain types of skin cancer also appears to represent a promising new type of immunologic therapeutic modality. Patients are sensitised by topical application of *DCNB* as an ointment. Following sensitisation, *DCNB* is applied to affected areas of skin. Thus, a specific cellular response surrounding the neoplasm may occur, with consequent lymphocytic infiltration of the affected region, and concomitant destruction of the neoplasm in the resultant type IV reaction (*vide supra*, introduction to Section II).

Tumour-Specific Antigens in Human Cancer

Many (perhaps most) related human tumours share certain specific antigenic components. This fact requires some explanation as to the possible mechanism(s) involved in this situation. Thus, a discussion of the possible biological derivation of such common tumour antigens is indicated.

To date, evidence for two distinct mechanisms for the occurrence of common group antigens in some tumours has accumulated:

(1) Certain antigens frequently associated with neoplasms are immunologically cross-reactive (or identical) with human foetal tissue antigens. These are termed *onco-foetal antigens*.

(2) Certain antigens from human tumours have been shown to be immunologically identical (or cross-reactive) to known viral antigens. Members of the herpes virus group have been clearly recognised in this context. For example, carcinomas of the cervix contain antigens of one herpes virus, and lymphoblasts from Burkitt's lymphoma contain antigens of another herpes virus, the *EB*-virus (*vide infra*).

Foetal Antigens in Cancer

A number of antigens occurring in neoplastic cells are identical to antigens found in the human embryo or foetus. These may or may not be associated with the cell membrane and may or may not stimulate humoral or cell-mediated immune reactions in cancer patients.

Carcinoembryonic Antigen (CEA): Gold and Freedman showed several years ago that a large percentage of malignant tumours of endodermal origin (*e.g.*, colon, stomach, pancreas, lung, liver) contained an antigenic material which cross-reacted with a similar material prepared from foetal digestive organs (but not the lungs). Immunofluorescent studies show that *CEA* is located on the surfaces of both cancer cells and foetal cells. It probably represents an extracellular material comprising part of the *glycocalyx*. By use of radioimmunoassay, it has been possible to demonstrate the presence of *CEA* in the serum of most patients with colonic tumours, and in some patients, before cancer of the colon could be demonstrated by other diagnostic procedures. Detectable circulating levels of *CEA*, however, are not always indicative of malignancy. Heavy smokers, alcoholics with hepatic cirrhosis, patients with ulcerative colitis, or individuals with (non-malignant) adenomatous polyps all have *CEA* in their serum, but nearly always less than the levels occurring in malignancy. *CEA* is immunogenic in humans; circulating antibody to it has been detected in both cancer patients and pregnant women. More will be said about *CEA* antibodies presently (*vide infra*, this Chapter).

α - Foeto Protein: Some human hepatomas (estimates differ from 30% to 80% of cases tested, depending on the assay employed) produce detectable levels of this protein in the plasma. It is synthesised in the foetus by perivascular hepatic parenchymal cells. In addition to its synthesis by hepatomas and by foetal hepatocytes, α-foeto protein is synthesised by gonadal teratoblastomas (malignant teratomas). α-foeto protein is not immunogenic in humans, and therefore, is of no potential interest as an agent for specific immunotherapy in human cancer.

Foetal Sulphoglycoprotein: This substance occurs in the gastric mucus of patients with gastric adenocarcinoma, as well as in extracts of foetal digestive organs. It is not immunogenic in man, perhaps because it is produced by normal enteric tissue in amounts sufficient to cause immunologic tolerance.

Regan Isoenzyme of Alkaline Phosphatase: This is a placental isoenzyme of alkaline phosphatase characterised antigenically, electrophoretically, and by its thermostability pattern. This isoenzyme occurs in a variety of carcinomas, as well as in placental trophoblast. It, too, is not immunogenic in man; perhaps, like foetal sulphoglycoprotein, because it is produced by adult tissue in amounts adequate to induce and maintain a state of specific immunologic tolerance.

Viral Antigens in Cancer

Information pertaining to the presence of virus-specific antigens in human cancer is increasing, though still somewhat scanty. Recent investigations have shown the presence of antigens specific for herpes viruses in cancer of the lip and invasive cancer of the cervix. Moreover, cultured lymphocytes from patients with Burkitt's lymphoma can be shown to contain antigenic components of a peculiar herpes virus known as the Epstein-Barr (*EB*) virus, the presence of which can also be demonstrated by electron microscopy.

Cellular Immunity to Neoplasms in Man

The T-cell division of the immune system has been established as being of paramount importance in resistance to experimentally-induced neoplasms in animals, and is believed to be of similar importance as a mechanism of resisting neoplastic growths in man.

Thus, the mechanisms of resistance to and destruction of neoplastic disease in man appear to be fundamentally similar to the mechanisms of rejection of transplanted tissue, discussed in the previous chapter (*vide supra*, Chapter 17), with tumour-specific transplantation antigens replacing the isoantigens of allogeneic donors as the principal antigens provoking an immune response.

It has been noted repeatedly that patients in whom cellular immunity is impaired or defective are at especially high risk to certain neoplastic diseases. Thus, it would seem that impaired T-cell function may favour the progressive growth of neoplastic cells.

Let us now examinc some of the general evidence supporting this concept:

(a) Malignancy and Lymphopenia: Patients with widely-disseminated neoplasms of many types tend to have levels of lymphocytes below normal.

(b) Malignancy and T-Cell Dysfunction: Patients with disseminated malignancies have lower than normal spontaneous responsiveness to skin-tests with candidin, tuberculin, histoplasmin, and other standard skin-test antigens (*vide supra*, Chapter 12). Moreover, such patients demonstrate impairment of their ability to be sensitised in the clinic to such strongly-sensitising substances as 2, 4-DNCB and Picryl chloride (*vide supra*, Chapter 12), and impairment of their ability to reject skin allografts (*vide supra*, Chapter 17). Finally, patients with continued demonstrable impairment of cellular immunity following surgical excision of their neoplasms generally have poor prognoses, whilst patients whose cellular immunity improves following surgery generally have good prognoses.

(c) As already discussed in Chapter 14 and above, many diseases of immunological deficiency are associated with a high incidence of certain types of malignancy.

(d) Finally, as noted in Chapter 17 (*vide supra*), patients receiving immunosuppressive therapy over long periods are at high risk to the development of certain types of malignancy. Moreover, withdrawal of immunosuppression may result in regression of the neoplasm in some cases.

Humoral Responses to Human Tumour Antigens

Circulating antibodies to tumour antigens are not generally detectable in human cancer patients. However, the demonstration of such antibodies may depend on the type of tumour, the presence (or absence) of metastases, and the sensitivity of the detection methods employed.

Carcinoembryonic Antigen: A large percentage of patients with non-metastatic adenocarcinoma of the colon and other tissues of endodermal origin develop circulating antibodies to *CEA*. However, antibodies of similar specificity for this antigen also occur in the sera of most pregnant women, in some individuals who are heavy smokers or alcoholics, and in many patients with intestinal polyposis or ulcerative colitis.

Upon excision of a colonic tumour, plasma *CEA* falls to a normal level, and the antibody disappears. If the patient is followed serially for plasma *CEA*, a rise in this parameter appears to be a reliable indicator of developing metastases - frequently occurring before metastases can be diagnosed by conventional means.

The observations discussed above are indicative that some tumour antigens may represent products of derepressed genes, related in some way to the embryonic or foetal state, rather than *de novo* products of mutation. These observations thus lend support to a widely-held concept of neoplasia; namely, that many neoplastic growths represent reversions to an embryonic state in which augmented proliferative activity represents one characteristic facet.

Viral Antigens: Although there has been little positive data showing the presence of specific viral antigens in human neoplasms, there is considerable evidence concerning the development of virus-specific antibodies by patients with a variety of cancers. High titres of antisera to Epstein-Barr (*EB*) virus were found in 87% of Burkitt's lymphoma patients, as opposed to 14% in controls. In women with carcinoma of the cervix, >80% have elevated antibody levels to type 2 herpes simplex virus, compared with <30% of controls.

Numerous efforts (generally unsuccessful) have been made to control human tumours by passive transfer of antibodies. The antisera employed have usually not been specific for tumour antigens. For example, if horses are immunised with human tumours, the antibodies produced are primarily directed against the strong species-specific antigens found on both normal and neoplastic cells. It is apparent that tumour-specific transplantation (membrane-bound) antigens comprise a very small percentage of the total cell-surface antigens of the tumour cell. Thus, tumour-specific antigens are generally weak stimulants of B-cells, and elicit little antibody formation when used to immunise animals of a different species. Furthermore, when (and if) strong tumour-specific antisera can be produced, it is not known whether such sera will enhance or inhibit the growth of the tumour. The observation that *in vitro* killing of tumour cells by specifically-sensitised T-cells can be abrogated by a serum factor from immunised individuals supports this possibility.

Enhancement of Tumour Growth: Enhancement of tumour growth by non-cytotoxic humoral antibodies has been described in the previous chapter (*vide supra*). Although the mechanisms of enhancement are not entirely understood, the coating of tumour cells by non-cytotoxic enhancing antibodies probably affects both the afferent and efferent limbs of the immune response. Thus, for example, enhancing antibodies which coat tumour-cells may mask tumour antigens, similarly to the way in which anti-*D* antiserum is believed to prevent the isoimmunisation of *Rh*-negative mothers by *Rh*-positive babies at time of delivery, (*vide supra*, Chapter 16). In addition, enhancing antibodies which coat tumour-cells may prevent the access of specifically-sensitised lymphocytes to surface antigens of tumour-cells. Since cytotoxic effects of sensitised lymphocytes require direct contact of sensitised cells and target-cells, cytotoxic effects would be inhibited by the interposition of enhancing antibodies, which would prevent cell-to-cell contact.

Whatever its mechanism, spontaneous development of enhancement in human cancer patients may enable certain tumours to overcome cell-mediated resistance mechanisms which might otherwise destroy them or suppress their progressive growth.

Although enhancement has been studied extensively only in experimental animals, there is good indirect evidence that it also occurs in man. For example, let us consider the situation occurring in chorioncarcinoma (chorionepithelioma) of the uterus in the human female.

Chorioncarcinoma of the uterus in the human female is an immunologically-unique neoplasm, since it is derived from trophoblastic tissue representing a composite of paternal and maternal genotypes and isoantigenic phenotypes. In spite of the fact that it is antigenically "foreign" to the patient (since half of its antigens are paternally-derived), it is amongst the most malignant of neoplastic diseases. Chorioncarcinoma may follow full-term pregnancy, ectopic pregnancy, abortion, or hydatidiform mole. Its course (if untreated) is usually fulminant, since growth is exceedingly rapid and metastases are both widespread and highly invasive. However, a small but consistent number of untreated cases regress spontaneously and completely, presumably as a result of an effective cell-mediated immune response developing in the patient.*

In one study, two groups of patients with chorioncarcinoma of the uterus were compared in an attempt to correlate the presence of antibodies to the husband's leucocyte antigens (*e.g.*, antibodies directed at the husband's *HL-A* antigens) with the prognosis of the disease. One group of patients lacked such antibodies in their sera, but another group did possess circulating antibodies of this type. The anti-leucocyte antibodies were assayed by means of an agglutination reaction occurring upon mixture of serial dilutions of the patients' serum with suspensions of peripheral blood leucocytes from the husbands.

The first group of patients (*i.e.*, the group in which serum leucoagglutinins could not be demonstrated) rejected skin allografts from their husbands readily, and were shown to have a better overall prognosis from their disease than patients of the second group.

The second group of patients (*i.e.*, those patients possessing demonstrable serum leucoagglutinins) were unable to reject skin allografts from their husbands. Moreover, they tended to have a poor overall prognosis in the face of rapidly-advancing disease.

These observations suggest that the leucoagglutinins observed in the second group of patients act as enhancing antibodies in at least one human tumour - *i.e.*, chorioncarcinoma of the uterus.

There is now little doubt that immune responses play an important or decisive role in the growth and development of neoplasms. Although single explanations cannot yet account for all of the phenomena relating neoplastic diseases to immune responses, continuing studies are increasing our understanding in many areas. Control of neoplastic growth by immunological means (immunotherapy) has not yet been achieved reliably in human cancer, but the hope of achieving it in the near future is quite realistic, and even highly probable.

* *The natural history of this tumour has been markedly altered by chemotherapy in recent years. Presently, a 74% cure rate is obtained by sequential use of Actinomycin-D and Methotrexate, with local radio-therapy and surgery where indicated.*

Chapter 19

AUTOIMMUNITY IN MEDICINE

Problems in Terminology and Definition

Antibodies and/or lymphocytes, capable of reacting against a patient's own tissue components or cells, occur in a number of human diseases. Such "autoantibodies" or "auto-sensitised (autoreactive) lymphocytes" are manifestations of autoimmunity; *i.e.*, immune reactions against "self". Certain human diseases, in which autoantibodies or autoreactive lymphocytes occur readily, have been frequently termed "autoimmune diseases"; such nomenclature, however, would imply that the autoantibodies or lymphocytes have primary pathogenetic significance. An autoimmune reaction has never been proven to be the initiating (primary) pathogenetic event in any spontaneously-occurring human disease, although autoimmune phenomena probably do represent important pathogenetic mechanisms. Oversimplified and blind acceptance of autoimmunity as a primary cause of many poorly-understood human diseases has undoubtedly obscured the true primary aetiology of many human diseases which demonstrate autoimmune phenomena. The use of the term "autoimmune disease" should probably be avoided at this time; its use would be more appropriate if (and when) autoimmune phenomena can be shown to be primary causes of disease.

Theoretical Mechanisms for the Development of Autoimmunity

Immunological tolerance to body components prevents the occurrence of autoimmune phenomena in most healthy individuals; however, this tolerance to "self" might theoretically break down under any of the following circumstances:

(a) Sequestered Antigen: An autologous antigen might never contact antigen-receptive lymphoid cells until after the period of embryological development in which tolerance to "self" normally develops (*vide supra*, Chapter 9 and 17). This mechanism has been postulated for autoimmune reactions against thyroglobulin (in *Hashimoto's struma*), seminiferous tubules (in *aspermia*), brain tissue (in *disseminated (multiple) sclerosis*) and the uveal tract of the eye (in *sympathetic uveitis (ophthalmia)*).

(b) Altered Antigen: Some chemical, physical or microbiological event might alter an antigen so that it is no longer recognised as "self" by the lymphoid system. The consequence would be an immunological reaction against the altered antigen. An example of a reaction of this type is contact dermatitis to the hapten, *DNCB*. This compound attaches itself covalently to free amino-groups of skin proteins, and induces cellular immunity to the complex (*vide supra*, Chapter 12).

(c) Release of "Forbidden" Clones: A mutation might occur in lymphoid cells, resulting in the production and proliferation of clones of immunocompetent cells, whose activity is directed against normal tissue antigens. Consequently, these normal tissue antigens could become prone to immunologic attack, since they would be no longer recognised as "self". This hypothesis has currently little direct evidence to support it in any particular disease (*vide supra et infra*, Chapters 9 and 23).

(d) Heterophile Antigen: An infecting organism might contain an antigenic determinant similar to some component of the host's body (*i.e.*, a heterophile antigen). In reacting against the invading organism, the host might thus produce antibodies which cross-react with its own tissues (*vide infra*, this chapter, discussion of *rheumatic myocarditis*).

Types of Observable Autoimmune Phenomena in Medicine

Antinuclear Antibodies (Antinuclear Factors, A.N.F.): These autoantibodies, directed against one or more components of cell nuclei, may be demonstrated by a variety of immunological techniques, *e.g.*, complement fixation, agglutination, precipitation, indirect immunofluorescence (*vide supra*, Chapter 6), or the unique *LE-cell test* in which nuclear material complexed with A.N.F. is phagocytosed by polymorphonuclear neutrophiles. The antibodies are usually of (*7S*) IgG type, and generally fix complement; occasionally, (*19S*) IgM or IgD antinuclear antibodies can be demonstrated.

Antinuclear antibodies are a prominent feature of *disseminated lupus erythematosus (DLE)*, and may be directed against nucleoprotein, nuclear membrane, *DNA*, or nucleolar antigens. Amongst the various types of *A.N.F.*'s, the anti-*DNA* antibody (and the *LE-cell* factor) are almost diagnostic of *DLE*, but the antinucleoprotein antibodies are less specific, and occur in other diseases. For example, *A.N.F.*'s of the latter type occur quite frequently in patients with long-standing *rheumatoid arthritis;* unlike those occurring in *DLE* they are mostly (*19S*) IgM in this disease. *Chronic active ("lupoid") hepatitis*, a disease of viral aetiology, is another disease often manifesting antinuclear antibodies. Antinuclear factors appear in the serum of patients following treatment with certain drugs; *e.g.*, *hydralazine (Apresoline®)* and *procaine amide (Pronestyl®)*. After prolonged administration of procaine amide, about 50% of individuals will develop antinuclear factors.

Antinuclear antibodies do not react with the nuclei of living cells, because of their inaccessibility to the antibodies. These antibodies may, however, complex with nuclear antigens of damaged cells in the presence of complement, and such complexes may injure endothelium or basement membranes when deposited in small arterioles or capillaries. For example, the glomerulitis occurring in *DLE* may result from the deposition of these complexes adjacent to the glomerular basement-membrane similarly to the way in which antigen-antibody-complement complexes are pathogenetic in post-Streptococcal glomerulonephritis (*vide supra*, Chapter 10).

Antigammaglobulin antibodies: These are prominent in *rheumatoid arthritis* and are commonly referred to as *"rheumatoid factors" (vide supra*, Chapter 6). Usually, they consist of (*19S*) IgM antibodies directed against γ-chain-specific antigenic determinants. Consequently, rheumatoid factors thus have the property of reacting with (*7S*) IgG. Rheumatoid factors most probably arise as by-products of prolonged antigenic stimulation. They have, in fact, been produced experimentally in animals by prolonged hyperimmunisation with bacterial antigens. Moreover, such antibodies occur naturally in patients with a variety of chronic infections which result in hypergammaglobulinaemia, and can be demonstrated in a majority of patients with *subacute bacterial endocarditis*.

Antigammaglobulin antibodies are normally demonstrated in the clinical laboratory by their ability to agglutinate particles (*e.g.*, red cells, latex, or bentonite) which have been coated with (*7S*) IgG, as noted in Chapter 6. They can also be demonstrated by immunofluorescence, or, in some cases, by complement-fixation. The latter method, however, is often insensitive and misleading. In some rheumatoid patients, serum rheumatoid factor titres above 1:5000 may be obtained. However, when very sensitive methods are employed for the demonstration of rheumatoid factors, low titres of antiglobulin antibodies can be demonstrated in many normal people, and are thus of little clinical significance *per se*.

As in the case of antinuclear antibodies, few direct harmful effects have been attributed to the mere presence of antiglobulin antibodies. It is possible, however, that complexes of such antibodies with IgG and complement may occur *in vivo;* these complexes may be responsible for certain inflammatory reactions occurring within the joints of patients with rheumatoid arthritis. For example, it has been shown that intra-articular injections of small amounts of purified IgG (3 mg.) into the knees of rheumatoid patients positive for rheumatoid factor can elicit acute arthritis in the injected joints. Furthermore, it is likely that arteritic or arteriolitic lesions occurring in patients with rheumatoid arthritis may be the result of deposition of such complexes adjacent to arteriolar endothelium.

Autoantibodies Against Blood Cells: Some patients with haemolytic anaemia have a positive direct Coombs' test (*vide supra*, Chapter 6) - indicating that these patients possess antibodies (IgG or IgM) attached to their red cell membranes. When antibodies to red cell membrane antigens react with a patient's own red cells and result in haemolysis, the diseases in which such antibodies occur are termed "autoimmune haemolytic anaemias".

Antiplatelet antibodies and antigranulocyte antibodies have been incriminated as causes of thrombocytopenia and neutropenia. In such cases, passive transfer of serum from patients with either condition to normal individuals may result in the development of transient thrombocytopenia or granulocytopenia in the recipient.

Although damage to the cell-membranes of circulating blood cells may result from non-specific absorption of preformed antigen-antibody-complement complexes onto the membranes, there is little doubt that the antibodies discussed above are usually directed specifically at actual antigens on respective target-cell membranes. Thus, haemolytic anaemias, thrombocytopenias, and granulocytopenias of this type may be designated justifiably as autoimmune phenomena of pathogenetic significance. However, the primary aetiology of the above conditions is usually not known; for this reason, classification of these entities as primary "autoimmune diseases" is not justified. Viral or mycoplasmal infections are reasonable candidates for primary aetiologic agents in some cases of haemolytic anaemia, granulocytopenia, or thrombocytopenic purpura. For example, *Mycoplasma pneumoniae* infections frequently initiate the development of "cold agglutinins", *i.e.*, antibodies which agglutinate erythrocytes at 0 - 5°C, but are inactive at 37°C. Some patients develop mild haemolytic anaemia following *Mycoplasma pneumoniae* pneumonia, but the relationship of clinical haemolytic anaemia to the presence of "cold agglutinins" remains rather tenuous at present.

<u>Antitissue Antibodies</u>: Serum antibodies reacting with tissue components or extracts are demonstrable in patients with a variety of diseases. Such antibodies have been demonstrated by complement-fixation, immunofluorescence, and agglutination. In certain diseases of obscure aetiology (such as *thyroiditis, ulcerative colitis, myasthenia gravis* and *pernicious anaemia*) antibodies which react with thyroglobulin, colonic mucosa, skeletal muscle, and gastric mucosa, respectively, have been demonstrated repeatedly. These findings understandably have aroused great interest. However, they do not in themselves suggest causality, since antibodies to cardiac muscle have been demonstrated similarly in myocardial infarction due to coronary atheroma, and antibodies to lung tissue have been recognised in pulmonary tuberculosis. Each of the latter findings suggests that the presence of autoantibodies may be a consequence rather than a cause of an underlying disease state.

In some infectious diseases, antibodies stimulated by exposure to certain antigens of invading parasitic organisms may cross-react with host-tissue antigens. Such cross-reacting antigens, occurring amongst unrelated or distantly-related species of organisms, are termed heterophile antigens, and have been discussed in Chapter 17 and previously in this chapter (*vide supra*). An example of a heterophile antigen shared by man and a microbial parasite is the M-protein of *Streptococcus haemolyticus* (Lancefield Group A) and a component of cardiac muscle sarcolemma. In rheumatic fever, cross-reacting antibodies to M-proteins which develop following Streptococcal infections have been implicated in the pathogenesis of rheumatic carditis, although there is yet a paucity of good supporting evidence for any aetiologic relationship.

As already described (*vide supra*, Chapter 10) some forms of glomerulonephritis demonstrate antibodies reacting with glomerular basement membranes. These glomerulonephritides are characterised by *linear* fluorescence of the basement-membrane when stained with fluorescent anti-human immunoglobulin serum - the most characteristic form occurring in Goodpasture's Disease (*vide supra*, Chapter 10).

It is often tacitly assumed that antitissue antibodies are harmful. However, such antibodies theoretically can be protective to tissue under certain circumstances, at least in experimental animals (*vide supra*, discussion of "enhancement", Chapters 17 and 18). At this time, it has not been proved unequivocally that the anti-tissue antibodies discussed above produce disease in humans.

Autosensitised Lymphoid Cells: In addition to autoimmune reactions dependent on the presence of autoantibodies, autoimmune reactions involving cellular immunity also occur. In certain diseases, (*e.g.*, *Hashimoto's thyroiditis*), both serum autoantibody to thyroglobulin and lymphocytes cytotoxic to thyroid cells in tissue culture are usually demonstrable. Stromal infiltrates of lymphocytes occur, which are sensitised to membrane antigens of thyroid cells; thus, the disease may be analogous to an "autograft rejection" phenomenon (*vide supra*, Chapter 17). Current investigations indicate that autoreactive lymphocytes are more important in the pathogenesis of this disease than are the anti-thyroglobulin autoantibodies.

Experimental Autoimmune Diseases in Laboratory Animals

(1) Normal rat brain tissue, mixed with Freund's adjuvant, and injected intramuscularly into healthy rats, will result in an acute demyelinating encephalitis occurring in the injected animals. This encephalitis can be transmitted serially to other rats by the transfer of sensitised lymphocytes from encephalitic animals, but not by passive transfer of serum antibodies. The encephalitis thus represents the result of an immunologic reaction between lymphocytes sensitised to rat brain antigens and the brain tissue of the animal in which it develops. Because the rat itself has produced the lymphocytes reactive to its own brain, the pathogenesis of the encephalitis may be regarded as autoimmune. This disease, *experimental allergic encephalomyelitis (EAE)*, represents an example of an autoimmune disease which is mediated by sensitised lymphocytes. Similar experimental diseases can be induced in other animal species; in fact, a similar disease (*acute haemorrhagic encephalomyelitis*) may occur (rarely) in man, following the use of Pasteur rabies vaccine (prepared from rabbit spinal-cord homogenate).

(2) A thyroglobulin-adjuvant emulsion injected intramuscularly into experimental animals will elicit an experimental thyroiditis, which has been compared with Hashimoto's thyroiditis in humans. In both "*autoimmune thyroiditis*" and "*autoimmune encephalitis*", lymphocytes from affected individuals can transmit the disease to normal isogeneic recipients. Such lymphocytes are cytotoxic to thyroid tissue and to embryonic neuroblast tissue in culture.

(3) In various species of animals, experimental autoimmune lesions of the testis (*autoimmune orchitis with aspermia*), adrenal (*autoimmune adrenalitis*), and

TABLE 1. HUMAN DISEASES WITH AUTOIMMUNE ASSOCIATIONS

DISEASE	AUTOIMMUNE ASSOCIATION
Acute Haemorrhagic Encephalomyelitis (post-viral and post-rabies vaccination)*	Occurs 10-14 days after acute viral infections or during course of rabies vaccination with formalised rabbit brain: May be analogous to experimental allergic encephalomyelitis when animals are injected with adjuvant and brain.
Peripheral neuritis, Guillain-Barré Syndrome	Probably multiple causation: Sensitised lymphocytes to Peripheral Nerve Antigen (PNA) in patients with Guillain-Barré Syndrome; (Irregularly) demonstrable antibodies to PNA in patients with peripheral neuropathies; Frequent demonstration of similar antibodies in peripheral neuritis following Mycoplasma pneumoniae infections.
Disseminated (Multiple) Sclerosis	Serum from patients may cause demyelination of axones in tissue culture preparations.
Pernicious (Addisonian) Anaemia	Antibodies against gastric parietal cells, intrinsic factor, and thyroglobulin are often present. Significance is questionable.
Ulcerative Colitis	Antibodies to colonic mucosa are often present. Significance is questionable.
Myasthenia Gravis	Antibodies to skeletal muscle are often present. Significance is questionable.
Idiopathic Addison's Disease	Antibodies to adrenal gland are often present. Significance is questionable.
Sympathetic Uveitis (Ophthalmia)	(?) Release of "Sequestered" uveal antigens from damaged eye causing immunological uveitis in other eye.
Aspermia*	Agglutinins to sperm are present in seminal fluid from some infertile male patients.
Glomerulonephritis with linear fluorescent staining (e.g., Goodpasture's Disease)	Circulating antibodies to basement membrane have been demonstrated in the sera of patients with the glomerulonephritis of Goodpasture's Disease.
Autoimmune Haemolytic Anaemia	"Warm" antibodies (reacting with Rh antigens at 37°C) "Cold" antibodies (reacting with I antigens at 5°C).
Autoimmune Thrombocytopenia	Anti-platelet antibodies demonstrable.
Autoimmune Granulocytopenia	Anti-granulocyte antibodies demonstrable.
Disseminated Lupus Erythematosus (DLE)*	Anti-nuclear factors; "autoimmune" haemolytic anaemia, granulocytopenia, thrombocytopenia; anti-coagulant antibodies; (?) renal and vascular lessions due to complexes of ANF + Nuclear Antigen + complement (C).
Rheumatoid Arthritis	Anti-gammaglobulin antibodies (rheumatoid factors - RF's); (?) Contribution of complexes of IgG + RF + C to arthritis and arteritis; in chronic cases, anti-nuclear factors also often present.
Chronic "Lupoid" Hepatitis	Chronic hepatitis, probably of viral origin, associated with anti-nuclear and anti-liver antibodies.
Rheumatic Fever	Cross-reacting antibodies between Streptoccoccal cell-wall antigens and cardiac sarcolemma antigens: (?) contribution to pathogenesis of myocarditis.
Hashimoto's Thyroiditis*	Infiltration of gland with plasma-cells and lymphocytes: Anti-thyroglobulin antibodies and sensitised lymphocytes cytotoxic to thyroid cells in tissue culture.
Thyrotoxicosis (Graves Disease)	Presence of a (7S) gammaglobulin called "long-acting thyroid stimulator" (LATS) which might be autoimmune in origin and a cause of the thyroid overactivity.

uveal tract of the eye (*autoimmune uveitis*) have been produced by similar immunisation procedures. It is, however, frequently necessary to use Freund's (or other) adjuvants to produce these lesions with any degree of consistency. These laboratory-induced diseases are thus somewhat artificial entities, without precise counterparts in naturally-occurring human disease.

Human Diseases with Autoimmune Associations

As already discussed, many different diseases (even those with well-defined microbiological aetiology) may demonstrate autoimmune phenomena. There are certain diseases, however, in which autoimmune manifestations probably contribute to the pathogenesis of lesions. Such pathogenetic mechanisms include:

(a) damage to cell membranes resulting from the action of autoantibodies and complement (*e.g.*, in *autoimmune haemolytic anaemias*),

(b) the induction of inflammatory reactions by autoantigen-antibody-complement complexes (*e.g.*, in the glomerulonephritis of *DLE*), and

(c) cytotoxicity resulting from the reactions of sensitised lymphocytes with autoantigens of cell membranes (*e.g.*, in *Hashimoto's thyroiditis* and *acute haemorrhagic encephalomyelitis*).

These diseases and their chief autoimmune associations are given in Table 1.

Disseminated Lupus Erythematosus (*DLE*)

DLE is a human disease characteristically-associated with numerous autoimmune phenomena. Of unknown aetiology, *DLE* occurs most commonly in younger women and derives its name from a characteristic erosive red facial rash.* *DLE* is, however, a generalised mesenchymal disease which may affect any organ of the body. The primary lesions occur in the endothelium of small blood vessels, giving rise to a diffuse vasculitis in which the protean clinical features depend upon the organs in which blood vessels are most extensively involved. For example, *DLE* may present as a *pyrexia of unknown origin*, *arthritis*, *glomerulonephritis*, *haemolytic anaemia*, *pericarditis*, or *pleuritis*. Any combination of these and many other manifestations may arise at any time during the course of this disease, which may be acute, fluctuant, or chronic.

* *Lupus = wolf, erythematosus = red. The rash is likened to a hungry red wolf, eating away at the face.*

The diagnosis of *DLE* is made from the association of a constellation of clinical manifestations with the finding of antinuclear (especially anti-*DNA*) autoantibodies. In addition to antinuclear factors, other autoantibodies often occur. These may include *autoimmune haemolysins*, *leucocyte* and *platelet-lysins*, *autoimmune anticoagulants* and *rheumatoid factors*. At this time, there is no entirely satisfactory understanding of the aetiology and pathogenesis of *DLE*, and the prominence of its associated autoimmune phenomena. As already noted in the discussion of antinuclear factors, (*vide supra*), it appears probable that complexes of nuclear antigen with antinuclear factors and complement may contribute to the development of renal lesions.

As noted above (*vide supra*), certain drugs can induce autoimmune phenomena in man similar to those encountered in *DLE*. Procaine amide (Pronestyl®), employed frequently for long-term management of cardiac arryhthmias, appears to have the greatest potential to induce a *DLE*-like syndrome. Although estimates of the percentage of patients developing *DLE* on long-term procaine amide therapy have varied, the value may be as high as 50% of patients so treated. Moreover, positive *ANF*- and *LE-cell* tests may develop as early as 2-3 months following the initiation of therapy; furthermore, the likelihood of a given patient developing stigmata of *DLE* is not necessarily related either to the doses of the drug employed in the treatment regimen or to the time period for which the patient was treated. Procaine amide-induced *DLE* is clinically-indistinguishable from idiopathic *DLE*. Furthermore, drug-induced *DLE* can develop into progressive, potentially life-threatening disease, unless it is recognised early in its development. Treatment with the offending agent must be stopped immediately. Unless the *DLE* begins to resolve upon withdrawal of the drug, a regimen of treatment appropriate for *DLE* must be initiated. Early recognition is usually possible by screening all patients on long-term procaine amide therapy at monthly intervals for serological conversion to positive *ANF*- and *LE-cell* tests, since serological conversion usually precedes the development of clinical disease.

Although the ways in which procaine amide-induced *DLE* are related to the "idiopathic" form of *DLE* are obscure, it is hoped that study of the pathogenetic mechanisms of the former may shed light on those of the latter. Unfortunately, there is little presently known about the early pathogenetic mechanism of either form of *DLE* at present.

The situation regarding our understanding of this enigmatic and intriguing disease, however, is not quite as hopeless as it may have sounded from the foregoing remarks.

A model disease has been described, which occurs in hybrid mice of the New Zealand strains (*NZB/NZW*)*. These mice develop a disease characterised by *positive ANF-tests*, both *Coombs' positive* and *negative haemolytic anaemias*, *splenomegaly*, *glomerulonephritis*, and a high incidence of *positive LE-cell preparations*. The glomerulonephritis is of the typical immune complex type, displaying a typical "lumpy-bumpy" pattern when kidney sections are stained with fluorescent anti-mouse immunoglobulin serum.

Genetic, immunologic, and viral factors are all involved in this disease, as will be seen from the following remarks:

(1) F_1 hybrid mice (*NZB/NZW*) are much more susceptible to the full-blown form of this disease than are homozygotes of either parental strain. Females are affected more frequently and more severely than males of the same hybrid strain. (In humans, *DLE* similarly tends to be more common and more severe in females.)

(2) The humoral autoimmune aspects of *NZB/NZW* disease tend to be polydispersed, in that they involve all classes of immunoglobulins, whilst extensive lymphocytic infiltrates found in many organs, including the salivary glands, probably indicate a relative functional deficit in the expression of (thymus-dependent) cellular immunity. Lymphocytic infiltrations may proceed to development of malignant lymphomas, especially when the mice are treated with long-term immunosuppressive agents (*e.g.*, azathioprine and prednisone).

There are a number of specific points wherein *NZB/NZW* mice differ in their immune responses from mice of other strains. Generally, they respond to antigenic stimulation with antibody production at an earlier age than most other mice, and the antibody titres to many (perhaps most) antigens are excessively high. Moreover, it is difficult to achieve immunologic tolerance to many antigens in mice of this strain; even where tolerance is achieved by injections of antigen during the neonatal period, it tends to be transitory and short-lived. Finally, these mice respond overwhelmingly to synthetic polynucleotide antigens with antibody production.

(3) New Zealand mice harbour the Gross virus (an oncogenic virus) transmitted vertically in certain mouse strains, and able to induce lymphomas in carrier mice when their immune surveillance mechanisms fail. However, whilst other strains of mice known to carry Gross virus are (and remain) tolerant to it, *NZB/NZW* break tolerance and produce antibodies to it by the age of

* *New Zealand black (NZB) by New Zealand white (NZW) F_1 cross.*

several months. At present, it is not thought that Gross lymphoma virus is responsible for disease in the *NZB/NZW* (except, perhaps, for the expression of lymphomas in older mice), but the fact that they respond unusually to a known viral agent may well be significant. For example, viral nucleic acid may be the immunogen for the antinuclear antibodies produced by New Zealand mice. In other words, a virus may not produce disease in an *NZB/NZW* mouse by establishing infection, but by initiating an autoimmune process (in this case by eliciting antibodies to viral *DNA* which cross-react with the animal's own *DNA*).

Thus, in summary, study of an experimental disease of New Zealand mice which resembles *DLE* in man indicates that a combination of genetic, immunologic, and viral factors may be involved in producing the disease. Susceptible mice are abnormal in that they mature rapidly in developing B-cell immunocompetence, and cannot be rendered immunologically-tolerant to most antigens by injection during a period of development when mice of other strains readily develop lasting tolerance. Furthermore, their T-cell immunocompetence is impaired, and the result is an animal with an "immunologic imbalance" of B-cells-to-T-cells. Exposure to and/or infection by one or more viruses may then initiate a series of "autoimmune phenomena", the culmination of which is the development of a clinical disease state resembling that of *DLE* in man.

It would not be unreasonable to envision a similar sequence of events occurring sporadically by a series of chance events converging on a susceptible human being. Perhaps we are at the threshold of understanding this most enigmatic but interesting of human diseases, *DLE*.

SECTION III

MOLECULAR IMMUNOLOGY

INTRODUCTION

Although the material discussed in this section is not directly related to clinical medicine and cannot be considered part of the "core curriculum" of undergraduate medicine, it is the fascinating story of a rapidly-expanding frontier of medical science.

The previous chapters have described the gross behaviour of the lymphoid system; here, the relationship between the function of an antibody and its molecular structure will be discussed. Moreover, the ways in which genetic evolution has produced the exceedingly specific and incredibly versatile antibody system will be examined.

Chapter 20 deals with the molecular structure of antibodies and endeavours to relate this to biological functions. The steric configuration and amino-acid sequence of the antigen-binding sites as well as the location of this site on the antibody molecule are described. Considerable emphasis has been given to the amino-acid sequences of immunoglobulin molecules because their definition has begun to clarify their biosynthesis and its genetic control.

Chapter 21 outlines the biosynthesis of immunoglobulins.

Chapter 22 attempts to describe how the exquisite specificity of antibody protection can be explained in terms of current genetic concepts. Two basic questions are - "How can the extraordinary number of specific antibodies, presumably each with an unique amino-acid sequence, be encoded and produced by the usual DNA-RNA mechanisms?" and "How can a reasonable amount of DNA accomplish the production of a myriad of differing antibodies?" It is hoped that this section of the book will arouse interest, not only in antibodies themselves, but also in the science of molecular genetics.

Chapter 20

THE ANTIBODY: STRUCTURE AND FUNCTION AT THE MOLECULAR LEVEL

The Antigen-Binding Site of the Antibody Molecule

Intense interest over many years has revolved around the nature of the antigen-binding sites of antibody molecules. It has been realised for a long time that antigens and antibodies are bound together by weak physical forces which act over short distances only, rather than by strong covalent bonds. Because the individual binding forces are weak, and incapable of acting at a distance, it follows that many such weak forces must act in a summated way in order to achieve the relatively stable bonds observed between an antigen and its antibody. In order for these weak forces to summate effectively within a limited binding-site area, the stereochemistry of both the antigen and the binding site on the antibody molecule must be highly complementary to each other. In other words, an antigenic determinant must fit the binding site of an antibody as a key fits its lock.

Location of the Antigen-Binding Site on the Antibody Molecule

Antigen-binding sites reside on the *Fab*-portions of antibody molecules. Both H-chains and L-chains are involved in the formation of binding sites. When antibody molecules are reduced and alkylated, and the H-chains are separated from the L-chains, the isolated H-chains retain more antigen-binding activity than isolated L-chains. The total antigen-binding activity of the isolated H- and L-chains, however, is always less than the antigen-binding activity of the intact or reconstituted antibody molecule. Nevertheless, both H- and L-chains do contribute to the binding site, a synergistic relationship appearing to prevail between the contributions of these chains toward antigen-binding activity.

The Tertiary Structure of Antibodies

A complete steric picture of the antibody molecule can be achieved only by subjecting monoclonal immunoglobulins with antibody activity to exhaustive study by

X-ray crystallography. Although such work has already begun, it is a monumental undertaking, which will likely require several years to complete. Nevertheless, recent X-ray diffraction studies indicate that H- and L-chains form globular sub-regions or *domains*, the significance of which will be discussed below (*vide infra*).

Studies of antibody molecules by the use of high-resolution electron-micrography have also contributed to our present concept of antibody tertiary structure, and have been of value in establishing spatial relationships between the antigen-binding sites and the sites of other biological activities within antibody molecules. These studies have enabled accurate assessment of the size and overall shape of antibody molecules as well.

When free IgG antibody molecules were studied by high-resolution electron-micrography, clear pictures could not be obtained. This suggested that free antibodies were loosely-structured, plastic molecules, without definite shape.

However, when the same antibody molecules were allowed to react with antigen prior to electron-micrographic study, good pictures were obtained, which have been most useful in developing concepts of antibody tertiary structure.

Antibodies with specific binding-affinity for 2,4 - dinitrophenyl haptens can be prepared by injecting rabbits with a protein possessing substituted 2,4 - dinitrophenyl groups (*DNP*-groups). These antibodies can be purified by the method of "affinity chromatography". In this method, antisera are passed through a column composed of the *DNP* groups conjugated to an insoluble solid matrix such as the beaded agarose gel, Sepharose . After repeated washing of the column, the anti-*DNP* antibodies are eluted by addition of free hapten to the column. The antibody-hapten complexes are dissociated at pH 3 (*vide supra*, Chapter 6) and the purified antibody is recovered by gel filtration. The purified antibody is used for electron-micrographic studies.

A synthetic divalent dinitrophenyl compound was prepared, in which two dinitrophenyl-groups were attached to each other via a six-carbon aliphatic chain (as illustrated in Figure 1), which was able to link two or more antibody molecules together by allowing one antigen-binding site from each molecule to bind each of the oppositely directed *DNP*-groups. Although this compound could not form precipitates on reacting with antibody, electron-micrographs made from the reaction mixture revealed antigen-antibody complexes appearing as triangular structures with apical projections. These structures were identified as complexes of three antibody

Fig. 1 DIVALENT SYNTHETIC 2, 4 - DINITROPHENYL ANTIGEN USED IN ELECTRON - MICROGRAPHIC STUDIES OF IgG ANTIBODIES

A. Chemical Formula of Antigen

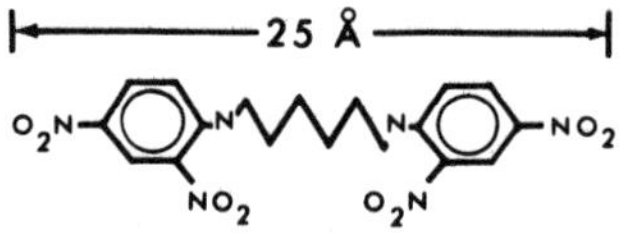

B. Symbol Used to Represent Formula

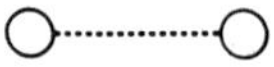

Fig. 2 STRUCTURE OF ANTIGEN - ANTIBODY COMPLEX OBTAINED BY REACTING DIVALENT DNP - ANTIGEN WITH ANTIBODY TO DNP OF IgG TYPE

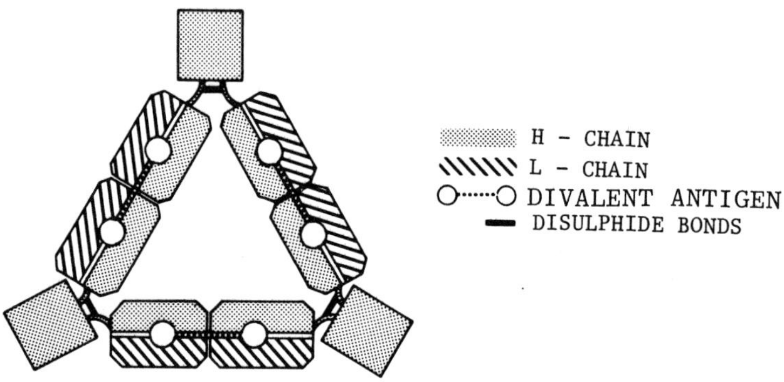

Fig. 3 STRUCTURE OF ANTIGEN - ANTIBODY COMPLEX WITH PEPSIN - TREATED ANTIBODY TO DNP OF IgG - TYPE OBTAINED BY REACTING DIVALENT DNP - ANTIGEN

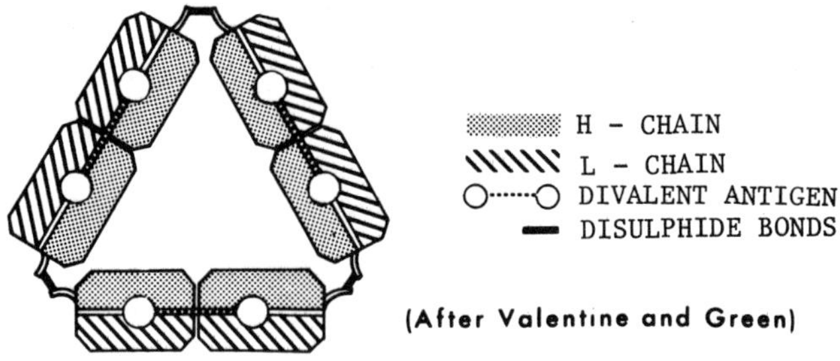

(After Valentine and Green)

molecules linked together by three molecules of the divalent *DNP*-antigen, as seen in Figure 2. (The antigen itself is invisible in the electron micrographs, because of its small size). Individual IgG antibodies thus are recognised as "Y"-shaped structures. Antigen-binding regions of adjacent IgG molecules are linked by divalent antigen into triangular complexes, in which the apical projections seen in the electron microscope represent those regions of the antibody molecules not directly involved in antigen-binding (*i.e.*, the *Fc*-fragments).

This interpretation is supported by another experiment, in which the antibodies were subjected to limited hydrolysis with pepsin prior to allowing them to react with the antigen. Pepsin hydrolysis of antibody molecules leads to the splitting off of a divalent antigen-binding fragment (denoted $(Fab')_2$) in which the two *Fab'*-regions are attached together by disulphide bonds. When pepsin-treated antibodies are reacted with the divalent *DNP*-antigen and examined by electron-micrography, triangular complexes lacking apical projections are seen, the nature of which is illustrated in Figure 3.

In summary, electron-micrographic studies have suggested that IgG antibodies are "Y"-shaped structures, in which the *Fc*-region acts as a swivel base, allowing the two *Fab*-arms to assume varied angles ranging from nearly 0° to 180°. They further suggest that flexible regions separate *Fab*-arms from *Fc*-base, and these flexible regions represent those portions of immunoglobulin molecules susceptible to limited hydrolysis by proteolytic enzymes (*e.g.*, papain, pepsin, and trypsin).

A gross steric model for IgG antibodies, based on the above experiments, is illustrated in Figure 4.

Models such as Figure 4 represent gross approximations of the tertiary structure of antibodies, which cannot be understood readily in terms of primary structure. Before we can relate the primary and tertiary structure of immunoglobulins, we must relate primary structure of immunoglobulins directly with their antigen-binding activity.

Affinity-Labelling of the Combining Site

An unique method of identifying amino-acid residues within the antigen-binding sites of antibody molecules has been developed by Dr. Leon Wofsy and his colleagues. This technique, called affinity-labelling, employs haptens possessing chemically-reactive groups which enable them to establish covalent bonds with certain amino-acid residues (*e.g.*, tyrosine, histidine, ly-

Fig. 4 STERIC MODEL FOR IgG ANTIBODIES

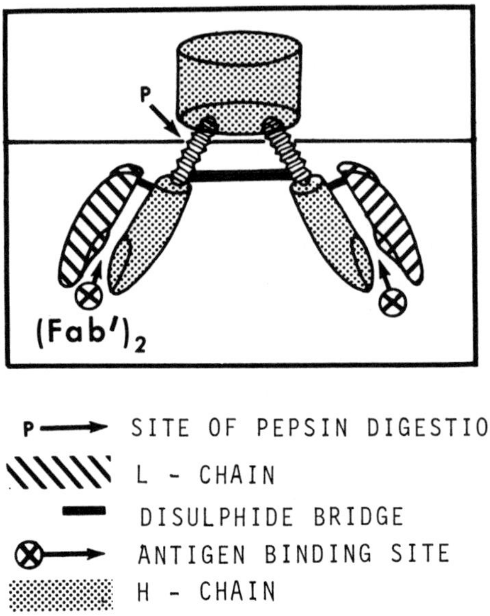

(MODIFIED FROM VALENTINE AND GREEN)

sine, and others) with which they come into direct contact. Thus, affinity-labelling haptens will attach themselves chemically to reactive amino-acid residues occurring within the combining sites of anti-hapten antibodies, but not to similar amino-acid residues occurring elsewhere within the antibody molecule. Thus, direct contact between hapten and amino-acid is required for attachment to occur. Affinity-labelling, then, provides a method for labelling and identifying certain amino-acid residues occurring within the antigen-binding sites of antibody molecules. If affinity-labelled antibodies are fractionated in various ways, the labelled amino-acid residues can be located subsequently on the appropriate fractions. Such studies have established that both H-chains and L-chains participate directly in antigen-binding, because both types of chains have had covalently-bound hapten associated with them in every case examined. H-chains, however, are often more heavily labelled than L-chains, which may reflect their relatively greater contribution to the antigen-binding site. If affinity-labelled antibodies are separated into H- and L-chains, and each of these fractions subjected to tryptic hydrolysis, it is possible to obtain short segments of polypeptide from the antigen-binding sites which can be recognised by their attached affinity label.

Interestingly enough, such affinity-labelled peptides from either H- or L-chains are always heterogeneous in their amino-acid composition and sequence, even when the antibodies employed are highly purified, and obtained from a single individual. This implies that antigen-binding sites are chemically heterogeneous (and therefore polyclonal), even within a population of antibodies to a single specific hapten, derived from a single individual.

Antibody Structure and Function

The linear immunoglobulin model of Porter will serve as a starting point in attempting to correlate the primary structure of immunoglobulins with the physiologic activities of antibodies. This model depicts the polypeptide chains of antibodies as linear structures, and shows the attachments of H- and L-chains to each other (*i.e.*, illustrates quarternary structure relationships). This model will be modified in a stepwise fashion in order to incorporate each new feature brought out in the discussion which follows.

Fig. 5 PORTER MODEL FOR THE IgG MOLECULE

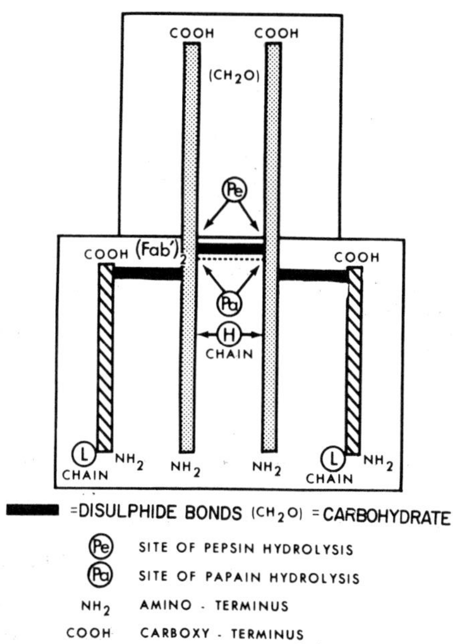

Figure 5 depicts the locations of the amino-termini and carboxy-termini of both H- and L-chains, and also the sites of hydrolysis by the proteases, papain and pepsin.

However, it has already been noted (in the previously-discussed electron-micrographic studies) that the region of the molecule susceptible to protease hydrolysis is a flexible area (between *Fab* and *Fc*) which permits the *Fc*-region to serve as a swivel base between the *Fab*-arms). This flexible region of the molecule will be represented in the linear model by drawing a bend between the *Fab*- and *Fc*-regions, as illustrated in Figure 6.

Figure 6 also illustrates two additional features, as yet not discussed:

Fig. 6 MODIFIED LINEAR MODEL FOR IgG ANTIBODY MOLECULES

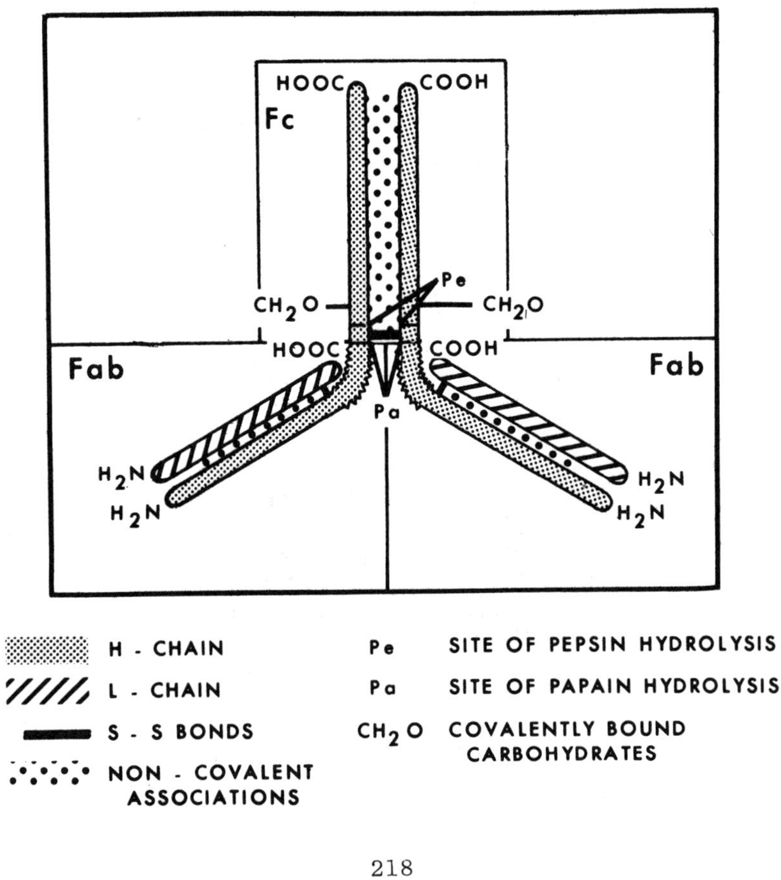

Firstly, the carboxy-terminal halves of the H-chains are associated with each other (to form the *Fc*-region) by both disulphide bonds and non-covalent interactions (*e.g.:* Van der Waal's forces, hydrogen bonding, hydrophobic bonding, etc.).

Secondly, most or all of the carbohydrate associated with IgG is bound covalently to each H-chain (via an aspartyl-residue located in the *Fc*-region).

Regions of Constant and Variable Primary Structure in Immunoglobulins

Both L-chains and H-chains consist of regions whose amino-acid sequence is virtually identical among all chains of similar isotype and allotype, and regions in which the sequence of amino-acid residues is unique for each immunoglobulin. The former are designated as *"constant"*, *"invariant"*, or *"C-regions"*; the latter as *"variable"*, *"specificity"* or *"V-regions"*.

The *C-regions* contain most of the antigenic markers which characterise immunoglobulins (including class-determinants, isotypic-determinants and allotypic-determinants). *C-regions* also determine the biological properties of immunoglobulin molecules other than antigen-binding (*e.g.*, complement-fixation, cytophilic affinity, transplacental transport, etc.).

The antigen-binding specificity of an immunoglobulin is a function of the primary structure of the *V-regions* of its component L- and H-chains (*i.e.*, the V_L-*region* and V_H-*region*). Thus, an individual's ability to respond to any antigen both reflects and is limited by his ability to generate immunoglobulins containing H-chain and L-chain *V-regions* (V_L- and V_H-*regions*) of appropriate sequence to react with that antigen.

The *V-regions* of H- and L-chains are of approximately similar size (*i.e.*, ∿ 110 amino-acid residues in length). Furthermore, both the *V-regions* of L- chains and the *V-regions* of H-chains are located at the amino-terminal portions of their respective chains. The *V-regions* of L-chains occupy about one half of the total length of the L-chain, whilst the *V-regions* of H-chains occupy about one quarter of the length of the H-chain, as illustrated in Figure 7.

The *C-regions* of L-chains (the C_L-*regions*) are approximately the same size as the L-chain *V-regions*, and occupy the carboxy-halves of the L-chains. The *C-regions* of H-chains (the C_H-*regions*), however, are three times the length of the *C-* or *V-regions* of L-chains.

Fig. 7 LINEAR MODEL FOR AN IgG ANTIBODY TO SHOW CONSTANT AND VARIABLE REGIONS

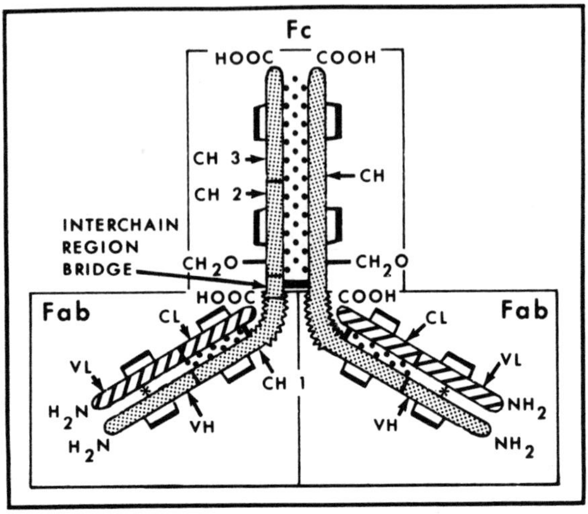

VL — VARIABLE REGION (SPECIFICITY REGION) OF L - CHAIN

VH — VARIABLE REGION (SPECIFICITY REGION) OF H - CHAIN

CL — CONSTANT (INVARIANT) REGION OF L - CHAIN

CH — TOTAL CONSTANT (INVARIANT) REGION OF H - CHAIN

CH1 — 1st CONSTANT REGION OF H -CHAIN

CH 2 — 2nd CONSTANT REGION OF H - CHAIN

CH 3 — 3rd CONSTANT REGION OF H - CHAIN

▬ — S -S BOND

* — ANTIGEN - BINDING SITE

:::::: — NON - COVALENT BONDS

CH_2O — CARBOHYDRATE

Moreover, H-chain *C-regions* can be divided into three sub-regions or *"domains"* of approximately equal length, denoted as C_H1, C_H2, and C_H3, which are remarkably similar in the sequence of their amino-acids. These *C_H-sub-regions* (or *domains*) are illustrated in Figures 7 and 9.

Genetic and Evolutionary Implications of Homology Within C-regions and V-regions

The term "homology", as applied to polypeptides and proteins, is an expression of the degree of similarity between different peptide molecules. Peptide homology is, of course, a reflexion of the underlying relationships of the genes encoding the peptides being compared. Its importance resides in the fact that homology is indicative of evolutionary and genetic relationships amongst different proteins.

Various degrees of peptide homology are illustrated in Figure 8. The following remarks which relate to the estimation of homology between peptides may be noted:

Fig. 8 PEPTIDE HOMOLOGY

IV IS EVOLUTIONARILY UNRELATED TO I, II, AND III BECAUSE:

1. DISPARATE LENGTH (DISPARITY = 50%)
2. NO AREAS OF COMMON SEQUENCE
3. DIFFERENT SIZED INTRACHAIN S - S LOOPS

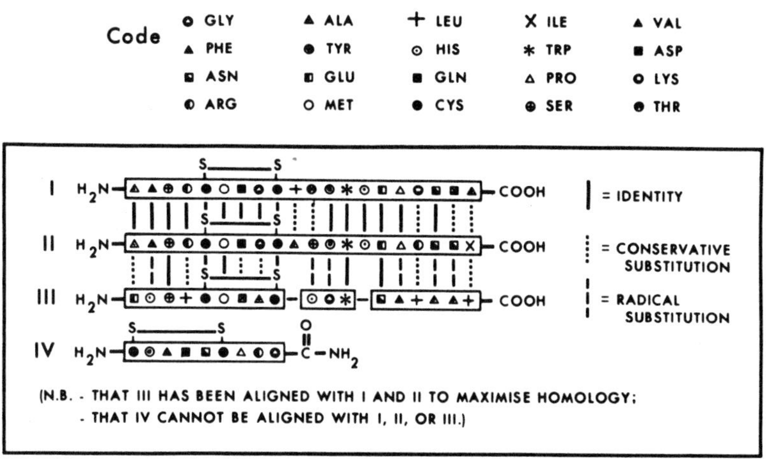

PEPTIDES	HOMOLOGY (% IDENTICAL RESIDUE POSITIONS)	
I - I	100%	(40/40)
I - II	70%	(28/40)
I - III	26.3%	(10/38)
I - IV	NIL	(0/30)
II - III	26.3%	(10/38)
II - IV	NIL	(0/30)
III - IV	NIL	(0/28)

Conclusions:

I AND II ARE CLOSELY RELATED IN EVOLUTION
I AND III ARE DISTANTLY RELATED IN EVOLUTION
II AND III " " " " "
I AND IV ARE EVOLUTIONARILY UNRELATED
II AND IV " " "
III AND IV " " "

(1) Peptides with identical amino-acid sequences are 100% homologous (by definition).

(2) Homology between non-identical peptides may be estimated in terms of the percentage of identical residues at comparable positions in the peptides compared.

(3) Peptides having no identical residues at comparable positions are not homologous.

(4) Certain amino-acid substitutions at individual positions alter the properties of peptides less than other substitutions; moreover, similar amino-acids are usually encoded by similar base sequences in *DNA*. Substitutions between such similar amino-acids are called conservative alterations, whereas substitutions involving dissimilar amino-acids are referred to as radical.

(5) In considering homology between two peptides, the amino-acid sequences may be identical or similar except that one or two amino-acid residues may be missing (deleted) or added (inserted) in one peptide or the other. When this occurs, the amino-acid chains may be realigned to adjust for these events prior to assessing the degree of homology. However, peptides should usually only be considered homologous if they are of approximately equal length.

(6) Certain structural features, as exemplified by intra-chain disulphide loops, are of special significance in evaluating homology. Thus, whereas chains of slightly disparate length may be broken and realigned to maximise the number of identical positions, such breaks should generally be avoided within the sequences of small disulphide loops because the results will likely be misleading.

All of the above remarks may be applied in considering the evolution and genetics of the immunoglobulins.

As already noted, immunoglobulin molecules contain regions of *constant (invariant)* amino-acid sequence (*i.e.*, the *C-regions*) and regions of *variable* sequence (*i.e.*, the *V-regions*). There is very little homology between the *C-* and *V-regions*. However, all *V-regions* and all *C-regions* (or sub-regions) contain one similar intra-chain disulphide bond, formed between two half-cystinyl residues, separated from each other by approximately 60 amino-acid positions, which causes the polypeptide chain to loop back on itself. The disulphide loops thus formed constitute globular regions called *"domains" (vide supra)*. They appear to be necessary features for both *V-region* and *C-region* function, and can be regarded as rather circumstantial evidence of a very minor degree of homology between *V-* and *C-regions*. In fact, the observed paucity of homology between *V-* and *C-regions* suggests that if, in fact, these regions are descended from a common ancestral gene, the split must have occurred very early in chordate evolution, with each gene subsequently evolving independently to serve different functions.

Homology of *V-regions*: Six positions (∿5% of the total positions) have been recognised to be always identical in all *V-regions* from both H- and L-chains - Appendix C-3. Considering the *V-regions* of L-chains alone, roughly 10% of the total positions are common to this group, as seen in Appendix C-3. A higher percentage of invariant positions (∿30% of the total positions) also occurs within the *V-regions* of H-chains.

Within the *V-regions* of light chains, the number of totally-invariant positions increases with successive sub-divisions of the group. Thus, ∿30% of the total positions are invariant within the *V-regions* of κ- or λ-chains, but ∿60% of the positions are invariant amongst members of a single sub-group (Appendices C-1 and C-2).

Unlike the *V-regions* of light chains, the *V-regions* of heavy chains have no equivalent of the κ- and λ-subdivision, and are thus unrelated to the H-chain class-determinants on the C_H*-regions* - Figure 10. They occur in at least 4 subgroups (designated V_HI - V_HIV). The subgroups of *V-regions* of κ-, λ-, and H-chains are based on very high degrees of peptide homology in the first 20 or so amino-acid positions from the amino-terminus. The similarities noted between members of single subgroups is illustrated in Figure 10 for all 13 known subclasses of *V-regions* (4 subclasses of V_κ-, 5 subclasses of $V\lambda$-, and 4 subclasses of V_H-).

Examination of the amino-acid sequences of any two individual *V-regions* reveals that the homology is always greater than the percentage of invariant positions common to their respective subgroups. For example, although the percentage of invariant positions common to subgroups *I* and *II* of κ-chain *V-regions* is only ∿30%, an individual member of subgroup *I*(*Eu*) and an individual member of subgroup *II*(*Cum*) have nearly 50% of their total *V-region* positions identical. Similarly, although *V-regions* of H- and L-chains have only 5% of their positions invariant and common to both groups, any individual H-chain *V-region* and any individual L-chain *V-region* will always demonstrate a much greater degree of homology (*e.g.*, ∿20%). This indicates that not only are the positions at which variance is permitted limited,

DIAGRAMS OF IMMUNOGLOBULIN PRIMARY STRUCTURE

Key to Figures 9 - 10

- PCA (Pyrollidone carboxylic acid, blocking amino terminus)
- Gly
- Ala
- Leu
- Ile
- Val
- Pro
- Phe
- Tyr
- Trp
- His
- Arg
- Lys
- Glu
- Asn
- Gln
- Asp
- Cys
- Met
- Ser
- Thr

- Asx
- Glx

Fig. 9 HOMOLOGIES BETWEEN C_L REGIONS AND C_H SUBREGIONS OF γ_1 SUBCLASS (DATA FROM Eu PROTEIN, ADAPTED FROM EDELMAN ET AL)

This figure illustrates the similarities between different C - REGIONS which has been offered as evidence suggesting the evolutionary origin of these regions by a mechanism of gene duplication and translocation.

Only homologous residues and identical residues are depicted in this figure.

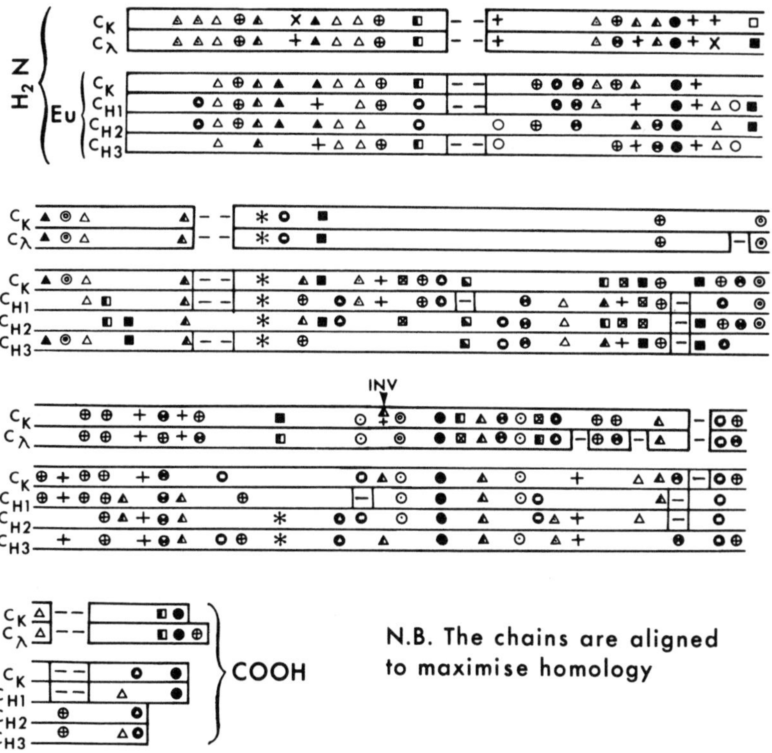

N.B. The chains are aligned to maximise homology

Fig. 10

N-TERMINAL SEQUENCES OF V-REGIONS OF K, λ AND H CHAINS SHOWING SUBGROUP VARIATIONS

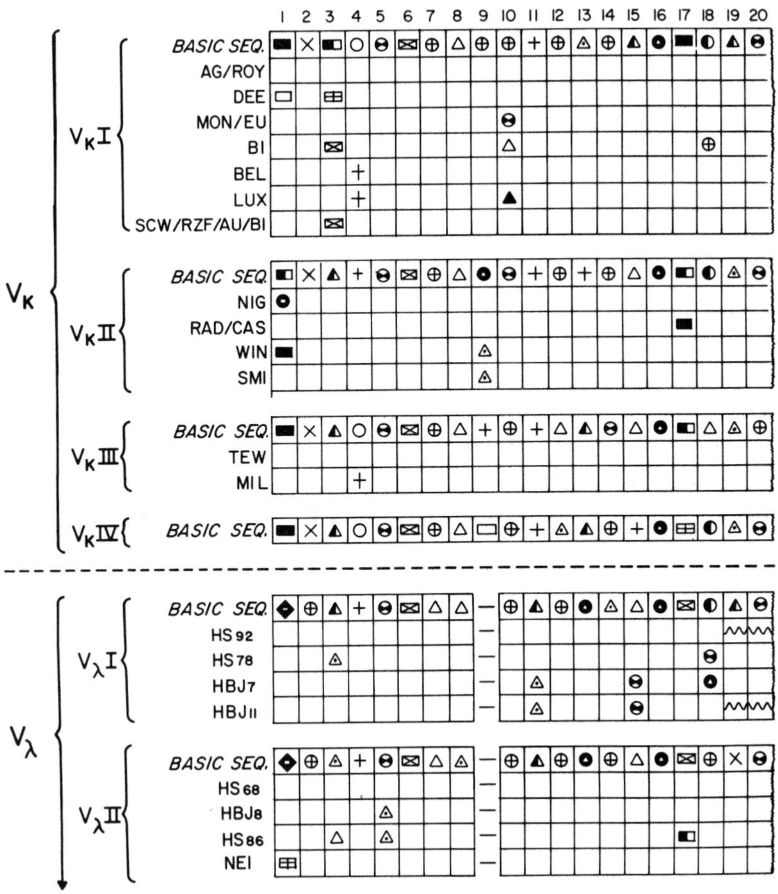

(NB: IDENTICAL RESIDUES APPEAR AS BLANK SPACES.)

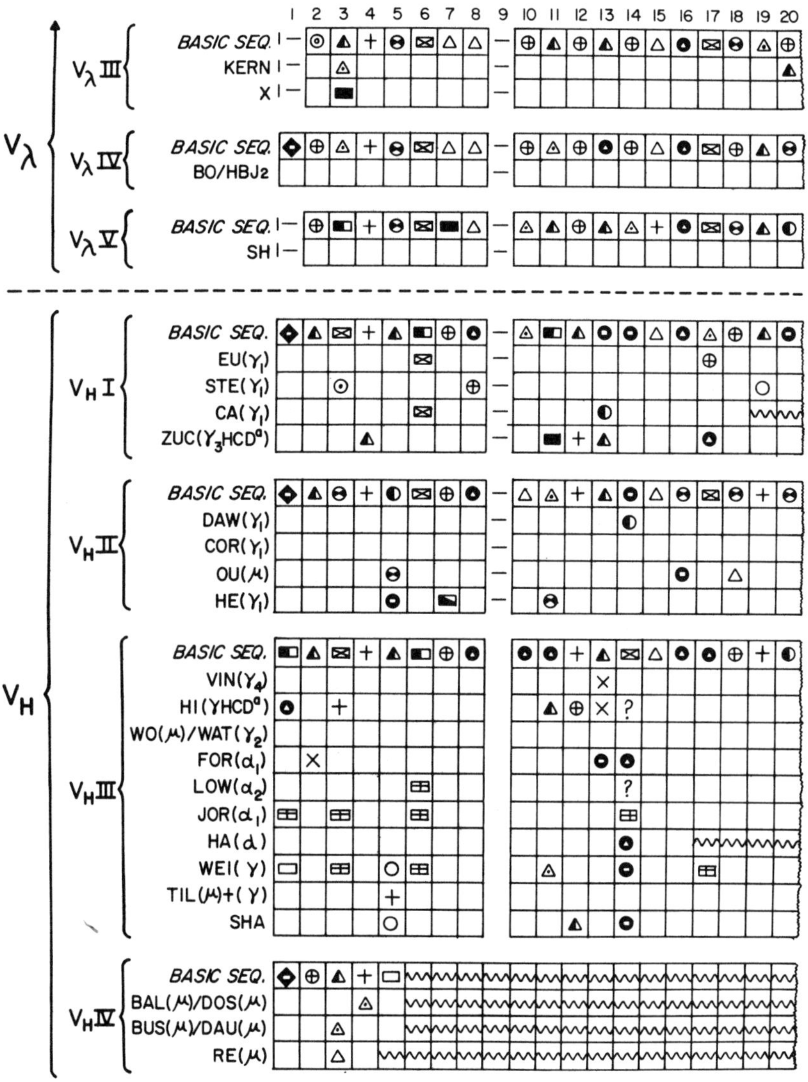
1 2 3 4 5 6 7 8 9 10 11 12 13 14 15 16 17 18 19 20
V_λ
V_λ III
BASIC SEQ.
KERN
X
V_λ IV
BASIC SEQ.
BO/HBJ2
V_λ V
BASIC SEQ.
SH
V_H
V_H I
BASIC SEQ.
EU(γ_1)
STE(γ_1)
CA(γ_1)
ZUC(γ_3HCD^a)
V_H II
BASIC SEQ.
DAW(γ_1)
COR(γ_1)
OU(μ)
HE(γ_1)
V_H III
BASIC SEQ.
VIN(γ_4)
HI(γHCD^a)
WO(μ)/WAT(γ_2)
FOR(α_1)
LOW(α_2)
JOR(α_1)
HA(α)
WEI(γ)
TIL(μ)+(γ)
SHA
V_H IV
BASIC SEQ.
BAL(μ)/DOS(μ)
BUS(μ)/DAU(μ)
RE(μ)

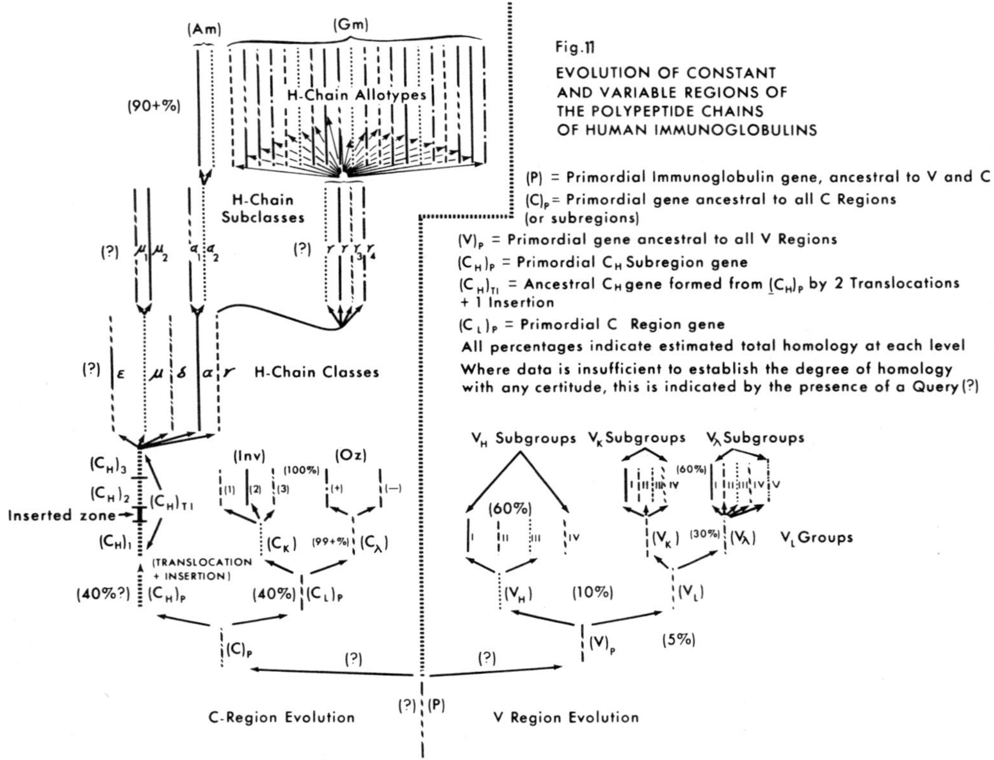

Fig. 11

EVOLUTION OF CONSTANT AND VARIABLE REGIONS OF THE POLYPEPTIDE CHAINS OF HUMAN IMMUNOGLOBULINS

(P) = Primordial Immunoglobulin gene, ancestral to V and C

$(C)_P$ = Primordial gene ancestral to all C Regions (or subregions)

$(V)_P$ = Primordial gene ancestral to all V Regions

$(C_H)_P$ = Primordial C_H Subregion gene

$(C_H)_{T1}$ = Ancestral C_H gene formed from $(C_H)_P$ by 2 Translocations + 1 Insertion

$(C_L)_P$ = Primordial C Region gene

All percentages indicate estimated total homology at each level

Where data is insufficient to establish the degree of homology with any certitude, this is indicated by the presence of a Query (?)

but the number of permissible alternatives at each variable position is also limited; thus, the same alternatives recur at corresponding positions in *V-region* peptides belonging to different groups. In other words, within *V-regions*, more positions with restricted variance have been conserved in evolution than have positions which are absolutely invariant. This suggests a closer evolutionary relationship between all *V-regions* than might be expected on the basis of homology between rigidly invariant *V-region* positions alone.

Homology in *C-regions:* Studies of homology in *C-regions* provide similar arguments supporting the evolution of immunoglobulins. The *C-regions* of H-chains contain three subregions or domains, any of which shows ∿30% homology to any other C_H*-sub-region* or to any L-chain *C-region* - Figure 9. This, plus one additional unrelated fact, is helpful in understanding the evolutionary development of H-chains.

A small region of the H-chain (less than fifteen residues in length) lies between sub-regions C_H1- and C_H2-. This region is the area where the interchain disulphide bonds linking the two H-chains together occur, and is dissimilar to all H-chain *C-sub-regions* and to any L-chain *C-region* in its amino-acid sequence.

These facts suggest that the H-chain *C-region* arose in evolution by an ancestral (H-chain *C-sub-region*) gene undergoing two translocations and one ∿15 amino-acid residue insertion to encode a complete H-chain *C-region*.

Evolutionary relationships discussed above are illustrated in Figure 11.

V-regions and Antigenic Specificity

In this section, the structure of immunoglobulin *V-regions* will be related to antigen-binding, since the specificity of an antibody depends on the amino-acid sequences of the *V-regions* of its H- and L-chains. As already stated, ∿ 5% of the amino-acids of *V-regions* are rigidly invariant; in addition, all *V-regions* contain an intra-chain disulphide loop comprising 60 amino-acid residues. These features would therefore seem to be necessary for the construction of the domains comprising the antigen-binding site.

In spite of the immense number of different antigenic configurations that can be recognised by antibodies, the variation in amino-acid sequence between immunoglobulin *V-regions* is (as already observed) limited - both in the number of variable positions and also in the number of permissible substitutions at any one position. Mechanisms proposed to explain the production and diversification of antibodies must take into account these limitations, whilst explaining the incredible versatility of antibodies for recognising diverse antigens. Therefore, such mechanisms must consider both the profound similarities and the profound differences amongst all individual *V-regions*.

It was noted earlier in this chapter that although individual light and heavy chains of specific antibodies are capable of binding antigen, an intact or reconstituted antibody (with conjoined light and heavy chains) can always be shown to have greater affinity for antigen than the summated affinities of the component heavy and light chains. The question thus arises as to whether a special structural relationship exists between the two types of chain to achieve this synergism. Because of the polyclonal nature of physiologically-produced antibodies, studies to answer this are best performed on monoclonal immunoglobulins, derived from myelomas. In a study of *V-region* homology between the heavy and light chains of a single myeloma globulin (by Edelman and his collaborators), 24% homology was found between the *V-regions* of the light and heavy chains, which proved to be no higher than would be expected to occur between any two *unrelated* immunoglobulin *V-regions*. There would seem, therefore, to be no special primary structural homology between the *V-regions* of the H- and L-chains within a single immunoglobulin molecule;* the mechanism of the observed synergism in antigen-binding between H- and L-chains of an antibody remains enigmatic, but it is thought that a common binding "Slot" is formed. An important conceptual advance in understanding the nature of the antibody combining site was provided by the finding that the variable regions of human H- and L-chains contain restricted areas with especially high variability. These *hypervariable regions* in L-chains occupy positions 24-34, 50-56, and 89-97. It has been suggested that these hypervariable regions make direct contact with antigen; indeed, L-chain residues 24-34 and 89-97 are probably brought into close proximity by the disulphide bond formed by the invariant half-cystines at positions 23 and 88. Similarly to the *V-regions* of L-chains, the variable regions of H-chains also have hypervariable segments, occupying positions 31-35, 50-65, 81-87, and 95-102. Close spatial proximity of the H- and L-chain hypervariable segments is permitted because of their symmetry;thus,a three-dimensional antigen-binding site can be formed in common by V_H- and V_L-*regions*. Further evidence relating hypervariable re-

* *N.B. that all of the molecules of a monoclonal immunoglobulin are identical to each other.*

gions to antibody activity is provided by affinity labelling studies using myeloma proteins with antibody activity. In experiments of this type, as well as in practically every study with conventionally raised antibodies, the affinity-labelled residues fall within one or both hypervariable regions.

If the hypervariable regions account for the required antigen binding specificity of antibodies it is reasonable to assume that antibodies with similar antigen-binding specificities might have similar sequences in their hypervariable regions. Certain human anti-gamma globulin antibodies (rheumatoid factors) from different patients show identical sequences for the first 40 residues of the L-chains, with unusual residues occurring at certain positions not previously observed in other L-chains. The H-chain sequences of two such antibodies also were identical, at least as far as residue 40. Thus, the first hypervariable areas of H- and L-chains derived from antibodies of similar antigen-binding specificities, showed striking structural similarity in at least one study.

The above discussion has referred to the recognition of antigen by immunoglobulins; the recognition of antigen by the cell membranes of sensitised T-lymphocytes has not been discussed. There is now some evidence that IgM monomers may confer the properties of antigen recognition on the membranes of sensitised lymphocytes (*vide supra*, Chapter 8). This has not yet been universally accepted, however, and will have to await confirmation or refutation by the immunologic community.

The Effect of Antigen-Binding on the Other Biological Properties of the Immunoglobulins and Lymphocytes

The reaction of antigen-binding initiates conformational (*allosteric*) alterations of the antibody molecule. These conformational changes begin in the region of the binding site, but rapidly involve other portions of the molecule. Conformational (*allosteric*) changes in the *Fc*-region of the molecule may activate this region, so that it becomes capable of exerting its biological functions (*e.g.*, complement-fixation, mast-cell degranulation, etc.), or, alternatively, may accomplish these activities by other mechanisms, as yet not entirely understood, but apparently involving the bridging of adjacent immunoglobulins by multivalent antigens.

Similar hypotheses have been offered to explain he initial processes involved in the specific activation of sensitised lymphocytes by contact with antigen. Thus, as the antigen-binding sites attached to the cell membrane react with antigen, they would induce conformational (*allosteric*) changes in the membrane receptors, or, alternatively, bridge adjacent membrane receptors, which would then initiate a series of reactions within the lymphocyte, the end result of which would be the development of a cell-mediated immune reaction. The entire process (*i.e.*, antigen-binding inducing conformational alterations, or bridging of adjacent receptors, in turn initiating a stereotyped sequence of biological reactions) would be entirely analogous to the mechanism of activation of complement by IgM or IgG antibodies following antigen-binding.

Chapter 21

THE MOLECULAR BIOLOGY OF IMMUNOGLOBULIN BIOSYNTHESIS

Neoplastic cells from the monoclonal gammopathies, such as multiple myeloma, are heavily committed to (or differentiated toward) the synthesis of a monoclonal immunoglobulin, which represents a significant fraction of their total protein synthesis. In this respect, these neoplastic immunocytes are comparable to the reticulocytes of the erythropoietic system, which are irreversibly differentiated toward the biosynthesis of a single protein (haemoglobin). Immunoglobulin biosynthesis by neoplastic cells in monoclonal gammopathies thus represents a nearly ideal model system for the physiologic synthesis of H- and L-chains, and their subsequent assembly into complete molecules of immunoglobulin.

Studies of immunoglobulin synthesis by neoplastic cells have enabled the following conclusions to be drawn:

(1) H-chains and L-chains are synthesised on separate strands of *m-RNA*, each from a single growing-point at the amino-terminus of the chain.

(2) The assembly process of immunoglobulins appears to be as follows: The separately-formed H- and L-chains associate to form 2-chain half-molecules of immunoglobulin. Two half-molecules associate to form the complete 4-chain molecule before release from the cells. Various degrees of disordered synthesis can occur in neoplastic disease. For example, free L-chains (Bence Jones Protein), or occasionally free half molecules, may be released prior to their incorporation into complete immunoglobulin.

(3) Finally, attachment of carbohydrate to nascent immunoglobulin appears to be a sequential process, beginning whilst polypeptide chains are still associated with polysomes, continuing after they are released from these organelles, and completed only after the nascent immunoglobulins are released from the cells. Because carbohydrate is added to the molecule in a stepwise manner, it has been suggested that carbohydrate may represent part of a mechanism whereby immunoglobulins are released from the cells that synthesise them. This is purely speculative; it is still not known what role carbohydrates play in the function of immunoglobulins; however, the ubiquity in these proteins suggests that they probably have some functions - Nature rarely se-

lects for evolutionary patterns conferring no advantages to the organism.

The Experimental Approach to H- and L-Chain Biosynthesis

Cells which actively synthesise immunoglobulin will incorporate radioactively-labelled amino-acids into the growing polypeptide chains of the immunoglobulin, when these cells are exposed to such labelled precursors. The amount of incorporation will be a function of the time of the exposure pulse (if the *m-RNA* encoding the polypeptide is stable). If a pulse of labelled amino-acids is followed by a chase of unlabelled (non-radioactive) amino-acids, one is able to allow the completion of the polypeptide chain to occur, with the amount of radioactivity in the completed chain a function of the time of pulse-labelling. If a mixture of radioactively-labelled amino-acids were provided in the pulse, and an enormous excess of a similar mixture of unlabelled (non-radioactive) amino-acids were provided in the chase, a linear relationship would be expected between specific radioactivity incorporated into the purified protein and the time of the pulse of labelled amino-acids. This theoretical relationship is illustrated in Figure 1.

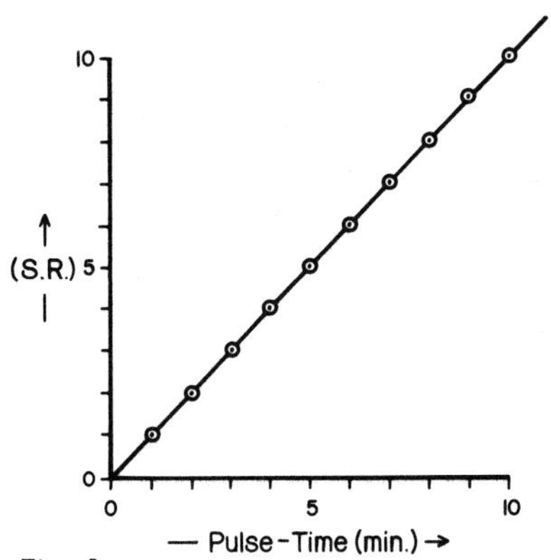

Fig. 1

Radioactivity associated with a Protein vs. Time of Exposure to Radioactive Amino - Acid Mixture. (Pulse – Time)

Having considered this relationship, one could then break the polypeptide chain at known sites, separate the fragments by appropriate means, and measure the amount of specific radioactivity in each peptide fragment. Knowing the order of the fragments in the intact polypeptide would allow the investigator to ascertain whether the amount of specific radioactivity incorporated into protein increased linearly as synthesis proceeded from amino-terminus to carboxy-terminus. A linear relationship would be expected if the polypeptide has a single growing-point at the amino-terminus (*i.e.*, if the entire chain were synthesised from a single strand of *m-RNA*),but would not hold if the polypeptide were synthesised from several growing-points and later joined into a single chain (*i.e.*, if several individual strands of *m-RNA* were translated separately). Consider for a moment the pattern of incorporation of labelled amino-acids into H-chains that would be obtained if these were synthesised from a single growing-point at the amino-terminus. It will be recalled that papain will cleave the H-chain into two fragments of similar size, the *Fd* (amino-terminal) half and the *Fc* (carboxy-terminal) half of the chain. Let T = the time required for the synthesis of a complete H-chain. Then, the label will increase linearly in the *Fd*-fragment from time 0 to $\frac{1}{2}T$, whilst no label will appear in the *Fc*-fragment during this time interval. During the interval $\frac{1}{2}T$ to T, the label in the *Fd*-fragment will remain constant, whilst the label in the *Fc*-fragment will increase linearly, until it equals the value in the *Fd*-fragment, at time = T. One can plot graphically the incorporation of labelled precursor into each half of the polypeptide chain as the specific radioactivity (*S.R.*) associated with each fragment (usually expressed as counts per minute on a scintillation counter, but expressed here in arbitrary units) against time of pulse-labelling. One can then plot the ratio of *S.R.* associated with the *Fc*-fragment to *S.R.* associated with the *Fd*-fragment against the time of pulse-labelling. Figures 2 and 3 show hypothetical data for such a system, where T = 10 minutes. It can be seen readily that the plot of S.R. *(Fc)* vs. time has certain peculiar properties. For example: *S.R. (Fd)*.

The ratio remains 0 until time = $\frac{1}{2}T$, whereupon it rises linearly to a maximum of 1.0 at time = T. It falls to a low of 0.5 at time = $1\frac{1}{2}T$, and again rises to 1.0 at time = $2T$.

This ratio plot stands in sharp contradistinction to the pattern obtained if the *Fd*-fragment and the *Fc*-fragment each had a growing-point within them. In the latter case, the *S.R.* associated with each fragment would rise synchronously, and the ratio of *S.R. (Fc) / S.R. (Fd)* vs. time would plot as a straight line of slope = 0 and ordinate = 1.0.

Data of this type have indicated that L-chains and H-chains are both synthesised from single growing-points

Fig. 2

Kinetics of H-Chain Synthesis based on single Growing-Point at Amino Terminus.

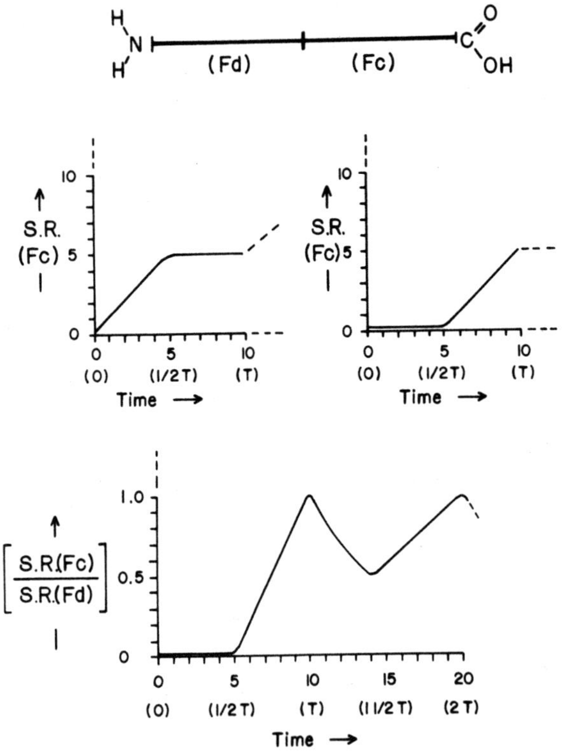

Hypothetical data is given in text.

Fig. 3

HYPOTHETICAL IDEALIZED DATA FOR INCORPORATION OF RADIOACTIVITY INTO GROWING IMMUNOGLOBULIN H-CHAINS.

(These data are consistent with 1 growing point per H-chain, in the Fd fragment at its amino-terminus)

It is assumed that : a) Fd and Fc are of equal length
b) 10 min. are required to synthesize 1 H-chain (i.e., T = 10 min.)
c) Chase completely dilutes pulse
d) Synthesis is initiated synchronously
e) S.R. = Specific Radioactivity, in arbitrary units

Time (min.)	S.R. (Fc)	S.R. (Fd)	$\frac{\text{S.R.(Fc)}}{\text{S.R.(Fd)}}$
0 (t = 0)	0	0	–
1	0	1	0
2	0	2	0
3	0	3	0
4	0	4	0
5 (t = 1/2 T)	0	5	0
6	1	5	0.20
7	2	5	0.40
8	3	5	0.60
9	4	5	0.80
10 (t = T)	5	5	1.00
11	5	6	0.83
12	5	7	0.72
13	5	8	0.63
14	5	9	0.56
15 (t = 1 1/2 T)	5	10	0.50
16	6	10	0.60
17	7	10	0.70
18	8	10	0.80
19	9	10	0.90
20	10	10	1.00

at their respective amino-termini, and, therefore, represent the translation products of single strands of *m-RNA*.

Since H-chains are approximately twice the size of L-chains, it would be predicted that if these are both synthesised on single strands of *m-RNA*, the *m-RNA* encoding the H-chain would be approximately twice the size of the *m-RNA* encoding the L-chain. In fact, it has been shown experimentally that H-chain polysomes are about twice as large as L-chain polysomes. The two classes of polysomes were identified serologically (using antisera directed against determinants specific for H-chain and L-chain) and separated according to size by sucrose density-gradient ultracentrifugation. Polysomes of the larger class precipitate with anti-H-chain serum, but not with anti-L-chain serum. The smaller class of polysomes behave exactly in the converse manner - precipitating with anti-L-chain serum, but not with anti-H-chain serum. H-chain polysomes contain ~18 ribosomes/polysome, whilst L-chain polysomes contain 8-9 ribosomes. These data agree with the data from pulse-chase experiments in suggesting the H- and L-chains are synthesised as complete units from single growing-points on separate strands of *m-RNA*.

The text and illustrations of this chapter were adapted from:

Gordon, B. L., Dyscrasias of Immunoglobulin Production, Philadelphia, Pa. (1969), with permission of the F. A. Davis Company

Chapter 22

MOLECULAR MECHANISMS OF ANTIBODY FORMATION AND FOR GENERATING DIVERSITY IN IMMUNOGLOBULINS

Mechanisms of genetic control in immune responses have no medical importance at present; but, nonetheless, are extremely interesting and widely discussed. Many aspects of such mechanisms are currently the subjects of heated controversy. Where alternative theories have been suggested, and neither alternative disproven by explicit experimental data, expert opinion is often polarised into conflicting camps. Under such circumstances, elaborate arguments have evolved in support of one or another theory, which are generally beyond the scope of this book. Current concepts have been outlined briefly without presenting a vast amount of detailed arguments in the discussion which follows.

The basic principles of biochemical genetics and molecular biology, which are prerequisite to understanding this discussion, have been reviewed in Appendix A, and familiarity with these concepts is assumed here.

The mechanisms by which an antigen stimulates the formation of antibodies will be considered first. For many years, it was hotly debated whether antigens provoked the synthesis of specific antibodies by serving as a template around which a plastic immunoglobulin molecule could be molded (*Instructional theories*), or whether an antigen merely selected a particular population of immunocytes (from a vast population present in the body) which were capable of producing an immunoglobulin with specificity toward that antigen, thereby inducing these cells to proliferate and increase their rate of antibody synthesis above a low basal level (*Selection theories*).

Although instructional theories have been useful in the past to explain serological specificity and the versatility of immune responses, they leave many aspects of immunity unexplained, and are totally incompatible with many experimental observations. Therefore, they are generally regarded as untenable at present.

Selection theories, on the other hand, have been useful in explaining nearly all of the aspects of immune responses incompatible with intructional mechanisms. Moreover, they have provided valuable stimuli for experimental work, and have lent themselves readily to modification and refinement to fit accumulating experimental data. A modification of the Clonal Selection Theory of Burnet is presented here, which, although compatible with most experimental data presently available, will likely require further modification as new data emerges in the future.

(1) An immunologically-competent individual possesses large numbers of inducible immunocyte clones,* each of which carries a single unique immunoglobulin on its surface which is capable of reacting with a single antigenic configuration. Each clone is committed to the synthesis of its unique immunoglobulin. Vast numbers of such clones are generated during development and maturation of the lymphoid system, and even, perhaps, in the mature lymphoid system. The mechanism by which immunocyte clones of differing specificities are developed remains controversial; this will be discussed in the next section of this chapter (*vide infra*).

(2) Reaction of an antigen with the immunoglobulin on the surface of a "committed" immunocyte may lead to either of two phenomena. For example, contact of this type may lead to mitotic proliferation of the clone and stimulation of antibody synthesis. Alternatively, such contact may lead to repression of both antibody synthesis and mitotic activity. Repression may involve the death of cells within the clone (*i.e.*, clonal deletion), or may occur in a potentially-reversible form; in either case, it results in the establishment of a state of immune tolerance to that antigen. When contact with antigen results in stimulation of the immunocyte clone, however, it initiates a specific primary response.

Tolerance is induced most readily during embryonic and foetal development, either because of a fundamental difference in immunocyte differentiation or because the immunocytes are less numerous.

(3) Where immunocyte stimulation results from contact with an antigen, the immunoglobulin product of a single clone is homogeneous in its primary structure.† Even in an individual heterozygous for immunoglobulin genetic markers (allotypes), a stimulated clone will produce an immunoglobulin product which possesses only one determinant at each locus; *i.e.*, only one genetic alternative at each locus is expressed in each mature plasma-cell, in spite of the fact that every cell contains the *DNA* for both alternatives at all loci for which the individual is heterozygous. (This phenomenon is referred to as *allelic exclusion*).

* *A clone is a single (genetically-homogeneous) cell and its progeny derived by mitotic proliferation.*

† *i.e., all molecules are identical to each other.*

(4) Although antigen-responsive immunocytes are already committed to the synthesis of one immunoglobulin product, a population of undifferentiated (and uncommitted) precursor cells probably exists even in developmentally-mature individuals, which continues to generate antigen-responsive clones *de novo*. Mutant clones may develop in the course of time which are committed to the synthesis of antibodies to self-antigens; these are called forbidden clones. If they should contact the antigen to which they are responsive, and the result of this contact is repression, tolerance to that antigen remains unbroken. Where stimulation results from autoantigen-contact, however, the development of autoantibodies will occur (*vide supra*, Chapter 19).

(5) Clonal redundancy is the rule for most antigens. That is, a number of clones, responsive to a single antigen, develop in the lymphoid system, all of which will respond to contact with the same antigen. Since serum antibodies represent a composite of all clonal products which are present in the circulation, even purified antibodies from a single individual with specificity for a single haptenic determinant are polyclonal in origin. Nevertheless, the product of any single antibody-producing cell and its progeny is structurally homogeneous (*i.e.*, monoclonal).

(6) During the course of a primary response, antigen-stimulated proliferating immunocytes give rise to long-lived progeny. These cells, morphologically small-to-medium lymphocytes, remain capable of antigen-recognition on subsequent contact. Such contact results in a flurry of proliferative activity and antibody synthesis, in turn resulting in the development of a secondary response to the antigen.

The Genetic Basis of Immunoglobulin Diversity

Some of the possible mechanisms by which the great diversity of structure in immunoglobulins might be generated and controlled genetically will now be discussed. Although this area is most controversial, the discussion will begin with those points on which there is general agreement, and proceed to the more controversial points.

(1) The *C-regions* (*vide supra*, Chapter 21) of both H- and L-chains are encoded by germ-lines* which

* *That is, genes which segregate in meiosis and are passed on to each individual as ordinary inheritable traits, encoded in parental DNA and transmitted via gametes to the progeny, according to Mendelian laws.*

segregate as expected for diploid organisms. This has been established by study of the inheritance of allotypic markers. *Inv*, *Gm*, and *Am* markers are located in $C\kappa$-, $C\gamma$-, and $C\alpha_2$-regions respectively, and are inherited as independently-assorting sets of germ-line alleles, in conformity with Mendelian laws.

(2) The *V-regions* are encoded by structural genes which are separate from the structural genes encoding the *C-regions*. The germ-line must carry at least 13 *V-genes* - one for each of the four subgroups of $V\kappa$, one for each of the five subgroups of $V\lambda$, and one for each of the four V_H subgroups. Thus, these 13 *V-region* genes occur in three known major linkage groups; *i.e.*, $V\kappa$, $V\lambda$, and V_H. The precise mode of inheritance of *V-region* genes, and the related question of genetic control of antibody specificity are not yet known in man, since genetic markers on human *V-regions* have not yet been reported. Genetic markers for V_H *regions* have been described in rabbits, however, which demonstrate that V_H*-regions* in that species are encoded by germ-line genes.

(3) The above has led to the conclusion that two genes code for a single polypeptide chain in immunoglobulin synthesis. Convincing evidence for this hypothesis was próvided by rare myeloma patients who simultaneously produce monoclonal IgG and monoclonal IgM M-proteins. Amino-acid sequences of the γ and μ chains were identical through the first hypervariable region even though the primary structures of the constant regions were different. Furthermore, the IgG and IgM M-proteins from the same patient's serum shared all idiotypic antigenic determinants - *i.e.*, the antigenic determinants on the variable region. These experiments of nature are the best evidence that the *V-regions* of each chain are under separate genetic control and that the *C-regions* of the μ and γ chains share the same V_H-gene.

(4) There are currently two types of hypotheses which have been proposed to explain genetic control of specificity regions.

- The first type suggests that there are a great number of specificity region genes carried in the germ-line of every individual, each specifying one particular *V-region* sequence. The origin of all of these *V-regions* would be via germ-line evolution. (Hypotheses of this type are referred to as *multi-gene* theories).

- The second type suggest that only a few specificity-region genes are carried in the germ-line of every individual, and that the high degree of variability observed in *V-regions* is introduced during somatic differentiation of the lymphoid system. This differentiation occurs during embryonic and foetal development, and probably continues throughout the life of the individual. Both somatic recombination and somatic cell hypermutability have been suggested as mechanisms for introducing this variability. (Hypotheses of this type are referred to as *pauci-gene* theories).

(5) Common to both multi-gene and pauci-gene theories is the concept of *VC-translocation*. One *V-region* structural gene (whether selected from a vast array of germ-line genes or generated *de novo* by somatic recombination of somatic mutation) is translocated onto an appropriate *C-region* structural gene, thereby forming a complete *VC-structural gene*. Similar translocations are thought to occur for H-chains and for L-chains. These two-gene complexes then transcribed single strands of *m-RNA*, specifying complete H- and L-chains. Translation of these *m-RNA* strands results in the synthesis of H-chains and L-chains from single growing-points at the amino-terminus of each chain - (*vide supra*, Chapter 22).

Translocation of *V-* and *C-* structural genes is thought to represent the mechanism of clonal expression and allelic exclusion (*i.e.*, synthesis of a single homogeneous immunoglobulin in which only one allele for each marker locus is expressed by any clone of immunocytes in heterozygous individuals). Irreversible differentiation and commitment of an immunocyte would thus occur at the time of translocation of *V-* and *C-* structural genes.

Finally, a few remarks will be made on the relative likelihood of multi-gene vs. pauci-gene theories of genetic control of immunoglobulin specificity regions.

Multi-Gene Theory for Control of Diversity in Immunoglobulins

Dreyer and his colleagues have suggested that separate single germ-line genes (alleles) encode the C_L*-regions* (invariant regions of L-chains), whilst V_L*-regions* (L-chain variable regions) are encoded by enormous numbers of individual germ-line genes, the diversity of which arose during the course of evolution. Synthesis of a complete L-chain or similarly, a complete H-chain is postulated to occur when a single specificity region gene (V_L or V_H gene) is chosen and spliced (translocated) onto an appropriate constant region (C_L or C_H gene).

This hypothesis explains the observed amino-acid sequence diversities in L-chain variable regions by assuming that a separate germ-line gene exists for each individual variable region. The observed similarities between *V-region* peptides of different immunoglobulins are explained in part by assuming that all *V-region* genes are the evolutionary descendants of a single primordial *V-region* gene, and are therefore related to each other.

During immunocyte differentiation, a single specificity gene (*V-gene*) is spliced to one invariant region gene (*C-gene*); the two-gene complex then transcribes a single strand of *m-RNA* which is translated into a complete L-chain or H-chain. The theory is thus consistent with observations of polysome size and the kinetics of L- and H-chain formation, which indicated that a single strand of *m-RNA* appears to be the template for translation of a complete L- or H-chain, since both chains are synthesised from single growing-points (*vide supra*, Chapter 21).

Since this theory postulates relatively small numbers of *C-region* genes, it is compatible with the observed Mendelian inheritance of allotypic markers located on the *C-regions* of H- and L-chains.

V-region diversity, *V-region* similarity (to some extent), the presence of allelic markers on *C-regions*, and the observations on the kinetics of H- and L-chain biosynthesis can all be explained by a multiple-gene theory in which diversity is introduced during germ-line evolution, and in which translocation of a *V-region* gene onto a *C-region* gene occurs. Nevertheless, other data and observations are not explained in a satisfactory manner.

(a) Multi-gene theories demand the assumption that an enormous amount of germ-line *DNA* must be devoted to encoding immunoglobulin variable regions. This mechanism seems far too expensive (in terms of germ-line *DNA* required) to have allowed its selection in vertebrate evolution - it would seem to the author that a less wasteful system for generating immunoglobulin diversity would have preferentially evolved.

(b) Allotypic markers have been identified on the *V-regions* of heavy chains in the rabbit. The allotypic markers on these rabbit *V-regions* arise from particular amino-acid sequences within a restricted area of heavy chain *V-regions*. Moreover, these markers are inherited in simple Mendelian fashion, which implies that all V_H *-genes* of individuals homozygous for this allotypic marker share one or the other allele. It is difficult to believe that every one of a vast number of

V_H-genes could share a common allelic marker (*i.e.*, that a common allelic marker would be conserved in all-or-none manner amongst a vast number of genes).

It is the author's opinion, therefore, that *V-region* variability is controlled genetically by a pauci-gene system.

Pauci-Gene Theories for Immunoglobulin Diversity

Two pauci-gene theories have been introduced to explain the genetic control of immunoglobulin *V-regions* by a small number of *V-region* genes.

The first suggests that a small number of *V-region* genes are "hypermutable" and undergo an enormous number of point mutations within somatic cells. These mutant cells (and their gene products) are selected for or against, depending on the nature of the product. Although this type of theory is extremely simple, it would require an incredibly high mutation rate to generate sufficient diversity within a small number of generations, so that appropriate genes could be distributed amongst the fairly large number of cells necessary to explain polyclonal antibody responses to single antigens. After commitment to an antigen, these hypermutable genes would have to be stabilised to discourage further mutation. Furthermore, a mechanism is required to confine the mutations to *V-regions* (and even to restricted positions within the hypervariable portions of *V-regions*). Such a mechanism is difficult to envision. In addition to the difficulties enumerated above, a pauci-gene theory based on somatic mutation fails to account for the non-random nature of the variance within *V-regions*. For example, this theory does not explain why the same limited alternative substitutions recur at comparable (homologous) positions amongst different individual *V-regions*, since mutation is nearly universally regarded as a random process. For the above and other reasons, theories of this type are considered to be incompatible with presently-available data.

The second category of pauci-gene theory suggests that a small number of *V-region* genes undergo controlled somatic-cell recombination, which generates diversity by producing a large number of diverse *V-regions* pursuant to genetic recombination. The *V-regions* generated in this manner would be translocated onto an appropriate *C-region* and transcribed into single segments of *m-RNA*, encoding an entire *VC-polypeptide* (either as a complete L-chain or as a complete H-chain). The author currently favours the version of this theory proposed by

Edelman and Gally as being the most acceptable mechanism for genetic control of *V-region* diversity amongst the immunoglobulins; for this reason, it is developed here in some detail. The following discussion refers to the model illustrated in Figure 1.

A set of structural genes exists for each *V-region* subtype. The individual members of each set are similar, but not identical, having many positions in common, but differing in many others. The positions of identity would permit synapsis of *DNA* to occur between the members of a sub-group gene set, whilst the positions of non-identity would be aligned appropriately to permit somatic-cell crossover to produce *de novo* recombinants, the peptide products of which would have new sequences of amino-acid residues. As suggested in Figure 1, the individual members of each gene set are envisioned to be situated in tandem on the same chromosome, and the somatic cell crossover which would generate new *V-region* peptides would be intra-chromosomal. For this to occur, the individual members of each gene set would be arranged in opposite configuration to each other (*i.e.,* 3'-ends adjacent or 5'-ends adjacent). The number of individual genes within a single set is not specified, although a single pair per set would be sufficient to account for all (or nearly all) of the observed variance within *V-regions*. For example, two alternative base pairs at n positions would yield 2^n possible recombinant nucleotide sequences.

Somatic crossover would be restricted to members of the same gene set (*i.e.,* to genes encoding *V-regions* of the same sub-type). Synapsis and crossover would thus not occur between *V-region* genes belonging to different sets.

Frequent pairing and recombination amongst tandemly-linked genes would tend to maintain the similarity of individual genes within a set during the course of evolution, whilst, at the same time, selecting for mutations tending to increase the number of antigen-binding sites and selecting against mutations producing useless (non-antibody) gene products.

The theory outlined above offers the following advantages:

(a) It is conservative in terms of the minor degree of novelty in its underlying mechanism; it does not require entirely new or unprecedented biochemical or genetic processes to occur in order to allow its operation.

(b) It is economically feasible in terms of germ-line *DNA* required to maintain immune responsiveness

Fig. 1

DIAGRAM OF A SPECIFICITY REGION GENE PAIR
(Adapted from Edelman and Gally)

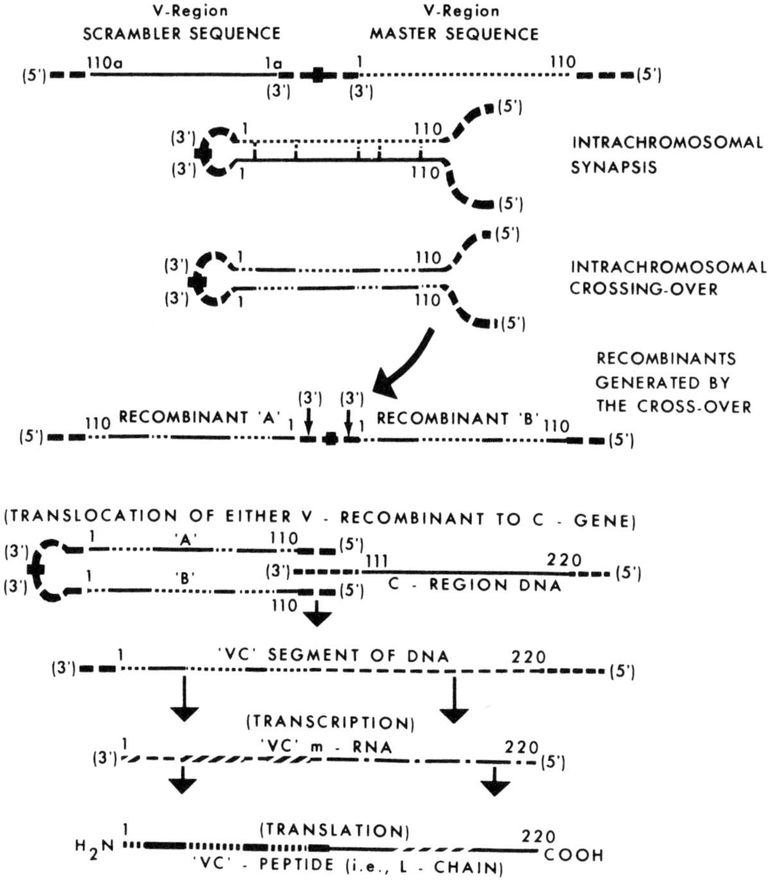

For example, if there were two *V-region* genes per set, less than 250 codons would be needed to encode an entire sub-group of *V-regions*.

(c) It explains both the striking similarity and the striking diversity amongst individual *V-regions*.

(d) It is compatible with the Mendelian inheritance of *C-region* allotypic determinants in man.

(e) It is also compatible with the Mendelian inheritance of *V-region* allotypes in rabbits, since only a small number of genes would be required to bear the allotypic markers in homozygous individuals, and the markers could occur in areas of *V-regions* where all of the members of any single gene set are identical.

(f) This theory is entirely compatible with the observed data on the kinetics of H- and L-chain synthesis.

However, in spite of the compatibility of this mechanism with all major experimental data accumulated to present, this theory cannot be accepted as fact until it has been proven directly to be valid. Until such direct proof appears, the matter of genetic control mechanisms in immune responses is likely to remain controversial.

APPENDICES

Appendix A

MOLECULAR BIOLOGY: REVIEW OF BASIC PRINCIPLES

The genetic material, *Deoxyribonucleic acid* (*DNA*), encodes the information for the synthesis of all proteins produced by organisms. *DNA* consists structurally of two polynucleotide chains, wound about each other in the configuration of a double helix. There are four types of basic building blocks which occur in *DNA*, differing from each other according to their component organic bases. These bases are of two generic types - the *purine* bases in *DNA* are *adenine* and *guanine*, and the *pyrimidine* bases in *DNA* are *thymine* and *cytosine*. The bases are attached to the sugar 2'-*deoxy-D-ribose* in the β-configuration at carbon 1', and each sugar unit bears a molecule of phosphoric acid at carbon 5'. The basic building block constituted by the organic base, sugar, and phosphoric acid is called a *nucleotide* Figure 1.

Fig. 1

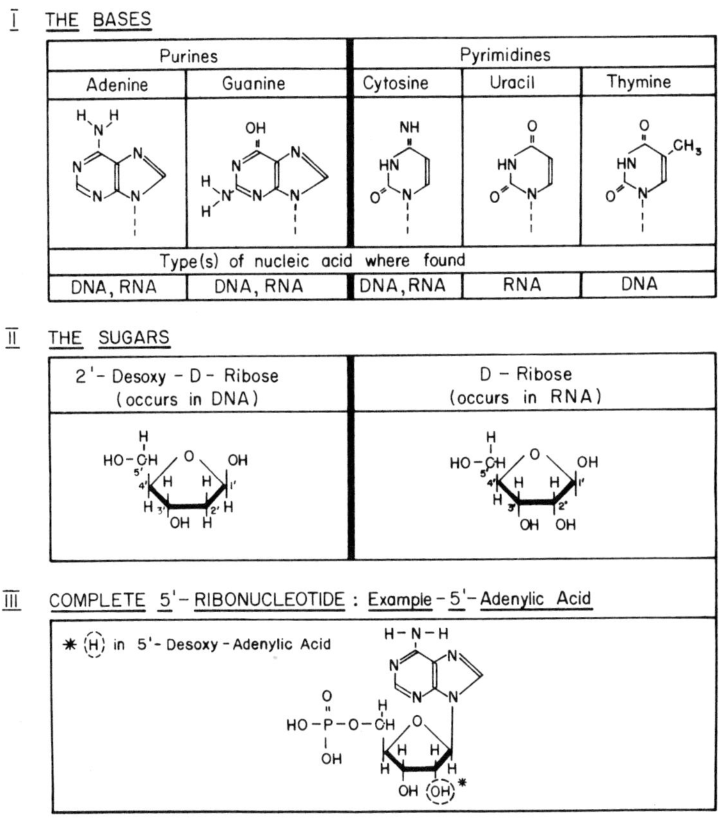

Nucleotides are joined to form polynucleotide chains* by linkage of the 5' phosphate of one to the 3' hydroxyl group on the sugar of the next nucleotide, and so on - Figure 2. The sequence of nucleotides on each strand of *DNA* varies greatly from molecule to molecule.

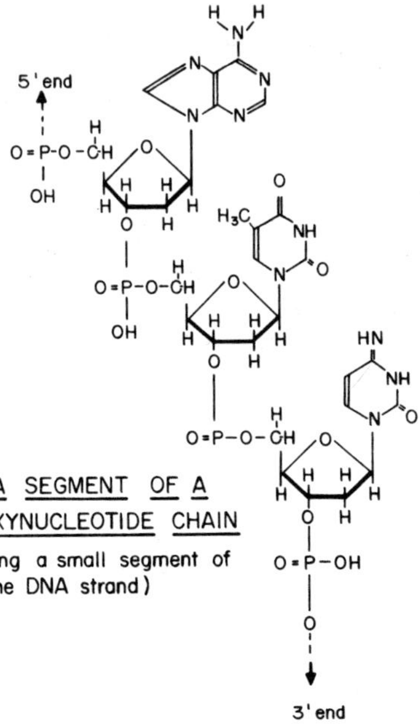

Fig. 2 A SEGMENT OF A POLYDESOXYNUCLEOTIDE CHAIN

(representing a small segment of one DNA strand)

The two associated polynucleotide chains of *DNA* are not identical, but complementary to each other, and joined together by hydrogen bonds between the bases of each chain. Hydrogen bonding is possible between *adenine* on one chain and *thymine* on the second (or *vice versa*), and similarly, between *quanine* on one chain and *cytosine* on the second (or *vice versa*), but in no other combination. In this way, the nucleotide sequence on one chain automatically determines the sequence of nucleotides on the complementary chain - Figure 3.

When *DNA* replicates, the two strands separate, and each builds a new complementary chain. In this way, the stable characters of each organism are passed on to the progeny via the germ plasm. Genetic information in *DNA* resides in the sequence of nucleotides. Groups of

* *Polynucleotide chains form the backbones of two types of nucleic acids (DNA and RNA), which differ from each other in the chemistry of the sugar which constitutes their nucleotides, and in one of the pyrimidines. For DNA, the sugar is 2' – deoxy-D-ribose, and the nucleotides referred to as "deoxynucleotides". For RNA, the sugar is D-ribose, and the nucleotides denoted as "ribonucleotides". In DNA, the two pyrimidines are cytosine and thymine; in RNA, they are cytosine and uracil.*

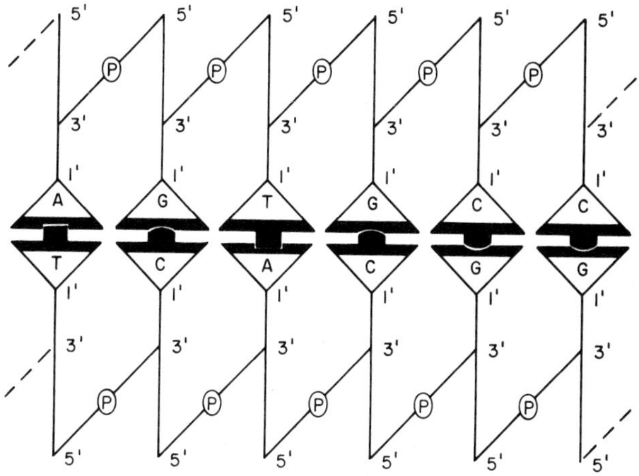

Fig. 3 DIAGRAM OF BASE PAIRING IN COMPLEMENTARY STRANDS OF DNA

G = GUANINE A = ADENINE
C = CYTOSINE T = THYMINE

Note : A strand of DNA can serve as a template for the synthesis of RNA, with Uracil (U) pairing with Adenine on DNA ...(i.e., U replaces T)

three nucleotides (*triplets*) encode the individual amino-acid residues in polypeptide gene products. *DNA* and polypeptide chains are co-linear, in that the sequence of *DNA* code triplets specifies the sequence of amino-acid residues in a polypeptide chain.

Ribonucleic acid (*RNA*) is synthesised (transcribed) from information encoded in a *DNA* strand - Figure 4.

Fig. 4

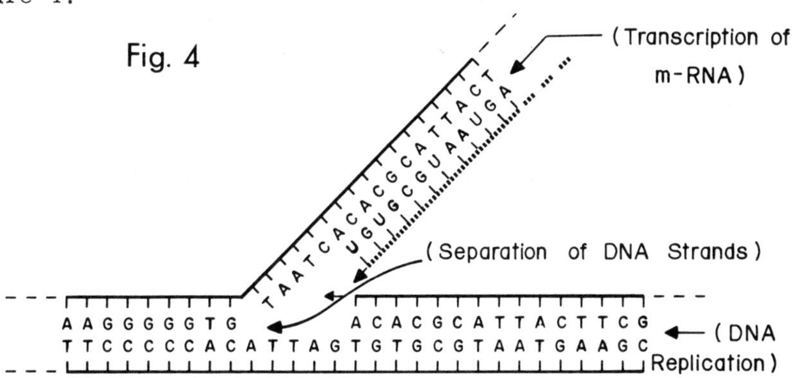

REPLICATION OF DNA AND TRANSCRIPTION OF m-RNA

(Schematic Representation)

When *RNA* is being formed, the strands of *DNA* separate, and one strand serves as a template for the synthesis of a complementary strand of ribonucleotides. As noted, ribonucleotides differ from deoxyribonucleotides in the component sugars (*D-Ribose* replaces *2'-deoxy-D-ribose* in *RNA*) and in one of the bases (*Uracil* replaces *thymine* in *RNA*). However, neither change affects the base-pairing properties; *uracil* and *thymine* have identical pairing properties, and the two sugars are stereochemically similar. The process whereby a segment of *DNA* encoding a complete polypeptide chain directs the synthesis of a complementary strand of *RNA* - *i.e.*, transcription - generates an *RNA*-chain called *messenger RNA* (*m-RNA*). Transcribed *m-RNA* is released from the nucleus into the cytoplasm of the cell. This *m-RNA* associates with sub-cellular organelles termed ribosomes, which represent the structures allowing the translation of a series of nucleotide code triplets into a specific sequence of amino-acid residues on a polypeptide chain - Figure 5.

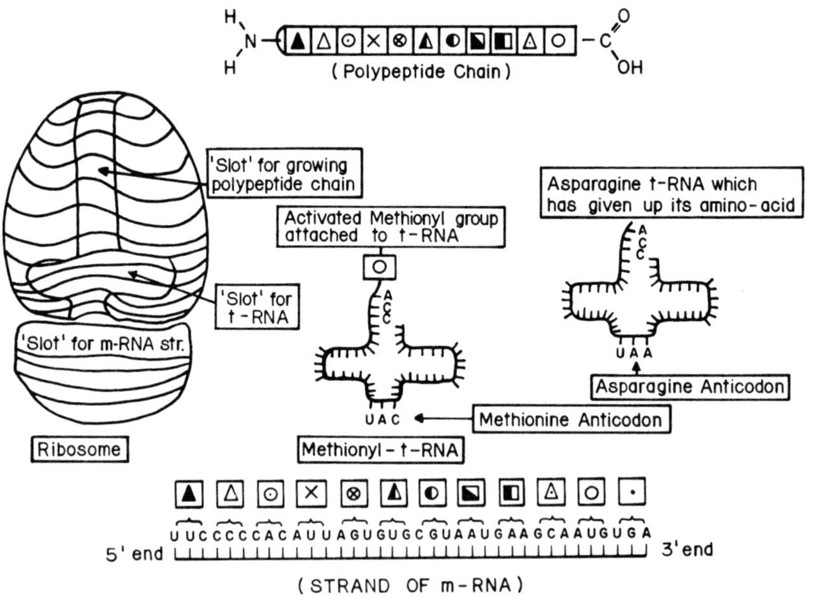

Fig. 5

A single *m-RNA* strand is usually associated with several ribosomes at a given time - the complex is termed a *polyribosome* or *polysome*. Each ribosome on a polysome contains a partially-completed polypeptide chain. The ribosomes traverse the *m-RNA* strand from 5'-end to 3'-end, adding amino-acids to the growing polypeptide chain from amino-terminus to carboxy-terminus.

The amino-acids being added to the polypeptide chain are attached to adaptor molecules of *RNA*, termed *transfer RNA* (*t-RNA*): these contain recognition sites (complementary triplets to *m-RNA* triplets). Nucleotide triplets on *m-RNA* specifying a specific amino-acid on a polypeptide chain are called "*codons*"; the complementary triplets on *t-RNA* serving as recognition sites for codon triplets are called "*anticodons*". The process of translation of *m-RNA* into a polypeptide chain, on the ribosomes, is depicted in Figure 6. In summary, the complementarity of *m-RNA* codons and *t-RNA* anticodons enables *aminoacyl-t-RNA* complexes to line up in the correct order along a strand of *m-RNA*. As this occurs, the aminoacyl groups are detached from the *t-RNA* and joined together in peptide linkages on ribosomes as these organelles traverse the *m-RNA* strand.

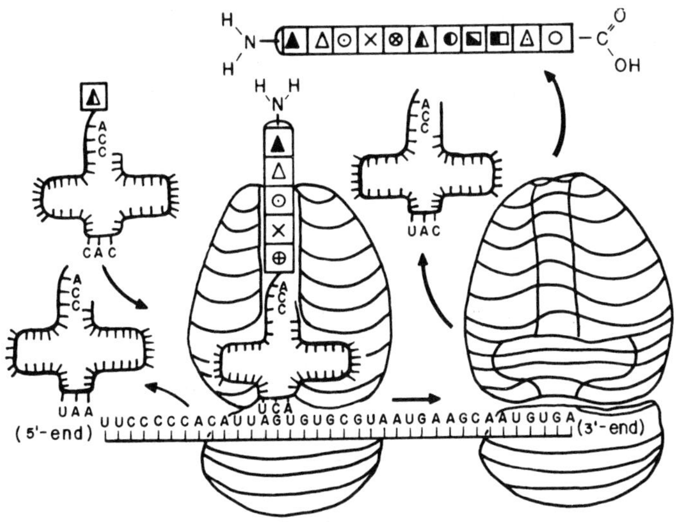

Fig. 6 THE TRANSLATION OF m-RNA (SCHEMATIC)

The genetic code for each amino-acid is known - all 64 possible triplets have been assigned a meaning - either as a codon for a specific amino-acid or as a codon specifying the end of a polypeptide chain. The genetic code, depicted in Figure 7, is universal; it appears to be identical in all organisms.

This universality of the genetic code has many biological implications. For example, in the laboratory, a protein-synthesising system from human erythrocytes can translate bacterial *m-RNA* into bacterial proteins, whilst human *m-RNA* can be employed to synthesise human proteins with a bacterial protein-synthesising system.

Fig. 7 THE GENETIC CODE

Amino-Acid	Letter Code	Symbol	m-RNA Codons (5'→3')
Cysteine	CYS	●	UGU, UGC
Methionine	MET	○	UAG
Serine	SER	⊕	UCU,UCC,AGU,AGC,AGC,AGU
Threonine	THR	●	ACU,ACC,ACA,ACG
Proline	PRO	Δ	CCU,CCC,CCA,CCG
Aspartic Acid	ASP	■	GAU,GAC
Asparagine	ASN	⬔	AAU,AAC
Glutamic Acid	GLU	◧	GAA,GAG
Glutamine	GLN	⊟	CAA,CAG
Arginine	ARG	◐	CGU,CGC,CGA,CGG,AGA,AGG
Lysine	LYS	o	AAA,AAG
Histidine	HIS	⊙	CAU,CAC
Alanine	ALA	Δ	GCU,GCC,GCA,GCG
Phenylalanine	PHE	▲	UUU,UUC
Leucine	LEU	+	UUA,UUG,CUU,CUC,CUA,CUG
Isoleucine	ILE	×	AUU,AUC,AUA
Valine	VAL	▲	GUU,GUC,GUA,GUG
Tryptophan	TRY	✳	UGG
Tyrosine	TYR	◎	UAU,UAC
Glycine	GLY	◉	GGU,GGC,GGA,GGG

Chain — Terminating Codons = UAA,UAG,UGA

Codon Abbreviations

U - Uracil
C - Cytosine
A - Adenine
G - Guanine

Note: The chain-terminating codons are analogous to "periods" at ends of code "sentences"---- releasing the nascent polypeptide chains from their ribosomes.

Since the foregoing facts are common to all known living organisms (irrespective of the system investigated), they should be accorded the status of scientific laws until such time as experimental data proves them invalid. Thus, when hypotheses are proposed to explain the biochemical and genetic mechanisms which operate in the immune system, these hypotheses should be compatible with the basic principles of molecular genetics as well as accounting for the known properties of immune responses.

The text and illustrations of Appendix A were adapted from:

Gordon, B.L., Dyscrasias of Immunoglobulin Production, Philadelphia, Pa., (1969), with permission of the F.A. Davis Company.

Appendix B

DETERMINATION OF THE PRIMARY STRUCTURE OF PROTEINS - EXPERIMENTAL METHODS EMPLOYED

The first step in determining the primary structure of a protein is to determine its amino-acid composition. This is usually accomplished by acid hydrolysis (using 6 N HCl at 100-110°C for 6-20 hours). This procedure will result in complete hydrolysis of the protein to amino-acids; however, tryptophan is destroyed by this procedure, as are the hydroxy-amino-acids (serine and threonine) to a lesser extent. Destruction of serine and threonine can be minimised, however, by analysis of the hydrolysate at various times of exposure to acid, which allows correction for destruction of these compounds. Tryptophan is usually determined separately by alkaline hydrolysis of the protein under study. Acid hydrolysis does not distinguish asparagine from aspartic acid, or glutamine from glutamic acid; both amides appear as the derivative acids in the hydrolysate. Alkaline hydrolysis suffers from even more severe drawbacks, however.

Amino-acids in acid hydrolysates are separated chromatographically and analysed spectrophotometrically. These operations are accomplished simultaneously on automated amino-acid analysers. On such an apparatus each amino-acid is eluted at a characteristic point specified by the conditions under which analysis is performed. Ammonia derived from amide-amino-acids (asparagine and glutamine) also elutes at a specific point.

Having determined an amino-acid composition for a protein, one can proceed to primary structure analysis. One of the most useful tools in this regard is amino-terminal analysis, which is accomplished by reacting the native protein with Dansyl chloride in alkaline solution. This reaction couples the "Dansyl" fluorochrome group onto free amino-groups in the polypeptide (both α- and ε-). The resulting *DNS*-derivatives are stable to acid hydrolysis, and can be identified in thin-layer chromatography as fluorescent spots on the chromatogram. The reactions involved in dansylation of a polypeptide chain are shown in Figure 1.

Dansyl chloride reacts with both α- amino-groups (amino-terminal residues of polypeptide chains) and ε-amino-groups (of lysine). Dansylated amino-acids (*DNS*-derivatives) are fluorescent, and are detected by exposing thin-layer chromatograms of a peptide hydrolysate to ultra-violet light. The chromatogram of the acid hydrolysate of a dansylated polypeptide is compared with a similar chromatogram of known *DNS*-amino-acids. The

AMINO-TERMINAL ANALYSIS: PREPARATION OF A DNS-AMINO-ACID

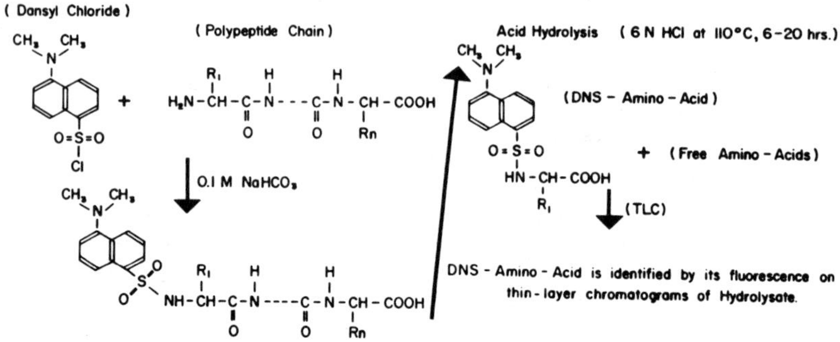

fluorescent spot in the chromatogram of the acid hydrolysate is compared with the spots of the known *DNS*-amino-acids and identified in this manner. ε-mono-*DNS*-lysines are obtained from internal lysines (*i.e.*, not at the amino-terminus), whilst α, ε-Di-*DNS*-lysine is obtained when lysine occurs at the amino-terminus of a polypeptide. When the amino-terminus of a peptide is blocked by the occurrence of pyrrolidone carboxylic acid (PCA), only ε-mono-*DNS*-lysines will be found, if the peptide contains any lysines. No *DNS*-amino-acids are found in peptides which contain no lysine and possess a *PCA*-residue blocking the amino-terminus of the polypeptide chain. Where two or more *DNS*-amino-acids (other than ε-mono-*DNS*-lysine) are identified in the hydrolysate of a protein, the protein can be assumed to possess more than one polypeptide chain. Multi-chain proteins are usually connected by interchain disulphide bonds - when these occur, the bonds may be broken by oxidising each cystine to two cysteic acids (by performate treatment) or by reducing each cystine to two cysteines (by mercaptoethanol-amine-urea treatment) followed by separation of the chains by electrophoresis of chromatography. Each chain can then be subjected to separate primary structure analysis.

Let us now consider primary structure analysis by the method of partial acid hydrolysis. This is accomplished by treatment of polypeptide chains with dilute acid at low temperature, followed by chromatographic or electrophoretic separation of the components of the hydrolysate. In this case, breakage of the polypeptide is random - the hydrolysate contains amino-acids, dipeptides, tripeptides, and oligopeptides which can be analysed individually and studied for overlaps. This is explained in Example 1.

Example 1: An oligopeptide suspected of having

pyrogenic activity was isolated from polymorphonuclear leucocytes. Complete acid hydrolysis of the peptide showed the following composition when the hydrolysate was subjected to amino-acid analysis:

Amino Acid	Symbol	No. of Residues	Amino Acid	Symbol	No. of Residues
Aspartic Acid or Asparagine		- 2	Valine		- 1
			Alanine		- 1
Glutamic Acid or Glutamine		- 1	Arginine		- 1
			Threonine		- 1
Methionine		- 1	Histidine		- 1
Phenylalanine		- 1	Ammonia	NH_3	- 2

Dansylation of the peptide followed by complete acid hydrolysis and thin-layer chromatography showed that phenylalanine was present as the *DNS*-derivative, and therefore represented the amino-terminal residue of the peptide. The peptide was then subjected to partial acid hydrolysis. The hydrolysate was treated with dansyl chloride, and separated by two-dimensional thin-layer chromatography. When the thin-layer chromatogram was examined in ultra-violet light, seventeen dansylated partial hydrolysis products were noted. Each of these was eluted from the chromatogram and subjected to complete acid hydrolysis. Each hydrolysed spot was again chromatographed and examined with ultra-violet light to detect *DNS*-amino-acids and sprayed with ninhydrin to identify the remaining free amino-acids. The following compositions were noted for each spot:

DESIGNATION OF SPOT AND COMPOSITION

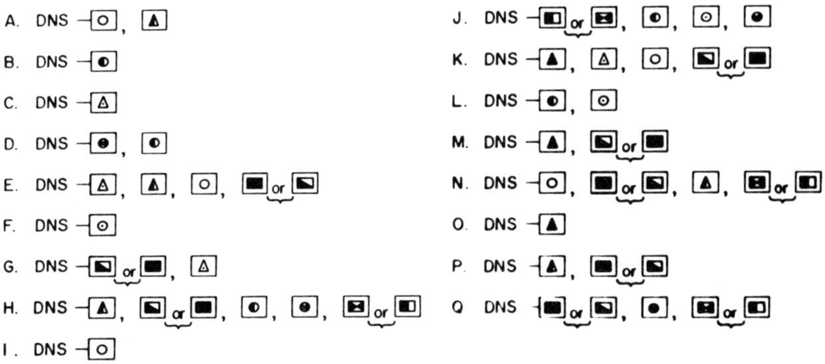

This enables us to derive partial sequences. For example:

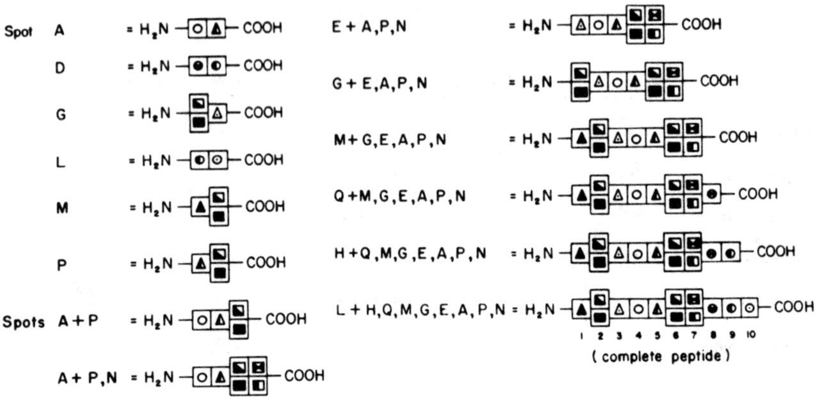

Note that positions 2, 6 and 7 could not be assigned precisely because this method does not discriminate between dicarboxylic-amino-acids and their amide-derivatives. Although the recovery of two moles of ammonia per mole of peptide suggested that two of the three dicarboxylic-acid residues were present as the amides, we are not able to decide on the basis of this data which residues were present in which form. The primary structure obtainable by this method alone is therefore ambiguous.

It thus can be seen that dansylation + partial acid hydrolysis enables the deduction of primary structure of polypeptides, although it is subject to certain limitations.

More powerful tools are available for primary structure analysis of polypeptide chains, which enable such analyses to be performed in much less time and remove some of the ambiguities inherent in the previous method.

Certain agents are capable of splitting polypeptide chains in specified positions. The first of these, trypsin, is a proteolytic enzyme that cleaves polypeptide chains on the carbonyl sides of arginine or lysine residues. Another enzyme, chymotrypsin, cleaves polypeptide chains at the carbonyl sides of phenylalanine, tyrosine, and tryptophan residues, and (more slowly) on the carbonyl sides of leucine, isoleucine, and methionine residues. Cyanogen bromide (CN-Br) hydrolyses polypeptide chains containing methionine at the carbonyl sides of their methionine residues, concomitantly changing these residues into homocysteine residues. Other enzymes (*e.g.*, papain, ficin, pepsin) will cleave polypeptides at other loci, but have not been as commonly employed as trypsin, chymotrypsin or CN-Br in primary structure analysis. Carboxypeptidases are enzymes which cleave the carboxy-terminal residues from polypeptides, provided these residues do not have their α-carboxyl groups blocked (*e.g.*, by amide groups).

A protein is dansylated, and subjected to acid hydrolysis and thin-layer chromatography to identify the amino-terminal composition. It may then be treated with carboxypeptidases followed by thin-layer chromatography to identify the carboxy-terminal residue. Following this, the peptide is then treated with trypsin, chymotrypsin and CN-Br, followed by separation on two-dimensional thin-layer chromatography or electrophoresis - chromatography to separate each peptide thus obtained.

Each peptide can then be analysed by a stepwise procedure called the Edman degradation. The Edman procedure is outline in Figure 2. This method enables the component amino-acid residues of a peptide to be released sequentially and identified as phenyl-thiohydantoin derivatives (PTH-AA),

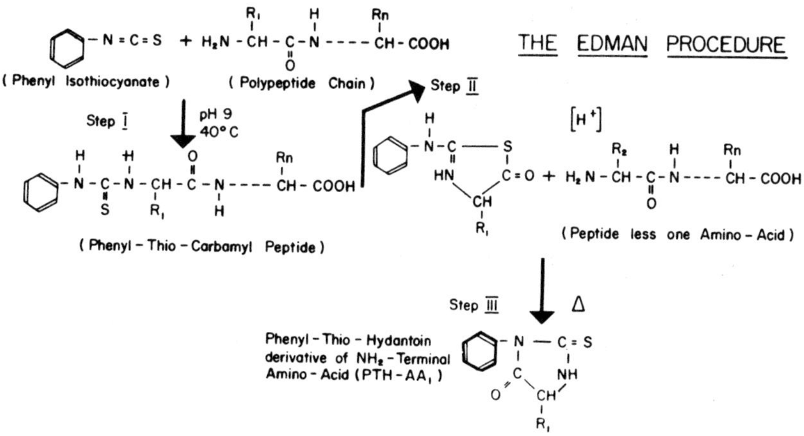

The combination of Dansylation + the Edman Procedure (Dansyl-Edman Procedure) represents an extremely powerful tool in primary structure analysis of proteins. Two examples will illustrate this combined method for primary structure analysis of peptides.

Example 2: A peptide hormone was subjected to amino-acid analysis after complete acid hydrolysis. The data obtained were as follows:

Amino-Acid	Symbol	No. of Residues	Amino-Acid	Symbol	No. of Residues
Aspartic Acid or Asparagine	■ / ◩	- 1	Phenylalanine	▲	- 1
			Histidine	⊙	- 1
Proline	△	- 1	Arginine	◐	- 1
Valine	◭	- 1	Tyrosine	●	- 1
Isoleucine	☒	- 1	Ammonia	NH_3	- 0
					(∴ residue A = ■)

Treatment with Dansyl chloride, followed by complete acid hydrolysis and chromatographic separation of the hydrolysate showed that only aspartate was dansylated (*DNS* -).

The complete peptide was treated with trypsin. Two peptides were obtained and separated by electrophoresis. Each of these were dansylated and hydrolysed with acid. The results obtained were:

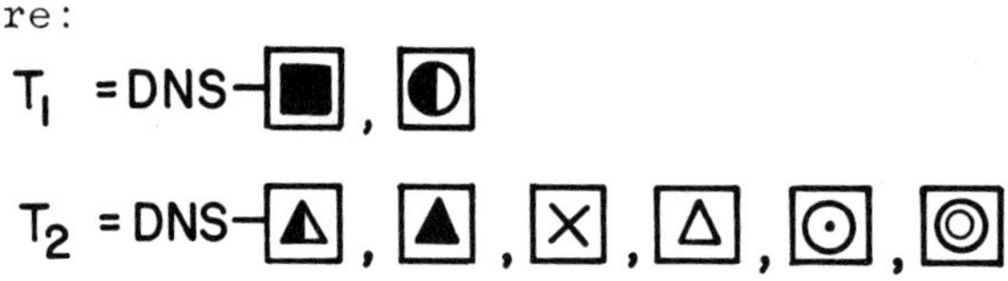

The complete peptide was then subjected to chymotrypsin digestion. Two peptides were obtained, separated and hydrolysed. The results were:

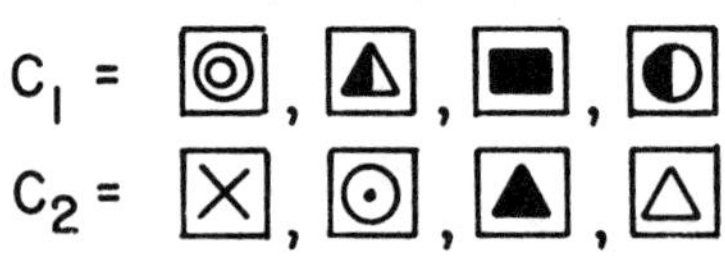

Peptide C_2 was subjected to the Edman procedure. This treatment yielded PTH - derivatives in the following order:

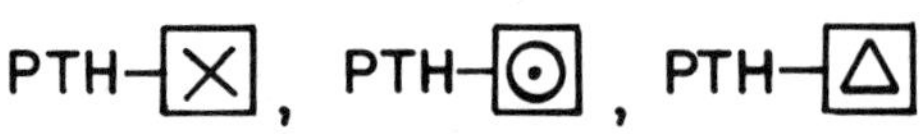

The fourth step was not conclusive. From these data, the primary structure of the peptide is deduced as follows:

The peptide contained eight residues, and the amino-terminus was aspartic acid, *e.g.:*

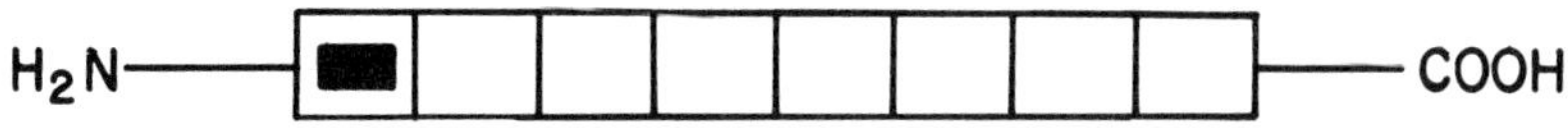

Since trypsin splits at carbonyl side of arginine, and T_1 contained one arginine and one *DNS*-aspartic acid, the second residue was arginine, *i.e.:*

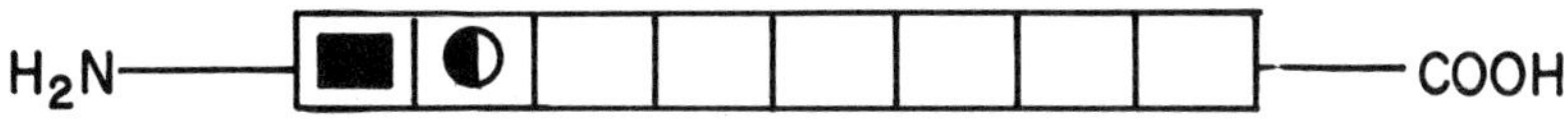

Since T_2 shows *DNS*-valine, this was the third residue, *i.e.:*

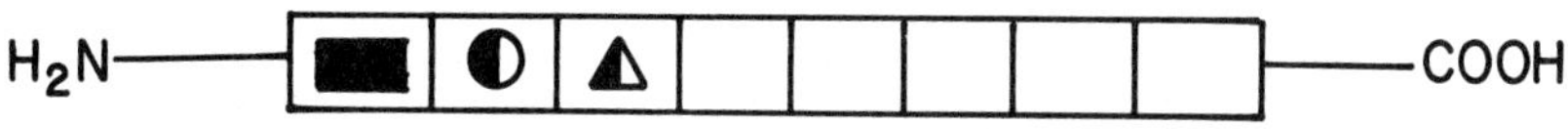

Chymotrypsin treatment resulted in two tetrapeptides. Since this agent has highest hydrolytic affinity for the aromatic amino-acids, it could cleave on the carbonyl side of tryosine or phenylalanine. Examination of the two peptides shows that C_1 was the amino-terminal peptide. Since the first three residues were already deduced, tyrosine was the fourth, and was cleaved by the enzyme at its carbonyl side, *i.e.:*

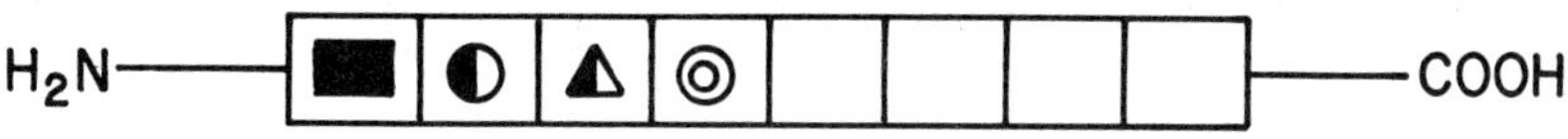

Application of the Edman procedure to C_2 indicates the order of the last four residues. Since the carboxyl-terminal residue was phenylalanine this explains why chymotrypsin failed to cleave the peptide into three fragments. Thus, the primary structure of the peptide was:

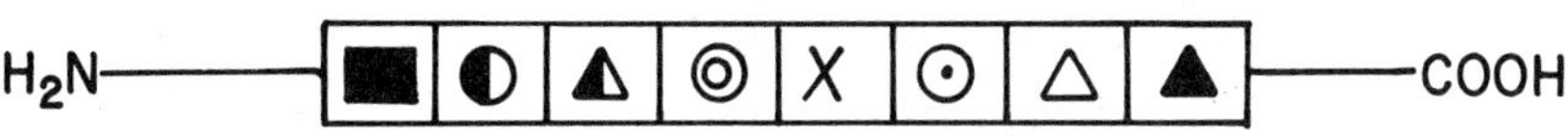

Example 3: A polypeptide hormone was isolated from the posterior pituitary, and found to have anti-diuretic activity. The hormone was subjected to acid hydrolysis and quantitative analysis. The results were as follows:

Amino Acid	Symbol	No. of Residues
Cystine	—S—S—	- 1 (= 2 Cysteines)
Proline		- 1
Glycine		- 1
Glutamic Acid or Glutamine		- 1
Aspartic Acid or Asparagine		- 1
Arginine		- 1
Tyrosine		- 1
Phenylalanine		- 1
Ammonia	NH_3	- 3

(∴ Both dicarboxylic amino-acids probably present as the amides)

The hormone was treated with Dansyl chloride, hydrolysed with acid and chromatographed. Mono-*DNS*-cystine was obtained. We conclude that one half of the cystine residue represented the amino-terminus of the hormone, and only one peptide chain was present in the hormone.

The hormone was then treated with performic acid (oxidising the cystine to two cysteic acid residues) and subjected to chymotrypsin digestion. Two peptides were thus obtained. These were separated by thin-layer chromatography, eluted, dansylated, and subjected to amino-acid analysis. The composition of each peptide was as follows:

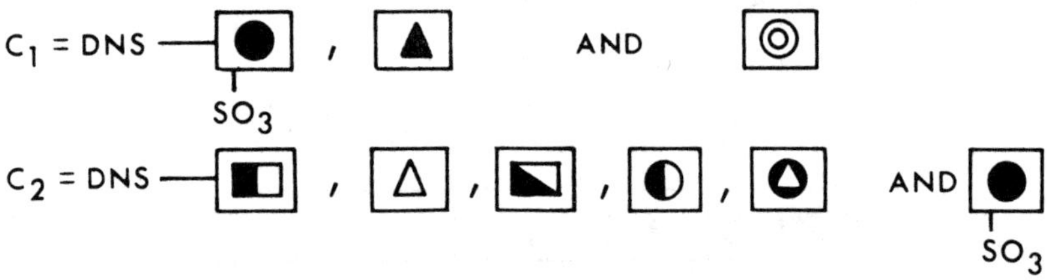

C_2 was then treated with trypsin. Two fragments were obtained, which were separated chromatographically, eluted, hydrolysed, and subjected to amino-acid analysis. One of the fragments thus obtained yielded only glycine and ammonia on acid hydrolysis.

The intact hormone was then treated with the carboxy-peptidases, both of which failed to release any amino-acid. This suggested that the carboxyl-terminus was blocked.

C_1 was then subjected to the Edman procedure, which yielded 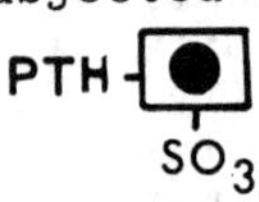

followed by 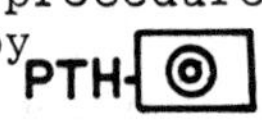

Therefore, the order of residues in C_1 was:

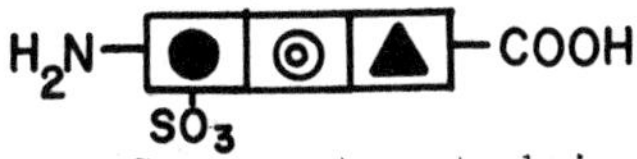

When C_2 was treated in the same manner, 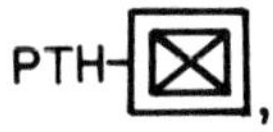, 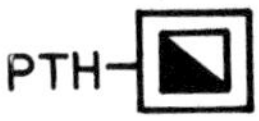 and 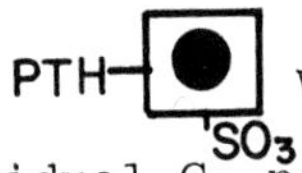 were sequentially released. The residual C_2 peptide was then treated with Dansyl chloride followed by acid hydrolysis and chromatography. The hydrolysate showed

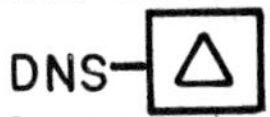 The order of residues in the C_2 fragment was therefore:

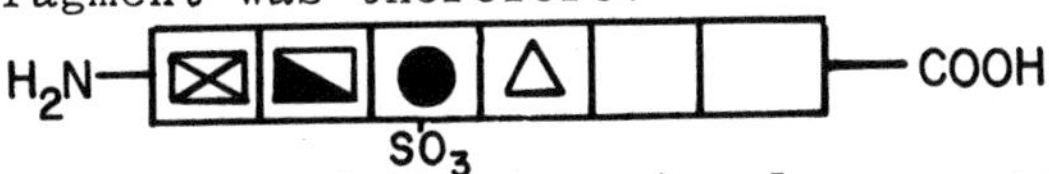

Making use of the trypsin cleavage products of C_2, the order of the fifth and sixth residues in C_2 could be deduced. We know that trypsin splits on the carbonyl side of arginine, and two products were obtained from each treatment, one of which was glycine and the other of which was ammonia. Thus we conclude that the C_2 peptide was:

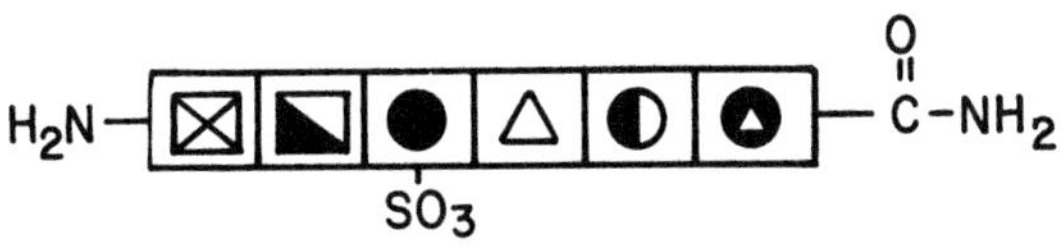

The carboxy-terminus was blocked by an amide-group attached to the α-carboxy group of glycine.

Since dansylation of the intact hormone yielded mono-*DNS*-cystine, and dansylation of the performate-treated chymotryptic fragment C_1 yielded *DNS*-cysteic acid, it is clear that the order of fragments in the hormone was H_2N-C_1-C_2-COOH. This was further substantiated by confirmation that carboxy-end of C_1 was phenylalanine, a residue preferentially split on its carbonyl side by chymotrypsin. Thus, the primary structure of the performate-treated hormone was:

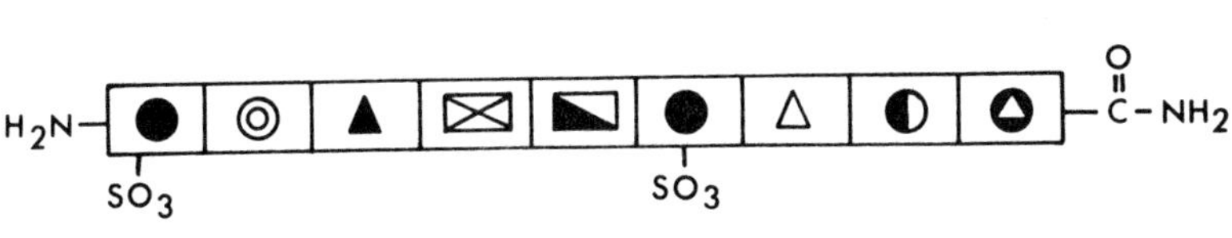

and the primary structure of the intact hormone was therefore:

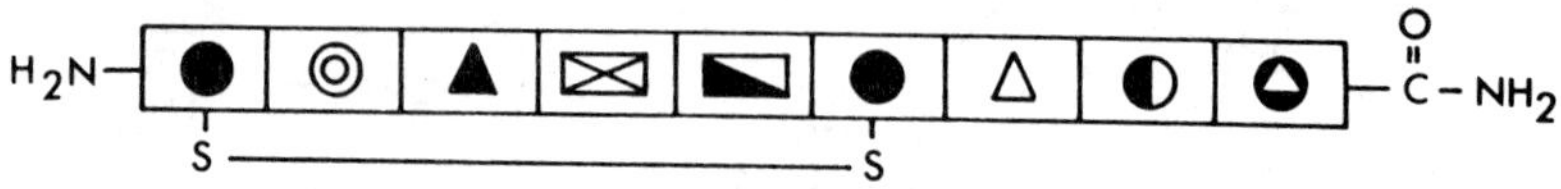

The preceding examples illustrate the basic operations and reasoning in peptide primary structure analysis. Although the examples used for illustration were small polypeptides, the reasoning employed in their solution is similar to that employed in the sequence analysis of much larger proteins, such as immunoglobulin H- and L-chains.

The text and illustrations of Appendix B were adapted from:

Gordon, B.L., Dyscrasias of Immunoglobulin Production, Philadelphia, Pa., (1969), with permission of the F.A. Davis Company

DIAGRAMS OF IMMUNOGLOBULIN PRIMARY STRUCTURE

KEY TO APPENDICES C-1—C-3

- PCA (Pyrollidone carboxylic acid, blocking amino terminus)
- Gly
- Ala
- Leu
- Ile
- Val
- Pro
- Phe
- Tyr
- Trp
- His
- Arg
- Lys
- Glu
- Asn
- Gln
- Asp
- Cys
- Met
- Ser
- Thr

- Asx
- Glx

C-1 INTERRELATIONSHIPS OF V_H REGIONS FROM DIFFERENT IMMUNOGLOBULINS (SHOWING SUBGROUP VARIATION), V_H AND V_L REGIONS IN GENERAL, V_K AND V_λ REGIONS IN GENERAL, AND V_H AND V_L REGIONS OF THE SAME IMMUNOGLOBULIN MOLECULE (Eu)

It is readily noted that the V - REGIONS of He, Daw, Cor, and Ou are members of one subgroup, while the V - REGION of Eu is a member of a different subgroup. The fact that all of the V - REGIONS are homologous structures is likewise evident.

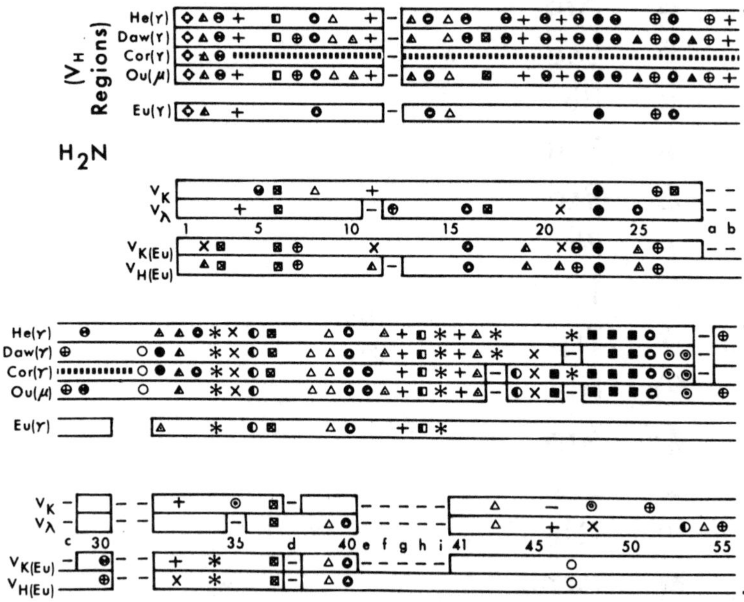

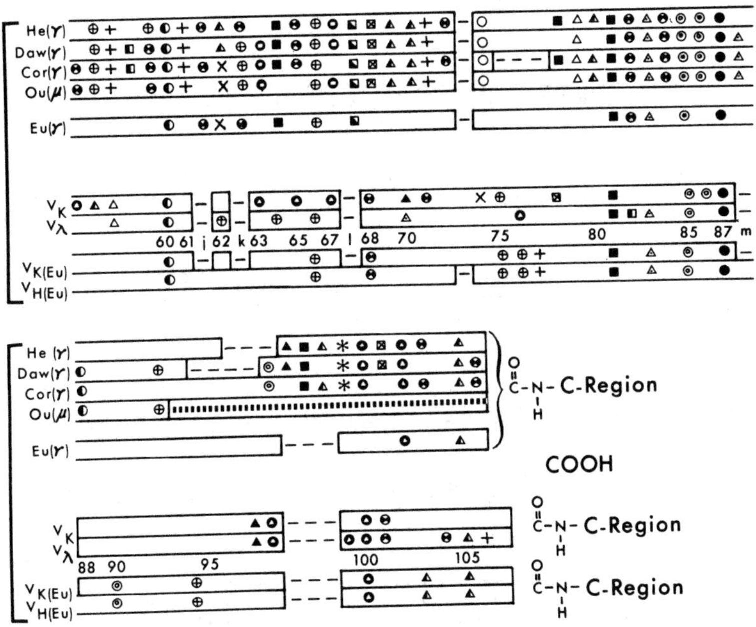

N.B. The chains are aligned to maximise homology

⁝⁝⁝⁝⁝⁝⁝⁝⁝ Sequence not available

C-2 VK REGIONS SHOWING SUBGROUP VARIATIONS

Complete or partial primary structures are illustrated for eight VK REGIONS, sorting into three subgroups based on sequence similarities within each subgroup, and broader variance amongst members of different subgroups. For example, the three V - Regions in the K_I subgroup (Eu, Ag, and Roy) are identical at 280/324, or 86.3% of their total amino acid positions. In contrast, Eu (K_I) and Cum (K_{II}) are identical at 108/221, or 48.9% of their total positions, while Eu (K_I) and Rad (K_{II}) are identical at 86/152, or 56.5% of their total homologous positions.

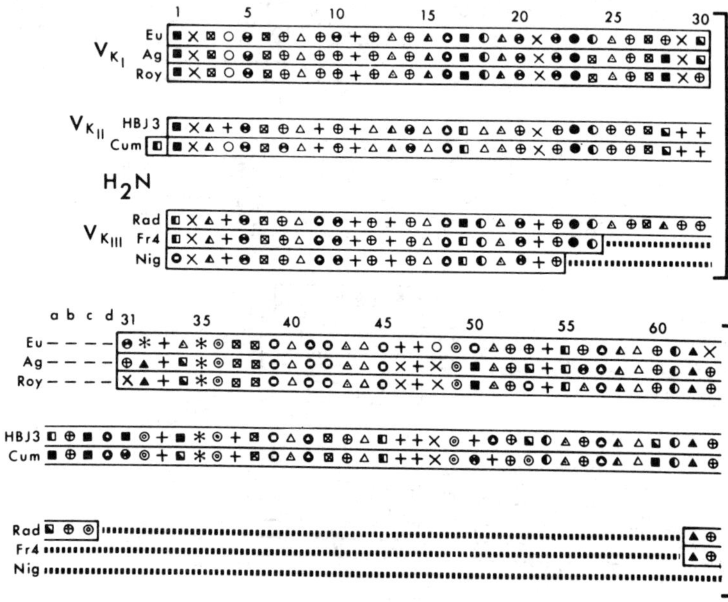

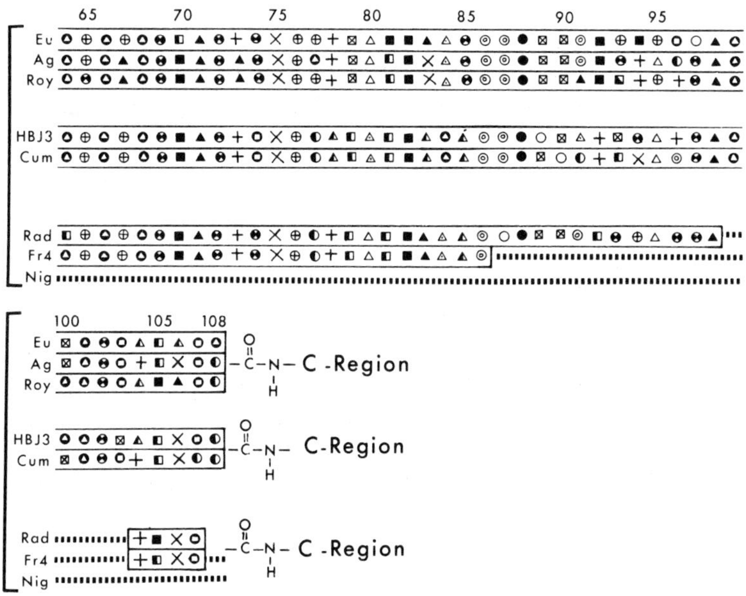

N.B. The chains are aligned to maximise homology

⋯⋯ Sequence not available

C-3 V_λ - REGIONS, SHOWING SUBGROUP VARIATIONS

Complete or partial primary structures are illustrated for seven V_λ - REGIONS, which sort themselves into four subgroups based on similarity of sequence within each subgroup and broader variance with respect to members of other subgroups. For example, the three V - REGIONS in the λ_I subgroup (New, Ha, and HBJ -7) are identical at 191/250 residues, or at 76.4% of their total positions. In contrast, New (λ_I) and Bo (λ_{II}) are identical at 134/225, or 59.5% of their total positions. Similarly, New (λ_I) and Sh (λ_{III}) are identical at 126/220, or 57.0% of their positions, and New (λ_I) and Kern (λ_{IV}) are identical at 118/218, or 53.8% of their total positions.

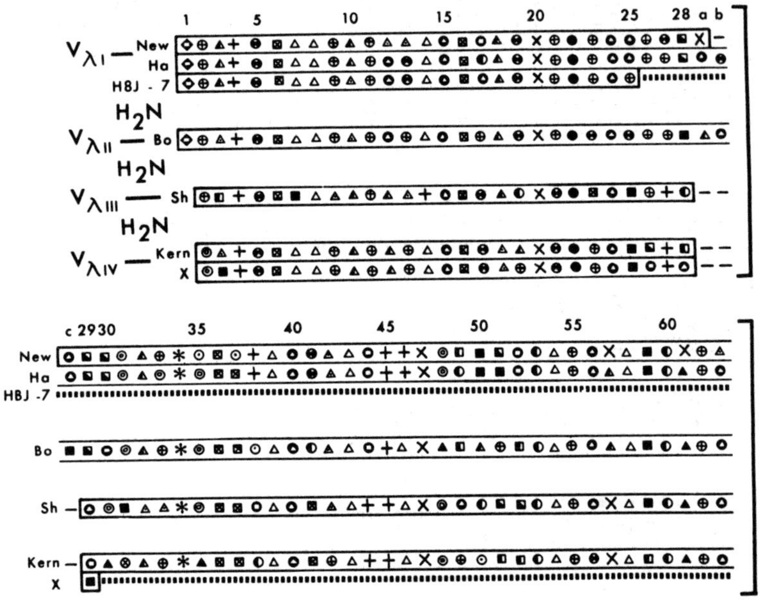

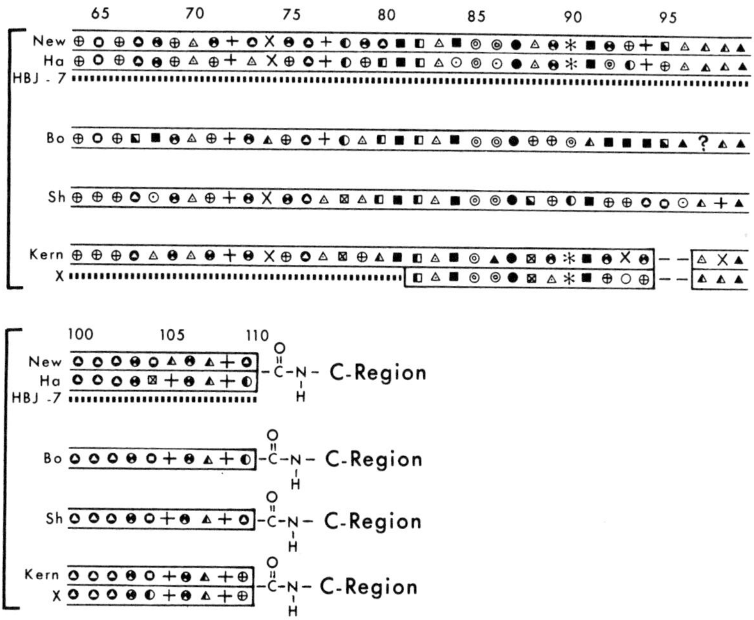

N.B. The chains are aligned to maximise homology

''''''''''' Sequence not available

INDEX

A

D

E

F

G

H

I

K

L

M

N

O

P

R

S

T

U

V

W

X